Cancer: Etiology and Prevention

Cancer: Etiology and Prevention

Proceedings of the Chicago Symposium on Cancer: Etiology and Prevention, Chicago, Illinois, U.S.A., October 4-6, 1982.

Editor:

Ray G. Crispen

Director of ITR Biomedical Research
University of Illinois at Chicago, Chicago, Illinois, U.S.A.

Sponsored by:
University of Illinois at Chicago and Illinois Cancer Council

Elsevier Biomedical
New York · Amsterdam · Oxford

Published by:

Elsevier Science Publishing Co., Inc.
52 Vanderbilt Avenue, New York, New York 10017

Sole distributors outside the USA and Canada:

Elsevier Science Publishers B.V.
P.O. Box 211, 1000 AE Amsterdam, The Netherlands

Library of Congress Cataloging in Publication Data

Main entry under title:

Cancer—etiology and prevention.

    Includes bibliographical references and index.
    1. Cancer—Immunological aspects—Congresses. 2. Cancer—Genetic aspects—
Congresses. 3. Carcinogenesis—Congresses. 4. Cancer—Prevention—Congresses.
I. Crispen, Ray G. II. University of Illinois at Chicago Circle. III. Illinois Cancer
Council. [DNLM: 1. Neoplasms—Etiology—Congresses. 2. Neoplasms—
Prevention and control—Congresses. QZ 200 C215155 1982]
RC268.3.C33   1983   616.99′4071   83-8889
ISBN 0-444-00785-7

Manufactured in the United States of America

Contents

Preface

Maturing evidence clearly supports the concept that cancer has a definite basis in the chromosomes of the cell and in the genetic makeup of the individual and that steps can be taken to actively prevent as well as treat cancer. This volume based on the 1982 Symposium, Cancer: Etiology and Prevention, presents current research on the alteration in genetic material that occurs prior to or as a consequence of cancer. Papers discuss chromosome structure, karyotypic abnormalities, and genetic theories of pathogenesis. The role of natural killer cells in immunogenetic regulation and their place in the host's defense against cancer are explored.

Theories on the mechanisms of carcinogenesis and approaches to prevention by use of chemical agents such as vitamins, vitamin analogues and immuno-restorators are presented. Characterized agents for immuno-manipulation, treatment and prevention are also discussed in their clinical application.

A special section is devoted to the hypothesis that BCG vaccination can prevent cancer. Nine retrospective studies from six countries throughout the world are presented. Some studies report a positive correlation between vaccination and reduction of cancer; while other studies do not show a change in the incidence rate of tumors in the vaccinated. A critique of the studies with suggestions for improving study design and analysis is given.

The construction of the text and the selection of outstanding contributors were designed to ensure a volume that would be of interest to clinical and experimental investigators, clinicians, medical students, public health officials and other health professionals.

Cancer: Etiology and Prevention

IMPLICATIONS OF PREMATURE CHROMOSOME CONDENSATION FINDINGS IN HUMAN LEUKEMIA

WALTER N. HITTELMAN, FRANCES M. DAVIS, AND MICHAEL J. KEATING
Department of Developmental Therapeutics, University of Texas System Cancer
Center, M.D. Anderson Hospital and Tumor Institute, Houston, Texas 77030

INTRODUCTION

The introduction of effective chemotherapeutic agents (e.g., cytosine arabi-noside and anthracyclines) has produced significant improvements in the remis-sion rate and duration of remission in patients with acute leukemia.[1,2] Remission can now be induced regularly in 60-70% of patients with acute myelog-enous leukemia (AML).[3,4] On the other hand, the overall cure rate or five year survival rate is only 20-25% of those who attain complete remission.[5] While the search for new, effective, and selective chemotherapeutic regimens will continue, significant further advances in the treatment of human leukemia (and other malignancies) require a better understanding of the biological principles involved in the malignant process.

This laboratory has found that the phenomenon of premature chromosome con-densation can be a useful tool in the study of malignancy. Normally, one can observe chromatin in the form of chromosomes only during mitosis when it has been packaged for cell division. However, in 1970, Johnson and Rao[6] reported that if one fuses mitotic and interphase cells, factors from the mitotic com-ponent induce the condensation of the interphase chromatin into discrete chro-mosomal units called prematurely condensed chromosomes (PCC). The morphology of these PCC is a reflection of the stage of the interphase cell in the cell cycle at the time of fusion. PCC from G1 cells exhibit a single chromatid per chromosome, whereas G2 PCC have two chromatids per chromosome. The PCC from S phase cells have a pulverized appearance yet one can see both unreplicated single chromosome pieces as well as replicated double pieces within chromosomal array. Thus, the PCC technique allows one to determine the cell cycle distribution of a population of cells. Further, since this technique allows one to visualize interphase chromosomes, cytogenetic analysis becomes possible even for nondividing cells.

The purpose of this paper is to review how the PCC phenomenon has been used to detect chromatin changes associated with cellular transformation and how this detection capability can be used in monitoring the disease process in patients with leukemia and in studying the biological basis for such changes.

MATERIALS AND METHODS

Many of the studies described here involved bone marrow cells from patients with leukemia, who were under treatment by the Leukemia Service of the Department of Developmental Therapeutics at U.T. M.D. Anderson Hospital. The mononuclear cells are concentrated by a single step[7] or double-step[8] Ficoll-Hypaque sedimentation technique.

The PCC technique involves the fusion of mitotic inducer cells with interphase cells (i.e. bone marrow mononuclear cells) resulting in the induction of premature condensation of the interphase chromatin. A detailed description of this methodology is presented elsewhere.[9]

In some cases, the bone marrow cells from patients with leukemia are probed for the presence of a nucleolar antigen usually associated with malignant cells. These studies employ rabbit antiserum raised against the nucleoli of HeLa cells and absorbed free of normal nucleolar antigens by incubation with human placental nucleoli.[10] The presence of the malignancy-associated antigen is then detected by indirect immunofluorescence staining of methanol-fixed cytocentrifuge preparations of cells using fluorescein-conjugated goat anti-rabbit immunoglobulin as the indicator antibody. The fraction of reactive cells can then be determined with the fluorescent microscope.

RESULTS AND DISCUSSION

PCC differences between normal and transformed cells

As described above, the morphology of the PCC indicates the cell cycle phase of the interphase cell at the time of fusion, i.e. G1, S, or G2 phase (Fig. 1). Moreover, early studies suggested that the conformation of the PCC also reflected a chromosome condensation cycle: mitotic chromosomes represent the most condensed state of chromatin and early S phase the least condensed chromatin.[11,12] Early G1 cells give rise to highly condensed G1 PCC whereas late G1 cells yield highly extended G1 PCC.[13,14,15] Similarly, unstimulated normal human peripheral blood lymphocytes give rise to condensed G1 PCC, whereas after mitogenic stimulation (but prior to entry into S phase), the G1 PCC appear highly elongated.[14]

For purposes of quantitation, G1 PCC are evaluated on a scale of 1 to 6, with a value of 1 representing the most condensed G1 PCC state and a value of 6 representing the most elongated G1 PCC state (Fig. 2). Since mitogenic stimulation of lymphocytes resulted in an increased fraction of cells in late G1, we defined the Proliferative Potential Index (PPI) as the fraction of G1 cells in late G1 (i.e. the fraction of G1 PCC with condensation values of 4,5 and 6). Thus a cell population with a high frequency of late G1 cells would have a high PPI value, regardless of the number of cells in S or G2 phase.

Most normal and tumor populations accumulate in G1 phase during periods of restrained growth.[16] In order to determine the accumulation point in G1 phase, normal and transformed cell populations were induced into a quiescent phase by medium depletion and their cell cycle distribution was determined by the PCC technique.[15] Normal cell population arrested in early G1 with condensed G1 PCC whereas transformed cell populations accumulated in late G1 with elongated G1 PCC (Fig. 3). Similarly, when solid tumor specimens were examined using the PCC technique, a high fraction of cells yielding late G1 PCC were observed, while normal cells infiltrating the tumor yielded early G1 PCC, with a normal chromosome complement.[17]

4

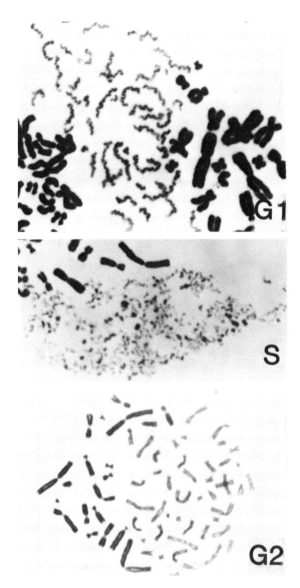

Fig. 1. Prematurely condensed chromosomes (PCC) of human bone marrow cells from various phases of the cell cycle after fusion with mitotic CHO cells. (a) G1 PCC exhibiting a single chromatid per chromosome. (b) S PCC exhibiting a pulverized appearance. (c) G2 PCC exhibiting two chromatids per chromosome.

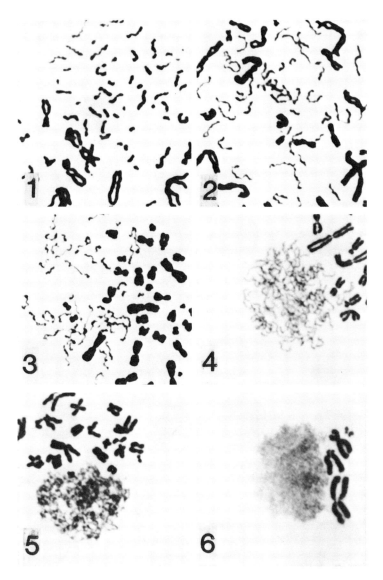

Fig. 2. G1 PCC of human bone marrow cells exhibiting varying degrees of chromosome condensation.

6

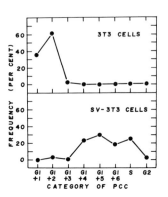

Fig. 3. Cell cycle distribution
of normal (3T3, top and transformed (SV-3T3, bottom) cells in
the plateau phase of growth.
Source: Hittelman, W.N., and
Rao, P.N.[15]

The molecular basis for the chromatin differences between normal and trans-

formed quiescent populations is not understood. A number of investigators have

suggested that there is a specific arrest point early in G1 phase where normal

cells accumulate.[16] Pardee has suggested that transformed cells do not recog-

nize this restriction point and proceed through G1 phase despite deprived growth

conditions.[18] Yet these cells might still be incapable of DNA synthesis and

might accumulate in late G1 phase. Studies using the premature chromosome con-

densation technique suggest that at least two generalized sets of reactions must

take place in the G1 to S transition. First, as described above, the chromatin

must decondense and become available for DNA replication. Second, the machinery

for DNA synthesis must become associated with the chromatin. The latter pro-

posal is based on the observations of Hanks and Rao[19] that if one adds tritiated

thymidine to the fusion mixture, G1 PCC from cycling cells will become labeled

whereas G1 PCC from quiescent cells will not. Different tumor populations might

differ in their ability to begin DNA synthesis despite growth restricting con-

ditions, and this might be reflected in their degree of malignancy or unre-

strained growth.

PCC characteristics in patients with leukemia prior to therapy

The mean PPI for bone marrow populations from normal individuals was found to be 11.7%.[20]   In contrast the mean PPI for patients with AML prior to remission induction therapy was approximately 35%, while that of patients with acute lymphocyte leukemia (ALL) was slightly higher at 42%.[21]   As shown in Figure 4 for a group of untreated patients with AML who were studied, the fraction of cells in S phase was generally decreased in marrow populations with a high PPI. This figure also illustrates the tremendous heterogeneity of PPI for different patients with the same disease.   The basis for these differences is not understood as there is no relationship between the apparent extent of disease (i.e. marrow blast counts or blast infiltrate) and PPI.

Fig. 4. Scatter diagram of the relationship between PPI and the fraction of cells in S phase for patients with AML. Open circles and triangles represent patients who failed to achieve complete remission due to infection or resistant disease, respectively. The closed symbols represent patients who achieved complete remission.

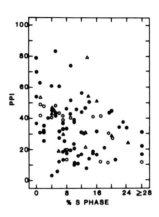

In this study, a predicted probability of response to therapy was calculated for each patient based on a previously developed linear regression model that takes into account various clinical and laboratory parameters.[22]   As shown in Table I, patients with lower PPI values did much better than expected, when both patients with AML and those with ALL were considered.

Bone marrow populations from patients with chronic leukemia showed different PCC characteristics.[21]   The PPI of patients with chronic myelogenous leukemia (CML) reflected the stage of disease. Newly presenting untreated patients with CML showed PPI values generally in the range 20-30%. After therapy, patients with clinically benign stages of CML show a low PPI around 12%, whereas patients

TABLE 1

RELATIONSHIP BETWEEN PRETREATMENT PPI AND RESPONSE TO REMISSION INDUCTION
THERAPY

PPI	# Patients	Observed CR No (%)	Expected CR* No	O/E
<20	21	16(78)	12.6	1.27
20-34.9	20	16(80)	13.4	1.19
35-50	28	18(64)	17.9	1.00
750	20	14(70)	13.2	1.06

*Based on pretreatment prognostic factors for each patient.

with CML in blastic phase exhibit PPI's similar to those observed in patients
with acute leukemia. In some cases where patients were observed serially, the
PPI was found to rise prior to clinical evidence of blastic transformation.
Patients with active chronic lymphocytic leukemia (CLL) exhibit high PPIs >40%,
even though the fraction of cells in S phase is low. This is an interesting
observation, since the bone marrow cells appear to be mature lymphocytes, yet
in the disease-free individual lymphocytes are in early G1. Thus morphology
alone is not a good indicator of the stage of the cell in G1 phase.

PCC characteristics after therapy: prediction of relapse

Following remission induction therapy, patients who responded to therapy
showed an initial drop in PPI, followed by a rise in both PPI to above 35%
and in S phase frequency during early bone marrow regeneration, followed by a decrease in PPI to under 35% as the peripheral blood counts began to rise. Considerable chromosome damage was also observed in the PCC during chemotherapy.
On the other hand, patients who did not respond to remission induction therapy
either showed no change in PCC characteristics or continued to show high PPI
as the peripheral blood counts rose.[23]

Early observations[20] suggested that a return to high PPI values during
remission might be useful in predicting relapse of disease. In order to test

this hypothesis, we serially followed a group of patients who were in complete remission and were to receive late intensification therapy in an attempt to eliminate residual disease. The late intensification therapy consisted of cyclophosphamide, zorubicin, oncovin, and predisone (CROP). Of the 19 patients followed, 14 relapsed during the course of study, and PPI above 35% was observed in 11 of the 14 relapsing patients prior to relapse. The median time from an elevation in the PPI to the development of clinical relapse was 3.5 months. Figure 5 illustrates how the mean PPI value for the group increased prior to relapse. On the other hand, the median time from a low PPI value to relapse or the end of the study was 8 months.[24]

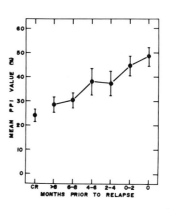

Fig. 5. Mean PPI of relapsing patients as a function of time prior to relapse. The single point marked CR is the mean of all the PPIs for the patients who stayed in complete remission. Source: Hittelman, W.N.[12]

One problem with the above study was that the patients had been in complete remission for different periods of time prior to late intensification therapy and thus had different expectations for relapse. In order to compare patients with similar expectations for continued complete remission (CR), we determined the PPIs of a totally separate group of patients with acute leukemia at specific intervals after CR was achieved. Patients were grouped into those having PPI $\geq$ 35% and those with PPI < 35%, and the subsequent duration of remission or time of follow-up in these two groups was compared. The results of such an analysis

for 25 patients studied between 9 and 15 weeks after achieving CR is shown in a

Kaplan-Meier plot[25] in Figure 6. In this case, 7 of the 9 patients exhibiting

high PPI values have already relapsed whereas only 4 of the 16 patients with low

PPI values have relapsed. The median time to relapse in the high PPI group was

13 weeks. Using a two-tailed Gehan-modified Wilcoxan analysis of this data[26]

these curves are significantly different at a p-value of 0.003. Similar trends

were observed at other time intervals during remission.

Fig. 6. Kaplan-Meier plot of the
proportion of patients remaining in
complete remission as a function of
time after either a high ($\geq$ 35%) or
low (< 35%) PPI for bone marrow
obtained at 9-16 weeks of complete
remission. NF, non-failure.

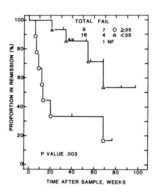

In some patients who were monitored serially during complete remission, the

PPI rose above 35% prior to relapse; however, it began to decrease once relapse

was clinically evident. Interestingly, in 22 patients studied both prior to

remission induction therapy and at the time of clinical evidence of relapse, the

PPI correlated slightly with a correlation coefficient of 0.45 (Fig. 7). This

is remarkable considering the fact that the two clinical situations were not

identical. Some patients were treated early in relapse before their bone marrow

reached the same infiltrate as it had prior to therapy.

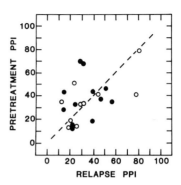

Fig. 7. A comparison of the PPI obtained prior to remission induction therapy with the PPI obtained at relapse for patients with acute leukemia. Open circles, AML; closed circles, ALL.

PCC characteristics of fractionated bone marrow cells

In order to characterize the PPI of different cell types, bone marrow cells of 30 patients at various stages of disease were fractionated using albumin gradient sedimentation and the fractions were analyzed by the premature chromosome condensation technique (2 normal, 11 untreated, 12 in remission, and 5 in relapse).[27] In general, normal bone marrow and marrow from most patients in complete remission showed lower PPIs throughout the gradients, with the most dense and most mature cells (Fraction 5) exhibiting the lowest PPI in the gradient (Fig. 8). On the other hand, bone marrow from newly presenting patients and from those in relapse showed higher PPIs, the highest PPIs were found in the most dense fraction containing the most mature cells (Fig. 9). Two of the patients who were studied in complete remission showed fractionation patterns similar to that shown in Figure 9, and these two patients relapsed clinically 2 and 5 months after these determinations. In contrast, the median time to relapse for the patients in CR who showed normal fractionation distributions was 9 months (range 3 to >67 months).

These fractionation studies again illustrate that the chromatin patterns

12

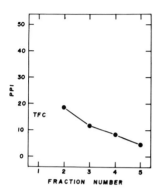

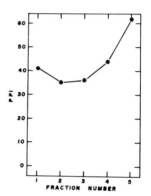

Fig. 8. PCC analysis of an albumin density fractionation of a bone marrow aspiration from a hematologically normal individual. Note the lowest PPI is found in the most dense fraction. Source: Hittelman, W.N.et al.[27]

Fig. 9. PCC analysis of a fractionated bone marrow from a newly presenting patient with ALL. Note the highest PPI in the most dense fraction. Source: Hittelman, W.N. et al.[27]

detected by the PCC technique reflect something other than the morphology of the cell. As is the case prior to remission induction therapy, the PPI of the least-mature cells varies from patient to patient and is more reflective of the patient's disease biology. However, the most mature cells of patients with active disease yield high PPI while those of healthy people and those of patients in good complete remission yield low PPI. Paradoxically, both populations are morphologically similar.

Biological implications of the PCC studies

The studies described above pose an interesting biological question. In normal individuals and in patients in good complete remission the mature cells arrest in early G1 phase. However, in newly diagnosed, relapsed, and about-to-relapse patients, the most mature cells arrest in late G1 phase. Two alternative hypotheses can be put forth to explain this puzzle. First, the morphologically normal mature cells might be derived from leukemic cells that have been induced to mature. This notion has gained support from situations where leukemic cells can be induced to differentiate _in vitro_ by a variety of agents.[28-36] Using the PCC technique, we have found that a human promyelocytic leukemia cell line, HL60, accumulates in late G1 phase (high PPI) when induced to mature in vitro with DMSO.[37] Thus, even though leukemic cells can be induced to mature with respect to morphology and function, the cells still retain the malignant characteristic of accumulating in late G1 phase.

Evidence is accumulating that leukemic cells can be induced to differentiate in the patient as well.[38-40] For example, Baker et al[41] have found that a high proportion of patients in complete clinical remission exhibit a high fraction of differentiated cells with leukemic surface markers in the months just prior to relapse. Similarly, others have cytogenetically detected residual leukemic cells during the time preceding relapse. Interestingly, the purported maturing leukemic cells often exhibit seemingly inappropriate cell markers both on the membrane and within the cell, and sometimes these cells appear to mature through inappropriate cell lineages (e.g. granulocytic pathway in a patient with lymphocytic disease).

Our laboratory has recently been pursuing this question by combing the PCC technique with a recently developed probe for malignant cells, an antibody against a human malignancy-associated nucleolar antigen (HMNA).[10,42] Rabbit antiserum has been raised against nucleoli isolated from the tumor cell line HeLa and has been extensively absorbed against human and bovine sera and extracts from normal human cells and tissues. The resulting antisera appear to be specific in staining nucleoli of neoplastic cells but not those of normal cells as revealed by indirect immunofluorescence (Fig. 10). The function of the HMNA is not understood; however it is species specific and might represent an oncofetal antigen that is involved in gene activation, either directly or through feedback mechanisms whose expression is intimately related to the cancer process.

All bone marrow specimens from patients with active acute leukemia have contained greater than 2% HMNA-positive cells, while none from nonleukemic

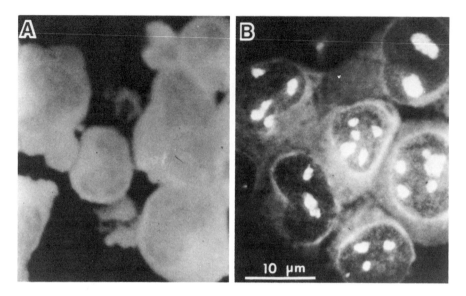

Fig. 10. Indirect immunofluorescence staining of human malignancy-associated nucleolar antigen (HMNA) in bone marrow cells from (A) normal individual and (B) patient with acute leukemia.

individuals has exceeded 2%, even when the normal marrows were enriched for immature cells by density fractionation. In bone marrow specimens from patients with leukemia, the fraction of HMNA-positive cells correlates well with the fraction of blast cells in the bone marrow (Fig. 11).[43] Occasionally, however, the fraction of HMNA-positive cells is higher than the percent blasts in the specimen, and HMNA positivity is observed in some cells progressing down the maturation pathway.

One of the problems with using the HMNA assay for detecting differentiating malignant cells is that cells of the myelocytic, monocytic, and erythrocytic series normally lose their nucleoli as they progress to the terminally differ- entiated state. Whether the antigen completely disappears or becomes diffusely distributed within the cell is not yet known. However, in a number of patients we have been able to detect residual HMNA positivity in morphologically

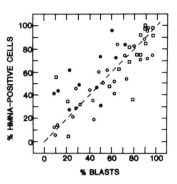

Fig. 11. Relationship of bone
marrow blast counts to percentage
of HMNA-positive cells in the bone
marrows of patients with acute
leukemia. Open circles, AML;
closed circles, AML with differentiation; open squares, ALL.

differentiating cells (Fig. 12). This has been observed in several clinical

situations, including the smoldering leukemic phase, very early in remission

induction therapy where the fraction of differentiated cells in the blood rises

quickly as the blast count falls, and in the period just prior to relapse. While

these studies are still early in development, they do suggest that in some

situations leukemic cells can differentiate in vivo.

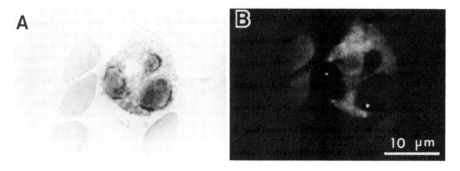

Fig. 12. Bone marrow cells of a patient with AML undergoing chemotherapy.
(A) Wright-Giemsa stained;   (B) positive fluorescence for HMNA.

The second hypothesis to explain the premature chromosome condensation findings described earlier (i.e. high PPI just prior to relapse and in mature cells) is that residual leukemic cells are capable of producing or inducing factors that can change the chromatin characteristics of resting normal cells. While the evidence supporting this notion is somewhat sparse in leukemia, studies in other tumor systems suggest that it might be a possible explanation. DeLarco and Todaro[44] found that tumor cells can produce factors that not only stimulate their own growth but can also induce normal cells to acquire phenotypic characteristics of tumor cells (e.g., the ability of normal fibroblasts to grow in semisolid agar). Such growth factors have been detected in a variety of tumors as well as in some normal cell lines.[45-50]

The role of this putative leukemic growth factor is not understood. However, stimulation of cells into the cell cycle has been suggested to be a multifactorial process.[51] The putative leukemia growth factor might stimulate bone marrow cells to pass beyond the restriction point, while differentiating or leukemic inhibitory factors might prevent the cell from entering S phase.[52] This sequence of events would result in the accumulation of normal maturing cells in late G1 and would result in a high PPI value for mature cells in leukemic situations.

At the present time, we cannot distinguish between these two hypotheses to account for the high PPI found in the morphologically normal cells of patients with active leukemia. It is possible, however, that both processes are taking place to different extents in patients with leukemia. Not only might this help explain the biological and clinical heterogeneity observed in patients with the same disease, but one might also view the course of disease within a single patient as an outgrowth of different leukemic clones with different abilities to differentiate and produce both positive and negative growth and differentiation factors.

Clinical implication of these studies

One of the problems in cancer therapy is that patients are treated with regimens that have proved to be the most beneficial for groups of patients with a particular type of tumor. However, each patient's disease is biologically distinct and will respond differently to the same therapeutic regimen. Further, during complete remission, one does not know whether to discontinue therapy, continue existing therapy, rotate therapeutic regimens, or introduce more drastic and aggressive therapy to delay or prevent the progression or onset of relapse. Similarly, at the first signs of progression, one does not know whether to treat aggressively immediately or whether to wait until the clinical manifestations of recurrent disease are life-threatening.

The results discussed above suggest that the premature chromosome condensation technique might be useful, in combination with other laboratory tests such as the detection of HMNA-positive cells, in the individualization of therapy based on each patient's disease. For example, at some point during complete remission we might want to identify a group of patients for whom therapy should be discontinued. These patients could be followed using these laboratory tests. If the patients showed early signs of relapse, therapy could be reinstated. The advantage of this approach is twofold. First, the patient would be relieved of toxicity associated with continued therapy and would face salvage therapy in a more healthy state. Second, the induction of new malignant clones and the selection of drug cross-resistant clones would be minimized. Similarly, these techniques might be useful in deciding when to change or intensify therapy for the patient in remission. Changing therapeutic regimens at the earliest signs of recurring disease might prolong remission and increase the chances for cure.

The results discussed here also suggest that the PCC and HMNA values might be useful in defining the biological characteristics of each person's disease. This information could then be used in deciding between alternative therapeutic approaches. In the past, therapy for malignant diseases has focused on

18

cytotoxic agents, which selectively kill tumor cells. However, the toxicity of these agents in normal tissues is routinely observed and can outweigh the beneficial effects of tumor cell kill. Recently, investigators have been focusing on potential therapies designed to both manipulate the tumor into a more benign state and to boost the body's ability to counteract the malignancy. As described above, there is accumulating evidence that certain leukemic cells can be induced to differentiate in the patient; however, this ability may vary with each person's disease. Mouse leukemia model systems have illustrated this point well[29] and therapies designed to induce leukemic cell differentiation in patients are now being reported.[53] The results described above suggest that the premature chromosome condensation and HMNA techniques will be useful in distinguishing whether morphologically normal mature cells are of normal or leukemic origin. This information would help not only in understanding the biological interactions underlying each patient's disease, but also in selecting the most beneficial therapy for each patient.

ACKNOWLEDGEMENTS

Supported in part by NIH grants CA 14528, CA 27931, and CA 28153 from the National Cancer Institute. We thank Josephine Neicheril for help in preparing the manuscript.

REFERENCES

1. Gale, R.P. (1979) New Engl. J. Med., 300, 1189-1100.
2. Cline, M.J., Golde, D.W., Billing, R.J., Groupman, J.E., Zigttelboim, J., and Gale, R.P. (1979) Annals Int. Med. 91, 758-773.
3. Weinstein, H.J., Mayer, R.J., Rosenthal, D.S., Camitta, B.M., Coral, F.S., Nathan, D.G.,and Frei, E. (1980) New Eng. J. Med. 303, 473-478.
4. Holland, D., Sotto, J.J., Berthier, R., Leger, J., and Michallet, M. (1980) Cancer, 45, 1540-1548.
5. Keating, M.J., Smith, T.L., Gehan, E.A., McCredie, K.B., Bodey, G.P., Spitzer, G., Hersh, E., Gutterman, J., and Freireich, E.J. (1980) Cancer, 45, 2017-2029.
6. Johnson, R.T., and Rao, P.N. (1970) Nature 226, 717-722.
7. Boyum, A., (1968) Scand. J. Clin. Lab. Invest. Suppl. 97, 9-108.
8. English, D., and Anderson, B. (1972) J. Immunol. Methods, 5, 171-179.

9. Hittelman, W.N. (1982) in Cytogenetic Assays for Environmental Mutagens and Carcinogens, Hsue, T.C. ed., Allanheld Osman, Totowa, New Jersey, pp. 353-384.
10. Davis, F., Gyorkey, F., Busch, R., and Busch, H. (1979) Proc. Natl. Acad. Sci. U.S.A. 76, 892-896.
11. Mazia, D. (1963) J. Cell. Comp. Physiol. 62, Suppl. 1, 123-240.
12. Hittelman, W.N. (1982) in Premature Chromosome Condensation:Application in Basic and Clinical Research, Johnson, R., Rao, P.N., Sperling, K. ed., Academic Press, New York, pp. 309-358.
13. Schor, S.L., Johnson, R.T., and Waldren, C.A. (1975) J. Cell Sci. 17, 539-565.
14. Hittelman, W.N., and Rao, P.N. (1976) Exp. Cell. Res. 100, 219-222.
15. Hittelman, W.N., and Rao, P.N. (1978) J. Cell. Physiol. 95, 333-341.
16. Lajtha, L.G. (1963) J. Cell Comp. Physiol. 62, Suppl. 1, 143-145.
17. Grdina, D.J., Hittelman, W.N., White, R.A., and Meistrich, M.L. (1977) Br. J. Cancer, 36, 659-669.
18. Pardee, A.B. (1974) Proc. Natl. Acad. Sci. U.S.A. 71, 1286-1290.
19. Hanks, S.K., and Rao, P.N. (1980) J. Cell. Biol. 87, 285-291.
20. Hittelman, W.N., and Rao, P.N. (1978) Cancer Res. 38, 416-423.
21. Hittelman, W.N., Broussard, L.C., and McCredie, K. (1979) Blood, 54, 1001-1014.
22. Freireich, E.J., Keating, M., Smith, T., Gehan, E., Estey, E., McCredie, K., and Bodey, G. (1982) Proc. Am. Soc. Clin. Oncol. 1, 125.
23. Hittelman, W.N., Broussard, L.C., McCredie, K., and Murphy, S.G. (1980) Blood, 55, 457-465.
24. Hittelman, W.N., Broussard, L.C., Dosik, G., and McCredie, K.B. (1980) N. Engl. J. Med. 303, 479-484.
25. Kaplan, E.L., and Meier, P. (1958) J. Am. Stat. Assoc. 53, 457-481.
26. Gehan, E. (1965) Biometrica, 52, 203-224.
27. Hittelman, W.N., Vellekoop, L., Zander, A.R., and Dicke, K.A. (1982) Blood, 60, 1203-1211.
28. Sachs, L. (1978) Nature (London) 274, 535-539.
29. Honma, Y., Kasukabe, T., Okabe, J., and Jozumi, M. (1979) Cancer Res. 39, 3167-3171.
30. Collins, S.J., Gallo, R.C., and Gallagher, R.E. (1977) Nature (London) 270, 347-349.
31. Collins, S.J., Ruscetti, F.W., Gallagher, R.E., and Gallo, R.C. (1978) Proc. Natl. Acad. Sci. U.S.A. 75, 2458-2462.
32. Collins, S.J., Bodner, A., Ting, R., and Gallo, R.C. (1980) Int. J. Cancer 25, 213-218.
33. Papac, R.J., Brown, A.E., Schwartz, E.L., and Sartorelli, A.C. (1980) Cancer Lett. 10, 33-38.
34. Rovera, G., Santoli, D., and Darnsky, C. (1979) Proc. Natl. Acad. Sci. U.S.A. 76, 2779-2783.
35. Huberman, E., and Callahan, M.F. (1979) Proc. Natl. Acad. Sci. U.S.A. 76, 1293-1297.
36. Regoraro, L., Abraham, J., Cooper, R.A., Levis, A., Lange, B., Meo, P., and Rovenag, G. (1980) Blood, 55, 859-862.
37. Hittelman, W.N. (1980) Eur. J. Cell. Biol. 22, 538.
38. Hoelzer, D., Kunale, E., Schmucker, H., and Harriss, E.B. (1977) Blood, 49, 729-744.
39. Lan, S., McCulloch, E.A., and Till, T.E. (1978) J. Natl. Cancer Inst. 60, 265-269.
40. McCulloch, E.A. (1979) J. Natl. Cancer Inst. 63, 883-891.
41. Baker, M.A., Falk, J.A., Carter, W.H., Taub, R.N., and the Toronto Study Group (1979) N. Engl. J. Med. 301, 1353-1357.
42. Busch, H., Gyorkey, F., Busch, R.K., Davis, F.M., Gyorkey, P., and Smetana, K. (1979) Cancer Res. 39, 3024-3030.

43. Davis, F.M., Hittelman, W.N., McCredie, K.B., and Rao, P.N. (1980) Cancer Res. 21, 229.
44. DeLarco, J.E., and Todaro, G.J. (1978) Proc. Natl. Acad. Sci. U.S.A. 75, 4001-4005.
45. Todaro, G.J., and DeLarco, J.E. (1980) in Control Mechanisms in Animal Cells (L.J. DeAsua, ed.) pp. 223-243.
46. Roberts, A.B., Lamb, L.C., Newton, D.L., Sporn, M.B., DeLarco, J.E., and Todaro, G.J. (1980) Proc. Natl. Acad. Sci. U.S.A. 77:3494-3498.
47. Heldon, C.H., Westermark, B., and Wasterson, A. (1980) J. Cell Physiol. 105, 235-246.
48. Knaver, D.J., Iyer, A.P., Banerjee, M.R., and Smith, G.L. (1980) Cancer Res. 40, 4368-4372.
49. Gajousek, C., DiCorleto, P., Ross, R., and Schwartz, S. (1980) J. Cell Biol. 85, 467-472.
50. Roberts, A., Anzano, M., Lamb, L.C., Smith, J., and Sporn, M.B. (1981) Proc. Natl. Acad. Sci. 78, 5339-5343.
51. Ruscetti F., and Gallo, R. (1981) Blood, 57, 379-394.
52. Broxmeyer, H., Jacobsen, N., Kurland, J., Mendelsohn, N., and Moore, M. (1978) J. Natl. Cancer Inst. 60, 497-511.
53. Housset, M., Danier, M.R., and Degos, L. (1982) Brit. J. Hemat. 51, 125-129.

SIGNIFICANCE OF PURE TRISOMY 12 COMPARED TO OTHER KARYOTYPES IN CHRONIC
LYMPHOCYTIC LEUKEMIA.

TIN HAN,+ HOWARD OZER,+ NAOKI SADAMORI,+ RATILAL GAJERA,+ GERMAN GOMEZ,+
EDWARD S. HENDERSON,+ MARVIN L. BLOOM++ AND AVERY A. SANDBERG+
+ROSWELL PARK MEMORIAL INSTITUTE, AND ++STATE UNIVERSITY OF NEW YORK AT
BUFFALO SCHOOL OF MEDICINE, BUFFALO, NEW YORK, USA

INTRODUCTION

Chromosome studies of phytohemagglutinin (PHA)-induced metaphases of
peripheral blood cells from patients with B-cell chronic lymphocytic leukemia
(CLL) have previously demonstrated normal karyotypes in almost all instances.[1,2]
Until recently, the cytogenetic aspects of CLL remained unclear, primarily
because of the very low spontaneous mitotic index of leukemic B cells; in
addition, these cells are very poorly stimulated by PHA, which is primarily a
T-cell mitogen. With the availability of techniques utilizing B-cell mitogens
or activators, such as Epstein-Barr virus (EBV), lipopolysaccharides (LPS),
protein A (PA) and pokeweed mitogen (PWM), cytogenetic analyses of leukemic B
cells can now be readily performed. We and others recently reported clonal
chromosome abnormalities in stimulated lymphocytes in patients with CLL.[3-9] An
extra chromosome 12 (trisomy 12) was the most frequent abnormal karyotype seen
in this malignancy.[3-6,9]

The present study was undertaken to determine the frequency and the
distribution of clonal chromosome abnormalities and to correlate abnormal
karyotypes with clinical and phenotypic data. The clinical results obtained
demonstrate significance of pure trisomy 12 in relation to trisomy 12 with other
chromosome changes or to other abnormal karyotype without trisomy 12 in patients
with CLL.

MATERIALS AND METHODS

Fifty-eight CLL patients with active disease were studied, of which 43 were
males and 15 females. The majority of patients were over 60 years of age.
Duration of disease ranged from one month to 17 years. Lymphocytosis ranged
from 10,000 to 310,000/cu.mm. Clinical staging (10) indicated that the patients
were widely distributed among the various stages (Stage 0, 11; Stage I, 2; Stage
II, 27; Stage III, 11; Stage IV, 7). Of 46 patients studied, 11 had
hypogammaglobulinemia, 3 had an elevation of IgG and 6 had a monoclonal IgM
gammopathy. Thirty-eight patients were previously untreated and 20 were pre-

viously treated (at least 3 months prior to analysis). The majority of patients' leukemic cell populations were immunologically classified as $\mu\delta$ or μ
heavy chain phenotype whereas light chain phenotypes were approximately evenly
distributed between κ and λ. Lymphocytes were isolated from heparinized venous
blood by centrifugation over Ficoll-Hypaque gradients. Separated lymphocytes
($1-2 \times 10^6$/ml) were cultured in RPMI 1640 culture medium with 10% fetal calf
serum and antibiotics (100 units of penicillin and 50µg of streptomycin/ml) with
EBV (supernatant from an EBV-producing permanent cell line B-95-8 at 1:9 V/V of
culture), LPS (40 µg/ml), PA (100 µg/ml) or PWM (0.1 ml of reconstituted
material) at 37°C in an atmosphere of 5% CO_2. After 3 days in culture the
cells were harvested. Colcemid (GIBCO Co., Grand Island, N.Y.) was added 2-18
hours prior to harvest. Karyotypic analyses of B-cell mitogen-stimulated
leukemic B lymphocytes were performed by G and/or Q-banding techniques.[11]

RESULTS

Of 58 patients studied, adequate metaphases were obtained in 48 (83%) and
no mitoses were observed in 10 (17%). Of those not forming metaphases 5 were
previously treated and the remaining 5 were previously untreated (Stage 0, 1;
Stage I, 1; Stage II, 6; Stage III, 2). An abnormal karyotype was seen in 24
(50%) of 48 patients with adequate metaphases induced by one or more of the
B-cell mitogens in these patients. Abnormal karyotypes were observed in over
80% of metaphases induced by EBV, LPS or PA and in only 60% of PWM-induced
metaphases.The distribution of specific clonal chromosome abnormalities among
those patients is shown in Table 1. Seven patients had trisomy 12 as the only
abnormality, 8 had trisomy 12 in combination with other karyotypic changes and
the remaining 9 had various karyotypic changes without trisomy 12. The
frequency of trisomy 12 with or without other changes was significantly higher
than other karyotypic changes without trisomy 12 ($p < 0.01$).

Table 2 demonstrates the correlations of clonal chromosome abnormalities
with clinical and phenotypic data in patients with CLL. There was no
correlation between the abnormal karyotype and sex, age, disease duration,
treatment status or leukemic phenotype. Among patients with adequate
metaphases, an abnormal karyotype was seen in 4 (36%) of 11 patients with Stage
0 or I, in 7 (33%) of 21 patients with Stage II and in 13 (81%) of 16 patients
with Stage III or IV, clearly indicating that karyotypic changes are more
frequently associated with advanced stages than with early stages of CLL
($p < 0.01$). Abnormal karyotypes were seen in 4 (80%) of 5 patients with a
lymphocytosis >100,000/cu.mm and in 5 (83%) of 6 patients with IgM gammapathies

whereas abnormal karyotype was seen in 11 (34%) of 43 patients with lymphocytosis <100,000/cu.mm and in 19 (45%) of 42 patients without IgM gammopathies, suggesting that the frequency of abnormal karyotypes may be higher in those with marked lymphocytosis or with an IgM gammopathy.

Correlations of several abnormal karyotypes with clinical stages in CLL are shown in Table 3. Six of 7 patients with pure trisomy 12 had Stage 0-II disease whereas all 8 patients with a complex karyotype including trisomy 12 plus other changes had Stage III-IV disease. The difference is statistically significant (p <0.02). However, patients with other abnormal karyotypes without trisomy 12 were equally divided; 5 had Stage 0-II and 4 had Stage III-IV disease. Of 5 patients with a monoclonal IgM gammopathy, 2 had pure trisomy 12 (single clone) and 3 had a complex karyotype involving both trisomy 12 and other abnormalities (two or more clones).

The follow-up period in these patients after cytogenetic study ranged from 4 to 32 months. Six patients had died of the disease at the time of evaluation . Of these, 4 patients with Stage III or IV had abnormal karyotypes (two with trisomy 12 plus other changes and two with other changes without trisomy 12), one with Stage III had no mitoses and the remaining one with an initial stage II subsequently progressing to Stage IV had a normal karyotype.

DISCUSSION

Our finding that 50% of active CLL patients with adequate metaphases had abnormal karyotypes is in agreement with those of others [6,7,9], confirming that cytogenetic abnormalities in CLL are not rare but rather frequent. Identical abnormal karyotypes were detected in metaphases induced by two or more mitogens, illustrating that these changes are not produced in normal cells by the mitogenic agents. Clonal chromosome abnormalities seen in untreated patients in the present study suggest that these changes are not treatment-related, but rather disease-related. It should be emphasized that although clonal chromosome abnormalities fail to correlate with sex, age, disease duration or leukemic phenotype, they are strongly correlated with clinical stage, degree of lymphocytosis and the presence of a monoclonal paraproteinemia. It has previously been demonstrated that abnormal karyotypes correlate with disease status.[5]

The present study and those of others[6,9] unequivocally indicate that trisomy 12 with or without other changes is the most frequent and specific chromosome abnormality in B-cell CLL. It has also been reported that trisomy 12 was observed in two patients with hairy cell leukemia [12, 13] which is now considered

to be a malignancy that is predominantly of B-cell origin.[14] Of interest is
the fact that the malignant population from one of these two hairy cell patients
was phenotyped as μδκ (identical to the surface immunoglobulin phenotype of most
B-cell CLL) although the other patient was not phenotyped.[12] The association
between trisomy 12 and other B-derived lymphoproliferative malignancies
including non-Hodgkin's lymphoma, Burkitt's lymphoma, acute lymphoblastic
leukemia, prolymphocytic leukemia and multiple myeloma has not been described.
However, the 14q+ abnormal karyotype, seen in two patients with CLL in the
present study and in a few patients reported by others,[6,7,9] has been frequently
or specifically associated with Burkitt's lymphoma,[15] B-cell acute lymphoblastic
leukemia,[16] non-Hodgkin's lymphoma,[17] and multiple myeloma.[18,19] It should be
pointed out that both of our patients with 14q+ had features not usually
associated with typical CLL. One had a γ leukemic phenotype and the other had a
lymph node histology of poorly differentiated lymphocytic lymphoma, diffuse
type. These observations lead us to speculate that B-cell CLL with 14q+ may be
closely related to other B-cell neoplastic diseases such as Burkitt's lymphoma,
non-Hodgkin's lymphoma and multiple myeloma rather than to CLL with trisomy 12.
In addition, the 14q+ anomaly has also been associated with a few cases of
chronic or adult T-cell leukemia.[20,21]

Our observations that pure trisomy 12 is usually associated with early
stages whereas trisomy 12 with other chromosome changes is exclusively associated with advanced stages of CLL lead us to hypothesize that trisomy 12 may be
the primary or the earliest karyotypic change in a majority of patients with CLL
and that other chromosome changes in addition to trisomy 12 may develop as a
result of clonal evolution, dedifferentiation or in response to chemotherapy.

TABLE I

TYPE OF CLONAL CHROMOSOME CHANGES IN CLL

Type of Abnormal Karyotype	No. of Patients (%)
Trisomy 12 alone	7[a] (29%)
Trisomy 12 with other changes	8[a] (33%)
Trisomy 16	2 (8%)
14q+	2 (8%)
Trisomy 18	2 (8%)
Trisomy 19	1 (4%)
Trisomy 1	1 (4%)
Minute Chromosome	1 (4%)
TOTAL	24

A frequency of trisomy 12 + other changes is significantly higher than others
without trisomy 12 p <0.01.

TABLE II

CORRELATIONS BETWEEN CLONAL CHROMOSOME CHANGES AND CLINICAL AND PHENOTYPIC DATA IN CLL

Clinical and Phenotypic Data	Total No. of Patients with Mitosis	No. of Patient with normal Karyotype	No. of Patients with abnormal Karyotype (%)
Sex: Males	36	18	18 (50%)
Females	12	6	6 (50%)
Age: <60 Yrs.	20	12	8 (40%)
60-87 Yrs.	28	11	6 (57%)
Duration of Disease:			
<5 Yrs.	35	17	18 (51%)
5-17 Yrs.	13	7	6 (46%)
Treatment Status:			
Untreated	33	18	15 (45%)
Treated	15	6	9 (60%)
Leukemic Phenotype [a]:			
$\mu\delta$, $\mu\gamma$	26	13	13 (50%)
μ	20	10	10 (50%)
γ	2	1	1 (50%)
κ	26	13	13 (50%)
λ	21	11	10 (48%)
Stage: 0 - II	32	21	11[b] (34%)
III - IV	16	3	13[b] (81%)
Lymphocytosis:			
<100,000/mm^3	43	23	20 (47%)
>100,000	5	1	4 (80%)
IgM Gammopathy:			
Absent	42	23	19 (45%)
Present	6	1	5 (83%)

[a] No light chain was detectable in one patient and only one patient had an $\mu\gamma$ heavy chain phenotype.

[b] p <0.01 by Yate's Chi-square Analysis.

TABLE III

CORRELATIONS BETWEEN VARIOUS ABNORMAL KARYOTYPES WITH CLINICAL STAGE IN CLL

Clinical Stage	No. of Patients Normal Karyotype	Pure +12	Complex +12	Others Without +12
0	7	2	0	1
I	0	1	0	0
II	14	3	0	4
	} 21	} 6^a	} 0^a	} 5
III	1	1	5	2
IV	2	0	3	2
	} 3	} 1^a	} 8^a	} 4
TOTAL	24	7	8	9

^{a} p <0.02 by Yate's Chi-square Analysis

ACKNOWLEDGMENT

This study was supported in part by NCI grant number CA-05834, CA-14555 and CA-27691, DHHS.

REFERENCES

1. Oppenheim, J. J., Whang, J. and Frei, E. (1965) Blood 26, 121-132.
2. Fleischman, E. W. amd Prigogina. E. L. (1977) Human Genet 35, 269-275.
3. Morita, M., Minowada, J. and Sandberg, A. A. (1981) Cancer Genet Cytogenet 3, 293-306.
4. Sadamori, N., Han, T., Minowada, J., Henderson, E. S., Ozer, H. and Sandberg, A. A. (1981) Blood 58, 151a, (Abst.).
5. Han, T., Ozer, H., Sadamori, N. Gajera, R., Gomez, G., Henderson, E. S., Minowada, J. and Sandberg, A. A. (1982) Proc. ASCO 1, 186 (Abst.).
6. Gahrton, G., Robert, K. H. Friberg, K., Zech, L. and Bird, A. G. (1980) Blood 57, 444-451.
7. Nowell, P., Shankey, T. C., Finan, J., Guerry, D. and Besa, E. (1981) Blood 57, 444-451.
8. Autio, K., Turunen, O. Penttila, O., Eramaa E., de la Chapella, A. and Schroder, J. (1979) Cancer Genet. Cytogenet 1, 147-155.
9. Robert, K. H., Gahrton, G., Friberg, K., Zech, L., and Nilsson, B. (1982) Scand. J. Hemat 28, 163-168.
10. Rai, K. R., Sawitsky, A., Cronkite, E. P., Chanana, A. D., Levy, R. M. and Paternack, B. D. (1975) Blood 46, 219-234.
11. Sandberg, A. A. (1980) The Chromosome in Human Cancer and Leukemia. Elsevier North Holland, pp. 31-414.
12. Golomb, H. M., (1978) Cancer 42, 946-956.
13. Golomb, H. M., Lundgren, V. and Rowley, J. D. (1978) Cancer 41, 1374-1380.

14. Jansen, J., Schuit, H.R.E., Meijer, C.J.L.M., Van Nieuwkoop, J.A. and Hijimans, W. (1982) Blood 59, 52-60.
15. Kakati, S., Barcos, M., and Sandberg, A. A. (1979) Med. Pedia Onc. 6, 121-129.
16. Roth, D. G., Cimino, M. C., Variakajis, D., Golomb, H. M. and Rowley, J. D. (1979) Blood 53, 235-243.
17. Mark, J. Ekedahl, C., and Dahlenfors, R. (1978) Hereditas 88, 229-242.
18. Liang, W. and Rowley, J. D. (1978) Lancet I:96 (Letter).
19. Gahrton, G., Zech, L., Nilsson, K., Loonquist, B. and Carlstrom, A. (1980) Scand. J. Hemat 24, 42-46.
20. Finan, J. B., Daniele, R. P., Rowlands, D. T., Jr. and Nowell, P. (1978) Proc. AACR 19,48 (Abst).
21. Ueshima, Y., Fukuhara, S., Hattori, T., Uchiyama, T., Takatsuki, K. and Uchimo, H. (1981) Blood 58, 420-425.

CYTOGENETIC ABNORMALITIES IN PATIENTS WITH ACUTE LEUKEMIA STUDIED WITH BANDING TECHNIQUES, INCLUDING THE HIGH-RESOLUTION BANDING METHOD

SHIN-ICHI MISAWA AND JOSEPH R. TESTA
Cytogenetics Section, University of Maryland Cancer Center, 655 West Baltimore Street, Baltimore, Maryland, USA

INTRODUCTION

Since the introduction of chromosome banding techniques, nonrandom patterns of chromosome changes have been revealed in many hematologic malignancies. Among these changes are certain chromosome rearrangements which are consistently associated with particular types of leukemia. Two examples are the 8;21 translocation in acute myeloblastic leukemia with maturation (AML-M2 according to the French-American-British, or FAB, classification[1]),[2] and the 15 and 17 translocation in acute promyelocytic leukemia (APL-M3).[3]

Overall, abnormal karyotypes have been reported in approximately 50% of the patients with acute nonlymphocytic leukemia (ANLL) de novo[4,5] and in approximately two-thirds of those with acute lymphoblastic leukemia (ALL)[6] whose bone marrow cells were examined with banding techniques. These chromosome findings have both diagnostic and prognostic significance.[4,6,7]

In this article, we review published data on adult patients with acute leukemia, especially with ANLL de novo, who were studied with banding techniques. Also included are findings obtained with improved culture methods. Finally, we present our own cytogenetic data on a series of 33 patients with acute leukemia.

MATERIALS AND METHODS

In many cytogenetic laboratories studies of leukemic cells are done by the traditional "direct" method. With this method, leukemic cells from freshly aspirated bone marrow or, if there is a considerable number of circulating immature cells, peripheral blood are processed after a 1-2 hour incubation period. The cells are briefly exposed to a mitotic arresting agent such as colchicine or Colcemid to accumulate mitoses. In some laboratories specimens are cultured in vitro for 1-3 days prior to harvesting mitotic cells ("short-term culture").

Recently, an improved short-term culture method has been developed which increases the yield of mitotic leukemic cells, particularly prometaphase or early metaphase cells which have elongated chromosomes.[8] Basically, cultured cells are synchronized by blocking them at a certain point in the cell cycle with methotrexate (MTX). After a large portion of the cells have accumulated at this point, the cells are released from the block and proceed in the cell cycle in synchrony. The cells are stopped with a brief (10 minutes) exposure to Colcemid at the time they are passing through the early stages of mitosis when chromosomes are elongated.

We did cytogenetic analyses of 24-hour cultures (both with and without MTX synchronization) on a series of 33 patients with acute leukemia, including 26 with ANLL, two with ANLL secondary to treatment for a primary malignancy, and five with ALL. Thirty patients were examined at the time of diagnosis (29 before initiating treatment for their leukemia), and three patients were examined in relapse. In 10 of the patients we also examined direct preparations. Chromosome analysis of phytohemagglutinin (PHA)-stimulated peripheral blood cultures was also performed when it was necessary to rule out the possibility of a constitutional abnormality. Giemsa-stained mitotic cells were photographed. The same cells were then stained and photographed with quinacrine fluorescence.[9] Chromosomes were identified and karyotypes described according to the International System for Human Cytogenetic Nomenclature, ISCN (1978)[10] and ISCN (1981).[11] Normal and abnormal clones were identified according to the criteria defined at the Second International Workshop on Chromosomes in Leukemia.[7]

CHROMOSOME ABNORMALITIES IN ADULTS WITH ACUTE NONLYMPHOCYTIC LEUKEMIA (ANLL)

There have been a considerable number of chromosome banding studies on relatively large series of unselected patients with ANLL. Table 1 summarizes data regarding the incidence of abnormal karyotypes from 11 reports on series of 25 or more patients, mostly adults, with ANLL who were analyzed with banding methods.[12-22] The incidence of patients with an abnormal karyotype ranged from 37%[13] to 73%[21], with an overall incidence of about 50%. Cells from most of the patients reported in these papers were processed by the direct method, whereas cells from some patients were processed by the short-term culture method. Patients examined by the high-resolution banding method are not presented in Table 1 except for some of the patients included in the report by Hagemeijer et al.[19] Therefore, results reported in those studies may not be comparable with the results obtained by Yunis et al.[23] with the high-resolution banding method.

Even though the karyotypic changes seen in patients with ANLL show substantial variation, certain nonrandom patterns are evident. Figures 1 and 2 summarize the chromosomal changes in 282 previously published adult patients who showed numerical or structural chromosome abnormalities. Included here are data on 249 abnormal patients reported by various investigators and summarized previously in Rowley and Testa[24] as well as data from several recent studies.[20-22] The nonrandom distribution of chromosome gains and losses is particularly evident in cases with a single abnormality (Fig. 1). Thus a

TABLE 1

KARYOTYPES ANALYSED WITH BANDING TECHNIQUES IN 11 SERIES OF 25 OR MORE PATIENTS WITH ANLL

Total number of patients	Number of patients with an abnormal karyotype	Number of patients with a normal karyotype	Percent abnormal	Reference
29	16	13	55	Mitelman et al.[12]
35	13	22	37	Oshimura et al.[13]
50	25	25	50	Rowley and Potter[14]
30	15	15	50	Alimena et al.[15]
88	37	51	42	Philip et al.[16]
36	20	16	56	Rowley[17]
34	20	14	59	Prigogina et al.[18]
74	34	40	46	Hagemeijer et al.[19]
31	13	18	42	Takeuchi et al.[20]
26	19	7	73	Shiraishi et al.[21]
60	28	32	47	Bernstein et al.[22]
TOTAL 493	240	253	49%	

gain of No. 8, the most frequent abnormality seen in ANLL, was found in 66 patients (23.4% of the 282 abnormal cases), in 33 of whom a +8 was the sole abnormality present. Similarly, loss of No. 7, another frequent numerical change, was observed in 32 patients, 14 of whom showed only this change in karyotype.   In contrast, gains or losses of other autosomes seldom occurred as the sole abnormality. Thus, these were likely to represent secondary events occurring in clonal evolution, rather than primary chromosome changes. Loss of Y, the second most frequent numerical change in this summary, and X often occurred in association with an 8;21 translocation.   Of the 10 females with a loss of X,

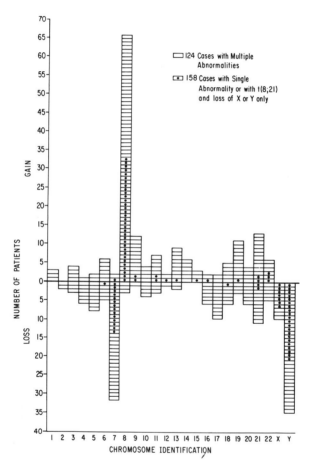

Fig. 1. Histogram of clonal gains and losses of chromosomes seen in initial cytogenetic samples from 282 adult patients with acute nonlymphocytic leukemia de novo.

seven had a t(8;21). Of the 35 males with a missing Y, 15 had a t(8;21); and in 11 of these 15 there were no further changes.

As with chromosome gains and losses, the nonrandom distribution of structural rearrangements is especially apparent in the cases with a single abnormality (Fig. 2). The most frequently rearranged chromosome was No. 17 which was observed in 51 patients, 30 of whom showed only one abnormality. Likewise, the majority of cases with rearrangements of Nos. 8, 15, or 21, the next three most frequently altered chromosomes, involved a single abnormality or, in some of the cases with a t(8;21), showed loss of a sex chromosome as the only accompanying change. Thirty-three of the cases with rearrangements of No. 15 and No. 17 involved an apparently identical 15;17 translocation; in 25 of these cases the t(15;17) was the sole abnormality present. An 8;21 translocation was observed in 37 patients, in nine of whom this was the only abnormality; in 17 of the 37 there was a t(8;21) with loss of an X or Y as the only other change. In contrast to Nos. 15, 17, 8, and 21, rearrangements of other chromosomes rarely existed as the sole abnormality in ANLL.

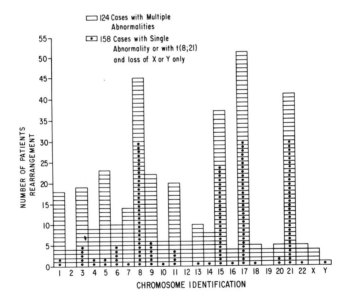

Fig. 2. Histogram of clonal structural rearrangements seen in initial cytogenetic samples from 282 patients with acute nonlymphocytic leukemia de novo.

The 8;21 Translocation and Acute Myeloblastic Leukemia (AML)

In 1968 Kamada et al.[25] recognized that a subgroup of AML patients may be characterized by an abnormality most likely representing a translocation between a C- and a G-group chromosome. The exact nature of this abnormality was resolved by Rowley who determined that it involved a balanced translocation between chromosomes 8 and 21, t(8;21)(q22;q22).[2] The frequency with which this translocation occurs seems to vary from one laboratory to another, but it amounted to 13% (37/282) of the abnormal cases summarized in Figure 2. The abnormality appears to be restricted to patients with a diagnosis of AML-M2 (acute myeloblastic leukemia with maturation) according to the FAB classification.[1] At the Second International Workshop on Chromosomes in Leukemia, all 43 cases with a t(8;21) and adequate bone marrow material available for cytological review had a diagnosis of AML-M2.[7] The incidence of this rearrangement among all patients with AML-M2 was 9.6% (41 of 429 patients). The median survival of the whole group with this translocaton was 11.5 months, which was much longer than patients with other chromosome abnormalities.

The 15;17 Translocation and Acute Promyelocytic Leukemia (APL)

A consistent structural rearrangement involving chromosomes 15 and 17 in APL was first recognized by Rowley et al.[3] There is considerable controversy about the breakpoints in this abnormality, but a translocation t(15;17)(q25?;q22) was suggested at the Second International Workshop on Chromosomes in Leukemia.[7] Of the 80 patients with APL who were reviewed at that workshop, 33 (41%) had a t(15;17) alone (23 cases), or in combination with other abnormalities, 7 had other types of chromosome changes, and 40 had a normal karyotype. The rearrangement was not found in patients with any other type of leukemia.[7] In our laboratory all six of our patients with APL, including all three from this study, had the 15;17 anomaly (unpublished data).

CHROMOSOME ABNORMALITIES IN ADULTS WITH ACUTE LYMPHOBLASTIC LEUKEMIA (ALL)

At the Third International Workshop on Chromosomes in Leukemia 330 patients with ALL were evaluated.[6] All of these cases were examined with chromosome banding methods at diagnosis; 173 patients were adults (older than 16 years). Among these 173 patients, 53 had a normal karyotype, and 120 patients (69.4%) had an abnormal clone. Thus, the incidence of patients with an abnormal karyotype appeared to be somewhat higher than that for ANLL. Among adults with clonal abnormalities, 57% had a modal number of 46. Hyperdiploidy was present in 31.7% of the patients. Translocations were reported in 37.6% of these patients. The most frequent structural rearrangements were:

Ph^1-translocation (17.3% of all adults); t(8;14) or 8q- (5.8%); other 14q+ (6.9%); t(4;11) (5.2%); and 6q- (1.7%).

PROGNOSTIC SIGNIFICANCE OF CHROMOSOME ABNORMALITIES IN ACUTE LEUKEMIA

Sakurai and Sandberg, using conventional staining methods, were the first to demonstrate a correlation between the karyotypic pattern of leukemic cells and survival in patients with ANLL.[26] Patients with only normal metaphase cells (NN) had a median survival of 11.5 months from the onset of symptoms as compared to 10.3 months for patients with a mixture of normal and abnormal metaphase cells (AN) and only 3.2 months in those with only abnormal metaphase cells (AA). Of the AML patients reviewed at the First International Workshop on Chromosomes in Leukemia, a substantially longer median survival (8 months) was found in patients who were NN as compared to that in patients who were AA (3.5 months). Patients who were AN had an intermediate survival (5 months).[4] However, one chromosome rearrangement, t(8;21), is not associated with a poor prognosis. Conversely, this abnormality is associated with a relatively long survival, particularly for patients who also have some normal metaphase cells.[7] The median survival time of all 46 patients with a t(8;21) who were reviewed at the Second International Workshop on Chromosomes in Leukemia, was 11.5 months which was comparable to that of patients with a normal karyotype.[7]

At the Third International Workshop on Chromosomes in Leukemia it was demonstrated for the first time that the karyotypic pattern is an independent prognostic factor in ALL.[6] In adults, remission was achieved in more than 84% of the patients without clonal abnormalities and in less than 55% of those with clonal abnormalities. Furthermore, the median duration of remission was longer in those who had a normal karyotype. Survival was longest for patients with all normal metaphases and shorter for patients with clonal abnormalities whether or not normal metaphases were present. An especially poor prognosis was noted for patients with either a t(4;11), t(8;14), 14q+, hypodiploidy, or hyperdiplody with a modal number of 47-50.

INFLUENCE OF METHOD OF PROCESSING SPECIMENS ON THE INCIDENCE OF CHROMOSOME ABNORMALITIES

Recent investigations have indicated that results obtained by different methods of processing specimens may not be comparable. Several reports have shown that the percentage of clonal abnormal cells in bone marrow in patients with various hematologic disorders may be significantly higher in preparations made after a 1-3 day incubation period than in those made by the direct method.[27,28] For instance, Knuutila et al. provided results on 32 samples from 21 patients, and in 18 of the samples cultures yielded

TABLE 2

INCIDENCE OF ABNORMAL CELLS DETECTED WITH THREE DIFFERENT PROCESSING METHODS

Laboratory case number	Diagnosis	Direct		24-hr culture		MTX-culture	
		No. of cells	Abnormal (%)	No. of cells	Abnormal (%)	No. of cells	Abnormal (%)
241	AML(M1)	9	0	12	0	43	0
242	APL(M3)	13	0	12	75	16	69
244	AML(M1)	10	0	17	29	12	17
260	AML(M1)	8	100	11	100	—	—
261	AML(M1)	13	0	26	0	5	0
262	AML(M1)	8	0	17	0	40	8
275	ALL(L2)	2	100	4	100	5	100
276	AMMoL(M4)	12	92	8	100	7	100
279	AML(M2)	8	38	13	62	6	33
283	AMoL(M5)	1	100	2	100	17	100

a higher percentage of abnormal cells than the direct method. In 10 of these instances the difference was statistically significant. Of greater interest, on four occasions the culture method revealed clonal abnormalities that would not have been detected if the direct method alone has been used.[27] Waghray et al. reported similar findings in a series of 14 patients; three of their 13 cytogenetically abnormal patients would have been incorrectly classified as being normal on the basis of the initial analysis of the direct preparation.[28] Our results on 10 patients are summarized in Table 2. Each of these 10 patients had acute leukemia. Bone marrow cells were examined at diagnosis, and clonal abnormalities were identified in eight of these patients. Abnormal clones were detected in five of the direct specimens as compared to seven of the 24h-culture preparations (without MTX). In case no. 262 a small clone was found only in the MTX-synchronized culture.

Overall, these results suggest that about 15-25% of patients with clonal abnormalities in culture preparations may show only normal karyotypes in direct marrow.

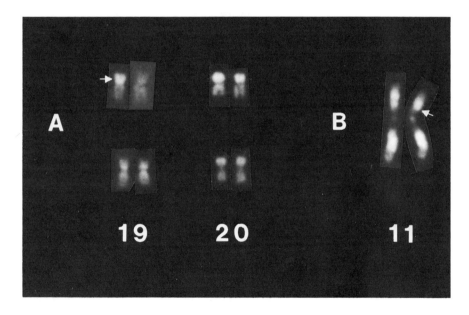

Figure 3. Partial karyotypes showing Q-banded chromosomes from two patients with ANLL. (A) Upper row: chromosome pairs 19 and 20 of metaphase cell from bone marrow culture. One No. 19 has abnormal, moderately bright band on short arm. Lower row: Normal pairs 19 and 20 of metaphase from PHA-stimulated peripheral blood. (B) Chromosome pair 11 of metaphase from bone marrow culture. One No. 11 has interstitial deletion of short arm, del(11)(p11p13).

TABLE 3

SUMMARY OF CYTOGENETIC FINDINGS IN OUR SERIES OF 29 PATIENTS WITH ACUTE LEUKEMIA

Diagnosis (FAB)	No. of patients	No. of patients with an abnormal karyotype	Percent abnormal
AML(M1)	11	8	73
AML(M2)	2	2	100
APL(M3)	3	3	100
AMMoL(M4)	5	4	80
AMoL(M5)	1	1	100
EL(M6)	1	1	100
ALL(L2)	4	4	100
Secondary acute leukemia	2	2	100
TOTAL	29	25	86%

HIGH-RESOLUTION BANDING ANALYSIS OF CHROMOSOMES IN ACUTE LEUKEMIA

We obtained an adequate number of mitotic cells for cytogenetic examination in 29 of 33 consecutive patients with acute leukemia. Twenty-five of 29 patients (86%) had detectable clonal chromosome abnormalities (Table 3). Of the 23 patients with ANLL, 19 (83%) were cytogenetically abnormal. No clonal abnormalities were detected in four patients (three with a diagnosis of M1; one with M4) even though 42 to 89 cells were fully karyotyped in each case; however, some single cell or non-clonal abnormalities were found. Previously reported nonrandom chromosome abnormalities in acute leukemia were identified, including +8 in four cases, and -7 in three cases.

One of the two patients with a diagnosis of AML-M2 had an 8;21 translocation which is specific for this type of ANLL. All three patients with an APL-M3 diagnosis had a t(15;17). Four of five patients with AMMoL-M4 showed clonal abnormalities, including one patient with a t(11;11)(q13;q23). Germane to this, Yunis et al.[23] recently suggested that abnormalities of band 11q23 may be specific for a new subtype of ANLL with monocytic involvement. All four of our patients with ALL-L2 showed abnormalities, and two of these patients had a 6q-. One had a del(6)(q21q25) and the other had a smaller deletion, del(6)(q21?q23?).

Results obtained with unsynchronized and MTX-synchronized culture methods were generally similar (Table 2). However, in one patient who had a small clone the abnormality was detected only in the synchronized cells (Table 2, case no. 262). Moreover, synchronized cultures often yielded more mitoses with high-quality, elongated chromosomes than unsynchronized cultures. On the other hand, on several occasions (4 of 29 cases) few or no mitoses were found in the synchronized culture, although an adequate number of mitotic cells was seen in the corresponding unsynchronized 24-hr culture. Thus, our experience suggests that it is advisable to use both of these culture methods in order to maximize the chance of detecting clonal abnormalities in acute leukemia. In two patients the only abnormality detected was a tiny structural rearrangement (Fig. 3). Although these abnormalities were identified in both the unsynchronized and the MTX-synchronized cultures in each case, these rearrangements would have been difficult to detect if not for the elongated chromosomes found in some cells with each culture method.

Table 4 summarizes the results from two series of patients examined with the high-resolution banding method, one by Yunis et al.[23] and the other, our present study. Yunis and his co-workers identified clonal abnormalities in every one of their 23 patients. We detected clonal abnormalities in 23 of 27 (85%) patients with acute leukemia de novo. These results indicate that chromosome abnormalities can now be detected in a much higher proportion of patients with acute leukemia than was thought previously. Our findings do not rule out the possibility that all patients with acute leukemia have a

TABLE 4

SUMMARY OF CYTOGENETIC FINDINGS IN TWO SERIES OF ACUTE LEUKEMIA PATIENTS EXAMINED WITH HIGH–RESOLUTION BANDING TECHNIQUES

Diagnosis	Yunis et al. (1981)*		Present Series**	
	No. of patients***	Percent abnormal	No. of patients***	Percent abnormal
AML(M1)	8 (3)	100	11	73
AML(M2)	6	100	2	100
APL(M3)	2	100	3	100
AMMoL(M4)	3 (1)	100	5 (1)	80
AMoL(M5)	3 (2)	100	1	100
EL(M6)	1	100	1	100
ALL	—	—	4 (1)	100
TOTAL	23 (6)	100%	27 (2)	85%

*One patient with erythromegakaryocytic leukemia is excluded in this table.
**Two patients with secondary acute leukemia are excluded in this table.
***Number in parentheses indicate subtotal of patients examined in relapse.

chromosome defect. It is possible that one or more of our four patients with normal karyotypes might actually have a tiny structural rearrangement which can only be delineated with even more finely banded chromosomes. However, as suggested by Rowley[30] at least some patients with leukemia will probably be found to have a normal karyotype, even when many mitoses with high-quality, elongated chromosomes are analyzed. In such cases the leukemia may result from the insertion of a DNA sequence far below the level of resolution of light microscopy.

Because the results obtained with high-resolution banding techniques do not appear to be comparable with those obtained with standard techniques, it will be important to re-examine karyotype/survival correlations according to the specific method used. As samples from more patients are analyzed with high-resolution banding, some specific subtle rearrangements that are associated with a relative favorable outlook, as well as others which may be associated with an especially poor prognosis, may be identified.

ACKNOWLEDGMENTS

The results presented in this article were obtained during research supported in part by PHS Grant No. 1P50CA-32107-01 awarded by the National Cancer Institute, DHHS; and by a grant from the Leukemia Research Foundation, Inc. awarded to J.R.T.

REFERENCES

1. Bennett, J.M., Catovsky, D., Daniel, M.T., Flandrin, G., Galton, D.A.G., Gralnick, H. and Sultan, C. (1976) Br. J. Haematol. 33, 451-458.
2. Rowley, J.D. (1973) Ann. Genet. 16, 109-112.
3. Rowley, J.D., Golomb, H.M. and Dougherty,C. (1977) Lancet 1, 549-550.
4. First International Workshop on Chromosomes in Leukaemia, 1977. (1978) Br. J. Haematol. 39, 311-316.
5. Testa, J.R. and Rowley, J.D. (1980) Cancer Genet. Cytogenet. 1, 239-247.
6. The Third International Workshop on Chromosomes in Leukemia (1980) Cancer Genet. Cytogenet. 4, 95-142.
7. The Second International Workshop on Chromosomes in Leukemia, 1979. (1980) Cancer Genet. Cytogent. 2, 89-113.
8. Hagemeijer, A. and Bootsma, D. (1979) Cytogenet. Cell Genet. 23, 208-212.
9. Caspersson, T., Lomakka, G. and Zech, L. (1971) Hereditas (Lund) 67, 89-102.
10. An International System for Human Cytogenetic Nomenclature (1978) Birth Defects: Original Article Series XIV (8), The National Foundation, New York.
11. An International System for Human Cytogenetic Nomenclature—High-Resolution Banding (1981) Birth Defects: Original Article Series XVII (5), The National Foundation, New York.
12. Mitelman, F., Nilsson, P.G., Levan, G. and Brandt, L. (1976) Int. J. Cancer 18, 31-38.
13. Oshimura, M., Hayata, I., Kakati, S. and Sandberg, A.A. (1976) Cancer 38, 748-761.
14. Rowley, J.D. and Potter, D. (1976) Blood 47, 705-721.
15. Alimena, G., Annino, L., Balestrazzi, P., Montuoro, A. and Dallapicolla, B. (1977) Acta Haematol. 58, 234-242.
16. Philip, P., Jensen, M.K., Killman,S.A., Divsholm, A. and Hansen, N.E. (1978) Leukemia Res. 2, 201-212.
17. Rowley, J.D. (1978) Clin. Haematol. 7, 385-406.

18. Prigogina, E.L., Fleischman, E.W., Puchkova, G.P., Kulagina, O.E., Majakova, S.A., Frenkel, M.A., Khvatova, N.V. and Peterson, I.S. (1979) Hum.Genet. 53, 5-16.
19. Hagemeijer, A., Hahlen, K. and Abels, J. (1981) Cancer Genet. Cytogenet. 3, 109-124.
20. Takeuchi, J., Oshima, T. and Amaki, T. (1981) Cancer Genet. Cytogenet. 4, 293-302.
21. Shiraishi, Y., Taguchi, H., Niiya, K., Shiomi, F., Kikukawa, K., Kubonishi,S., Ohmura,T., Hamawaki, M. and Ueda, N. (1982) Cancer Genet. Cytogenet. 5, 1-24.
22. Bernstein, R., Pinto, M.R., Morcom, G., Macdougall, L.G., Bezwoda, W., Dukes, I., Penfold, G. and Mendelow, B. (1982) Cancer Genet. Cytogenet. 6, 187-199.
23. Yunis, J.J., Bloomfield,C.D. and Ensrud, K. (1981) N. Engl. J. Med. 305, 135-139.
24. Rowley, J.D. and Testa, J.R. (1982) in Advances in Cancer Research 36, Klein, G. and Weinhouse, S. ed., Academic Press, New York, pp. 103-148.
25. Kamada, N., Okada, K., Ito, T., Nakatsui,T. and Uchino, H. (1968) Lancet 1, 364.
26. Sakurai, M. and Sandberg, A.A. (1973) Blood 41, 93-104.
27. Knuutila, S., Vuopio, P., Elonen, E., Sumes, M., Kovanen, R., Borgstrom,G.H. and de la Chapelle, A. (1981) Blood 58, 369-375.
28. Waghray, M., Eques, C., Rowley, J.D., Martin, P. and Testa, J.R. (1981) Amer. J. Hematol. 11, 409-415.
29. Hagemeijer, A., Hahlen, K., Sizoo, W. and Abels, J. (1982) Cancer Genet. Cytogenet. 5, 95-105.
30. Rowley, J.D. (1981) N. Engl. J. Med. 305, 164-166.

CHROMOSOMAL STUDIES ON DIRECT PREPARATIONS OF PRIMARY RETINOBLASTOMA: IMPLICA-
TIONS FOR THE FUNCTION OF THE RETINOBLASTOMA GENE

WILLIAM F. BENEDICT[1] AND A. LINN MURPHREE[2]
Clayton Ocular Oncology Center[1,2] and the Divisions of Hematology-Oncology[1] and
Ophthalmology[2], Childrens Hospital of Los Angeles, Los Angeles, California
90027, Department of Pediatrics[1,2] and Ophthalmology[2], University of Southern
California School of Medicine

INTRODUCTION

Retinoblastoma is a malignant intraocular tumor of childrens which exists
in hereditary, non-hereditary and chromosomal deletion forms. The gene loci for
both hereditary deletion[1,2] and non-deletion[3] forms of retinoblastoma have
recently been assigned to chromosomal region 13q14 implying that there may be
one retinoblastoma locus common to both hereditary forms of this tumor.

In this section we wish to emphasize some of our recent findings from
direct chromosomal preparations of primary tumors. In particular, we shall
present evidence from one patient which suggests that the retinoblastoma gene is
a recessive gene at the cellular level. A discussion of the chromosome findings
in retinoblastoma follows.

A PATIENT WITH THE 13 DELETION FORM OF RETINOBLASTOMA PROVIDES EVIDENCE THAT THE
RETINOBLASTOMA GENE IS A RECESSIVE CANCER GENE

The locus for esterase D, an enzyme of unknown function found in most
tissues, has been assigned to chromosomal region 13q14 by deletion mapping[2] and
is closely linked to the retinoblastoma gene.[1,2] Since the activity of this
enzyme is gene dose dependent, an individual with a deletion of chromosome 13
that includes region q14 has only 50% of normal esterase D activity constitu-
tionally. The patient presented here is described more completely elsewhere.[4]
She was admitted to Childrens Hospital with bilateral retinoblastoma and except
for these tumors no other physical or developmental abnormalities were present.
However, the esterase D activity in her red blood cells was 50% of normal. We
therefore initially considered this individual to have the hereditary deletion
form of retinoblastoma. However, neither peripheral lymphocytes, lymphoblastoid
cells nor skin fibroblasts exhibited a microscopically apparent deletion within
13q14 while each tissue had only half normal esterase D activity. Although independent mutations of the esterase D and retinoblastoma gene loci are possible, a
more likely explanation of the association of half normal esterase D activity
and retinoblastoma is a single submicroscopic deletion involving both loci.

Published 1983 by Elsevier Science Publishing Co., Inc.
Cancer: Etiology and Prevention, Ray G. Crispen, Editor

The direct chromosomal preparations from the retinoblastoma in one eye showed two distinct stem lines that were represented approximately equally. The first stem line showed a modal karyotype of 49, X, +2, +7, -13, +15, -16, -17, -18, -21, +M1, +M2, +M3, plus three other unidentifiable chromosomes.[4] None of the abnormal chromosomes appeared to contain any portion of a chromosome 13. The marker chromosomes M1, M2 and M3 were present in each karyotype from that stem line. The second stem line had a modal karyotype of 49, XX, -13 +19, +20, +22, +M4. The multiple differences in the karyotypic patterns between the two chromosomal lines and the lack of common marker chromosomes makes it impossible that they could have resulted from clonal evolution of only one transformed cell. A loss of one 13 chromosome was the only consistent chromosomal change found in both of the tumor stem lines. When the esterase D activity within the tumor was analyzed, a complete absence of esterase D activity was found. These results indicate that the non-deleted 13 chromosome was lost in both stem lines. Thus, this patient represents the first individual in which it has been possible to demonstrate at the tumor level a loss of both alleles at a chromosome locus known to contain a cancer gene for a specific malignancy, in this case retinoblastoma. These results also strongly suggest that the retinoblastoma gene is a recessive gene at the tumor level in that the loss of both alleles are required for tumor formation.

SPECIFIC CHROMOSOMAL CHANGES IN RETINOBLASTOMA

We have recently finished an extensive study on the chromosomal patterns of direct preparations from both hereditary and non-hereditary forms of primary retinoblastoma. Over 15 tumors have been analyzed and the results of these studies are reported in detail elsewhere.[5] Non-random chromosomal changes found in these tumors included a frequent loss of a 13 chromosome and the presence of an additional isochromosome which we believe to be an iso 6p. Balaban and her colleagues have also recently reported a deletion of a 13 chromosome including chromosomal region 13q14 in several direct tumor preparations,[6] but a statistically significant loss of a 13 chromosome was not found by other investigators.[7] It should be noted that the majority of these latter studies were not done on direct tumor preparations. This same group, however, was the first to identify an isochromosome in retinoblastoma tumors which was initially considered to be an iso 17.[7] We both now believe this chromosome is an iso 6p.

The importance of the loss or specific deletion of 13q14 at the tumor level in retinoblastoma can only be speculated upon at this moment. However, we would suggest that they may represent two mechanisms for inactivation of the second 13q14 retinoblastoma allele. The role of the iso 6p found in many of the retinoblastomas also can only be speculated upon, but it is possible that this region may contain genetic information for the expression of tumorigenicity.

ACKNOWLEDGEMENTS

We wish to thank Dr. Robert Sparkes for his contributions to many of the studies outlined, and Dr. Ashutosh Banerjee for making the majority of the direct chromosomal preparations of primary retinoblastomas. This work was supported in part by Grant EY-02715 from the National Eye Institute and was performed in conjunction with the Clayton Foundation for Research.

REFERENCES

1. Yunis, J.J. and Ramsey, N. (1978) Am. J. Dis. Child. 132, 161-163.
2. Sparkes, R.S., Murphree, A.L. Lingua, R.W., Sparkes, M.C., Field, L.L., Funderburk, S.J. and Benedict, W.F. (1983) Science, in press.
3. Sparkes, R.S., Sparkes, M.C., Wilson, M.G., Towner, J.W., Benedict, W., Murphree, A.L. and Yunis, J.J. (1980) Science, 208, 1042-1043.
4. Benedict, W.F., Murphree, A.L., Banerjee, A., Spina, C.A., Sparkes, M.C. and Sparkes, R.S. (1983) Science, in press.
5. Benedict, W.F., Banerjee, A. and Murphree, A.L. (1983) Cancer Genet. Cytogenet, in press.
6. Balaban, G., Gilbert, F., Nichols, W., Meadows, A.T. and Shields, J. (1982) Cancer Genet. Cytogenet., 6, 213-214.
7. Gardner, H.A., Gallie, B.L., Knight, L.A. and Phillips, R.A. (1982), Cancer Genet. Cytogenet., 6, 201-211.

A NON-RANDOM CHROMOSOMAL ABNORMALITY, del(3)(p14-23) in
SMALL CELL LUNG CANCER (SCLC)

J. Whang-Peng[+], D.N. Carney[++] E.C. Lee[+], C.S. Kao-Shan[+], P.A. Bunn[++],
A. Gazdar[++], and J.D. Minna[++]
[+]Medicine Branch, and [++]NCI-Navy Medical Oncology Branch, DCT, NCI
National Institutes of Health, Bethesda, Maryland 20205

INTRODUCTION

Each year in the United States, there are approximately 25,000 new cases of
small cell lung cancer (SCLC); these represent roughly 25% of all types of
lung cancer[1]. SCLC is an aggressive neoplasm with early metastasis, and
there is a dramatic response to combination chemotherapy and radiotherapy
in over 90% of the patients leading to a cure in about 10%. In contrast, non-
small cell lung cancer (non-SCLC) including adenocarcinoma, squamous cell
carcinoma, and large-cell carcinoma, have much lower response to current chemo-
radiotherapy regimens. Thus, accurate diagnosis and distinction of SCLC from
non-SCLC is essential. Here we would like to describe a specific chromosomal
marker, deletion(3)(p14-23) associated with and diagnostic of small cell lung
cancer.[2] In the most common form, an interstitial deletion is present in the
cytogenetic preparations of tumors taken directly from patients as well as in
cultures of these tumors. In the remainder of the patients studied, a large
deletion of 3p is found, such as deletion(3)(p11→pter). The demonstration of
this marker in patients with lung cancer represents a cytogenetic method of
distinguishing lung cancer types.

MATERIALS AND METHODS

A total of 68 patients with histologically confirmed SCLC were studied cytogenetically to determine whether or not a specific abnormality existed in this
disease. With the exception of one cell line established from a Japanese
patient (courtesy of Dr. Y. Shimosato, Toyko, Japan), all specimens were from
patients being evaluated for therapeutic protocols at the NCI-VA and later the
NCI-Navy Medical Oncology Branch.

Direct cytogenetic studies of bone marrow were performed on 54 patients (40
males and 14 females). In addition, a total of 16 continuous SCLC tissue

Published 1983 by Elsevier Science Publishing Co., Inc.
Cancer: Etiology and Prevention, Ray G. Crispen, Editor

culture lines (13 males, 3 females) derived from metastatic lesions, bone marrow, or pleural effusion; one short term (2-day) culture of pleural fluid and two lymphoblastoid lines from SCLC patients were analyzed karyotypically. Only one primary chest lesion (2 day culture) has been studied. Five tissue culture lines from patients with non small cell lung cancer served as controls.

The tissue culture lines were established from patents with documented histologic diagnosis of SCLC, and the tumors were grown in a serum-free defined medium supplemented with hydrocortisone, insulin, transferrin, 17-β-estradiol and selenium (HITES).[3] Thirteen of the lines have cytology and nude mouse tumor histology characteristic of SCLC. All of the 16 SCLC lines also have specific biochemical and immunological markers as well as unique ultrastructural properties.[4] Nearly all have high specific activity of the amine precursor uptake and decarboxylation (APUD) cell enzymes, L-dopa decarboxylase and neuron specific enolase. They also have high specific activities of creatine kinase BB isoenzyme and produce the peptide hormone bombesin. In addition, electron microscopy reveals dense core granules in all SCLC lines with high L-dopa decarboxylase activities. The non-SCLC cell lines lack these features.

Chromosome preparations of the cell lines, direct bone marrow, and tumor specimens were made according to the method of Tjio and Whang.[5] Air-dried slides were stained with conventional Giemsa stain, G-banded using a modified trypsin-Giemsa technique,[6] and C-banded.[7] Detailed chromosome analyses were carried out according to the criteria established by the Paris Conference.[8]

RESULTS

Cytogenetic studies of fresh tumor samples. Chromosome preparations were made of a primary chest tumor and a pleural effusion from two patients. Cytogenetic analysis of cells from the primary chest lesion, grown for two days in HITES medium showed a chromosome range from 35 to 85 although 90% were hypodiploid with a modal number of 42. All of the hypodiploid metaphases had a normal chromosome #3 and two abnormal #3 chromosomes, del(3)(p21), and del(3)(p14-23); in addition, all metaphases were missing one chromosome #21 and one #22. The pleural effusion had a modal chromosome number of 68, in the triploid region. All of the metaphases had the interstitial deletion (3)(p14-23).

Cytogenetic studies of fresh bone marrow samples. In the 54 patients
studied, no mitoses or inadequate banding analysis were found in 26. Of the
28 patients with successful cytogenetic studies, 19 had no tumor cells seen
histologically and all had a normal karyotype. One patient had normal histology but 20% of the mitoses had an abnormal karyotype. Eight were shown to
have tumor cells histologically, with seven having an abnormal karyotype.
One patient had tumor found histologically but in the 15 metaphases available
for analysis, only diploid normal cells were found. The percentage of aneu-
ploidy found in each of the 8 patients was 20%, 28%, 43%, 60%, 70%, 73%, 90%,
and 100%. Chromosome distribution is shown in Figures 1A, and 1B. One case
was hypodiploid (Figure 2), one was diploid, and the rest had chromosome
numbers in the triploid or tetraploid range (Figure 3). Structural abnormalities found in at least 50% of the metaphases are shown in Table 1. All eight
patients had a deletion of 3p, seven of them had the interstitial deletion in
more than 50% of the analyzed metaphases. The last patient also had the interstitial deletion but in only 35% of the involved cells. Chromosomal
aberrations were minimal in the aneuploid cells. Double minutes (DMs) or a
homogeneously staining region (HSR) were not seen in any of the direct
specimens. In summary, in every aneuploid or abnormal metaphase in every one
of the eight patients, direct cytogenetic preparations of the bone marrow
revealed some form of deleletion of chromosome #3p; the most common being an
interstitial deletion (3)(p14-23).

Table 1

STRUCTURAL ABNORMALITIES IN ≥ 50% OF THE BONE MARROW METAPHASES

Case	Cytology	Range	Modal #	%A	Karyotype
FB	+ ?%	45	45	100	1p+,1p++,+del(3)(p14-23),14q+
RB	+ 60%	69-97	70	28	t(1;3)(1q;3q),del(3)(p14-23),del(3)(p21q21), del(22)q
GE	+ ?%	40-46	45	90	1p+q21-,t(1;3;9),del(3)(p11-23),del(3)(p13q26)
WF	+ ?%	75-92	77	43	del(3)(p14-23),del(3)(p14-q21),del(3)(p13)
DF	+ <1%	62-67	63	70	del(3)(p21),del(3)(p14-23),del(3)(p14-23q21)
CM	−	46-47	46	20	del(3)(p14-23)
JS	+ 50%	62-96	77	60	del(3)(p14q21),t(13;14),del(22)(q11)
RT	+ 70%	70-156	156	73	del(3)(p14-23)

50

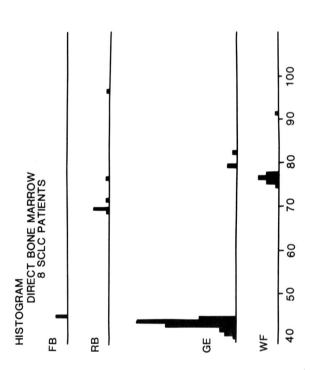

Figure 1A

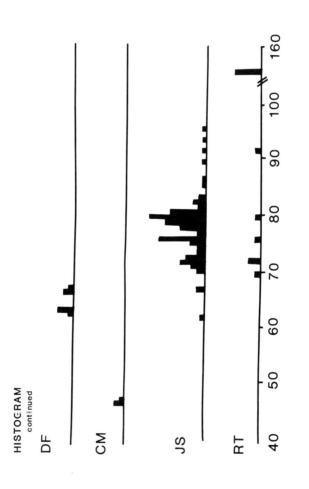

Figure 1B

52

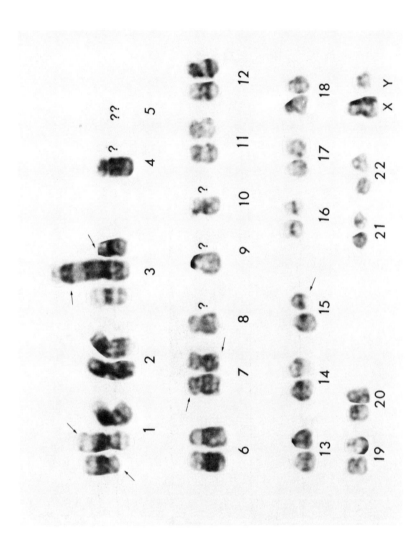

Figure 2. G-banded karyotype from a hypodiploid cell of involved bone marrow; arrows indicate marker chromosomes

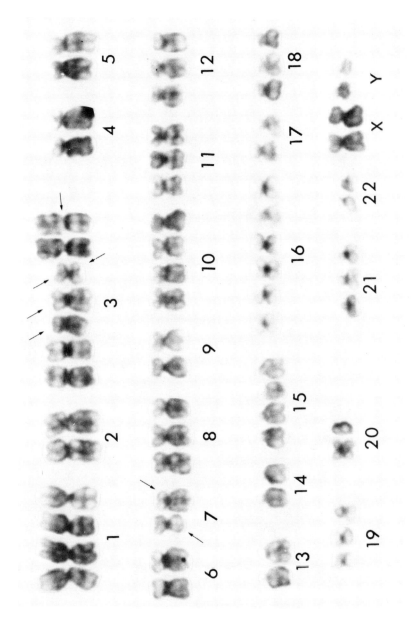

Figure 3. G-banded karyotype from a triploid cell of involved bone marrow; arrows indicate marker
chromosomes

54

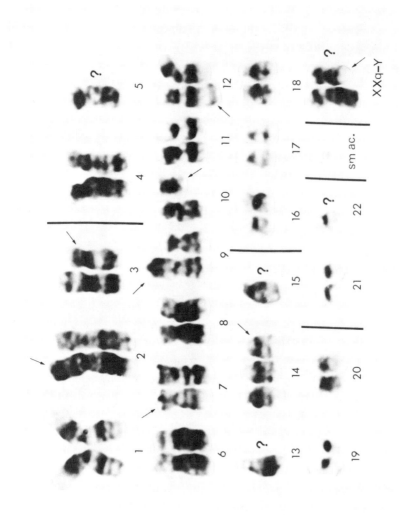

Figure 4. G-banded karyotype from the SCLC tissue culture line, H64; arrows indicate marker chromosomes

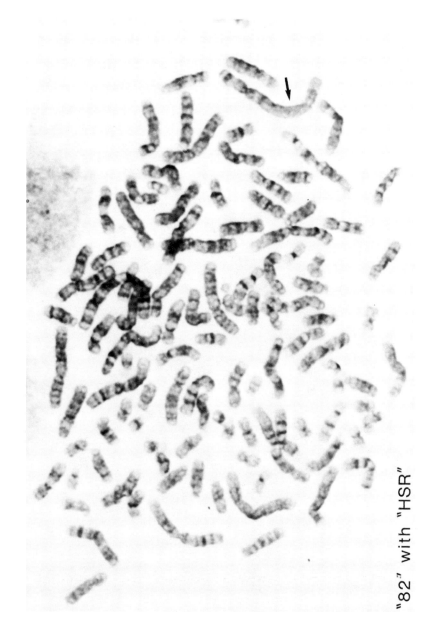

"82" with "HSR"

Figure 5. GTG banded metaphase spread from SCLC line H82 showing a HSR

56

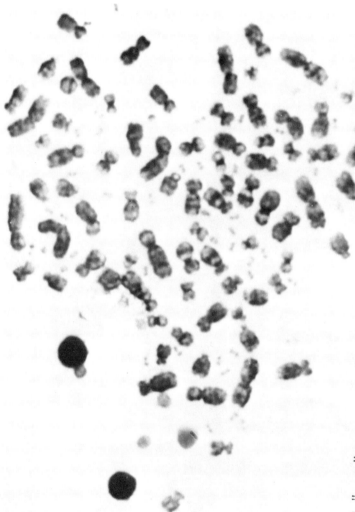

"" ""
60 with double minutes

Figure 6. GTG-banded metaphase spread from SCLC line H60 showing numerous double minute chromosomes

Cytogenetic studies of SCLC tissue culture lines. All of the 16 SCLC cell lines studied were aneuploid.[2] Chromosome numbers varied greatly for these 16 lines; ranging from hypodiploid to greater than tetraploid. Four lines were hypodiploid, although one of these had a second mode in tetraploid region as well. One line was near diploid (Figure 4), six had modal chromosome numbers between hyperdiploid and tetraploid, and five lines were tetraploid or greater. All of the lines had numerous structural and numerical abnormalities involving many chromosomes. Structural aberrations of chromosome #3 were found in all 16 lines with 100% of the metaphases having a 3p deletion, most usually the interstital deletion involving the p(14-23) region. The shortest region of overlap analysis showed all of the cell lines to have a deletion in this area of chromosome #3. Additional chromosomes involved in structural abnormalities were (in decreasing frequency) chromosome #1 (13/16), #10 (12/16), #2 (11/16), #9 (10/16), X (10/16), and #14 (9/16). All of the remaining chromosomes, with the exception of chromosome #18, were also involved in structural abnormalities in at least one of the cell lines. Chromosome #3 was the only chromosome to have a specific region of involvement in abnormalities. One line had a homogeneously staining region (HSR) on chromosome #15 involving 96% of the metaphases in that line (Figure 5); C-banding showed this HSR to be euchromatic. Two of the 16 lines had double minutes (DMs) in 2 and 30% of the metaphases respectively; these ranged from two per metaphase to numerous DMs in a single metaphase (Figure 6).

Cytogenetic studies in lymphoblastoid cell lines from SCLC patients. Two lymphoblastoid cell lines derived from SCLC patients had normal karyotypes.

Cytogenetic studies of non-SCLC lines. None of the metaphases of the five non-SCLC lines had a deletion of 3p below band 3p25.

Search for a translocation of the deleted 3p segment. Thus far no definite translocation of the deleted 3p segment to another chromosme has been found. However, the interstitial nature of the deleted region may hinder this type of analysis.

DISCUSSION

An acquired, specific deletion of chromosome #3p for small cell lung cancer is described here. In a total of 26 small cell lung cancer patients who had successful cytogenetic studies, direct chromosome preparations of involved bone marrow (eight patients), of a primary chest lesion (one patient),

and of pleural effusion (one patient); as well as chromosome analyses of 16
SCLC tissue culture lines showed that at least one chromosome #3 in every
metaphase had a deletion of 3p. Twenty-two of the 26 patients had an interstitial deletion(3)(p14-23) in at least some of the metaphases analyzed, and
this region of 3(p14-23) was shown to be deleted in all metaphases when shortest region of overlap analysis was applied to structural abnormalities of
chromosome #3. Studies of lymphoblastoid lines from two of these patients and
of five non small cell lung cancer lines did not show this abnormality.

At present, the knowledge of this specific, acquired chromosomal deletion
provides a new, cytogenetic method of distinguishing SCLC from other types of
lung cancer. The evidence is becoming strong enough to begin using the existence of this deletion of chromosome 3p to select patients for SCLC treatment
trials; and with confirmation from other investigators to eventually introduce
cytogenetic analysis into general clinical practice as a diagnostic aid.

It is possible that the deletion of 3p is related to chromosomal damage by
carcinogens such as cigarette smoke, or by other chemicals and radiation. Of
even greater interest is the possibility that this deletion points to a specific
genetic change leading to SCLC. It may be that the deletion allows expression
of a mutant gene on the "normal appearing" chromosome #3 or that translocation
of the deleted portion of #3 causes the cell to behave in a malignant fashion.

A recent report by Luthardt[9] showed expression of a genomic "hot spot"
at 3p14 which was induced in vitro. In the 23 of 39 patients studied, a
chromatid break (ctb) at 3p14 was found, ranging in frequency from one to
20%. The expression of ctb(3)(p14) was inversely related to the concentration
of folic acid in the medium and was partially suppressed by addition of BrdUrd
although not by addition of thymidine. The relationship between this fragile
site and the deletion(3)(p14-23) is not explored in this study. In the present
study, the use of the HITES medium and/or RPMI 1640 supplemented with 10% fetal
bovine serum as well as the very low frequency of chromosomal aberrations
found in the SCLC patients may make any correlation with the location of the
fragile site unlikely.

In recent reports of renal cell carcinoma, two families are described
with chromosomal abnormalities of 3p. One family had a translocation between
chromosomes #3 and #8 involving a break at 3p21;[10] and the second, a translocation between #3 and #11 involving a break at 3p13 or p14.[11] In neither
family was there a deletion of the 3p14-23 region; although the report of the

abnormality of chromosome #3 in these two families with renal cell carcinoma raises many interesting questions concerning the tumorigenicity of this region of #3. Whether or not the 3p abnormality described in renal cell carcinoma and its association with chromosme #8 or #11 is functionally related to that found in SCLC remains to be determined.

The importance of the homogeneously staining region (HSR) found in one cell line, and the double minutes (DMs) found in two of the cell lines has not yet been defined. These three cell lines are derived from tumors relapsing after chemotherapy which included methotrexate. Whether or not these abnormalities represent gene amplification or drug resistance developing in vivo is being studied.

In conclusion, we propose that the chromosomal abnormality del(3)(p14-23) is specific for small cell lung cancer. Routine cytogenetic studies of tumor, pleural effusion, lymph nodes or involved bone marrow with or without selection in HITES medium will facilitate diagnosis and permit quick institution of appropriate therapy that will increase long term survival and prognosis in these patients. In addition, further evaluation of the genes located on chromosome 3p should point to a specific, acquired, genetic cause for this type of lung cancer.

60

REFERENCES
1. Minna, J.D., Higgins, G.A., and Glatstein, E.J. (1981) in Principles and Practice of Oncology, DeVita, V.T. Hellman, S. and Rosenberg S. ed., J.B. Lippincott, Philadelphia, pp. 396-473.
2. Whang-Peng, J., Bunn, P.A., Kao-Shan, C.S., Lee, E.C., Carney, D.N., Gazdar, A., and Minna, J.D. (1982) Cancer Genetics and Cytogenetics, 6, 119-134.
3. Carney, D.N., Bunn, P.A., Gazdar, A.F., Pagan, J.A., and Minna, J.D. (1981) Proc. Nat. Acad. Sci. 78, 3185-3189.
4. Gazdar, A.F., Carney, D.N., Russell, E.K., Sims, H.L., Baylin, S.B., Bunn, P.A., Guccion, J.G., and Minna, J.D. (1980) Cancer Research, 40, 3502-3507.
5. Tjio, J.H., and Whang, J. (1962) Stain Technol. 37, 17-20.
6. Seabright, M. (1971) Lancet 2, 971-972.
7. Arrighi, F.W., and Hsu, T.C. (1971) Cytogenetics, 10, 81-86.
8. Paris Conference, 1971 (1972): Standardization in human cytogenetics. Birth Defects: Original Article Series, VIII: 7, The National Foundation, New York
9. Luthardt, F.W. (1982) Abstract, Thirty Third Annual Meeting, American Society of Human Genetics, Detroit, MI
10. Cohen, A.J., Li, F.P., Berg, S., Marchetto, D.J., Tsai, S., Jacobs, S.C., and Brown, R.S. (1979) N. Eng. J. Med. 301, 592.
11. Pathak, S., Strong, L.C., Ferrell, R.E., and Trindade, A. (1982) Science, 217, 939-941.

ON THE NATURE OF STEM LINES IN TUMORIGENIC CELL POPULATIONS

LARRY L. DEAVEN,[+] EVELYN W. CAMPBELL[++] AND MARTY F. BARTHOLDI[++]
[+]Office of Health and Environmental Research, U.S. Department of Energy,
Washington, D.C. 20545, [++]Life Sciences Division, Los Alamos National
Laboratory, Los Alamos, New Mexico 87545

INTRODUCTION

Elucidation of the role of chromosomal change in malignant transformation
and progression has been a challenge to cancer cytologists for over 60 years.
Since 1914, when Boveri[1] suggested that chromosomal imbalance may lead to
malignancy, numerous investigators have sought evidence necessary to support
or reject his hypothesis. Although the subject has received continual attention, including a period of intense research activity in the 1950s, our understanding of it remains incomplete. This record is not too disappointing if
one considers the technical problems inherent in the analysis of chromosomes
in tumor cells. Unique problems have been encountered in making cytological
preparations of tumor tissues, the mixtures of normal and malignant cells
commonly found in tumors make individual cells difficult to identify, and the
chromosomal rearrangements frequently found in tumor cells compound the difficult task of accurate and precise chromosomal analysis. Steady progress has
been made in solving these problems and new insights have accompanied each
improvement in technique. Chromosome banding methods and flow cytometry are
innovations in technique that can be applied to analyzing the relationship
between chromosomal changes and malignancy. The application of these new
approaches to studies of the chromsomal evolution that accompanies malignant
progression is the subject of this paper.

HISTORICAL CONSIDERATIONS

The literature concerning chromosomal evolution in tumorigenic cell populations has been extensively reviewed[2-4] and only the salient facts are
considered here. A few references appeared in the early literature on
chromosomes of cancer tissues[5-7]; however, it was not until the 1950s that
experimental systems were devised that had sufficient resolving power to shed
light on the problem. The extensive observations reported during this period
were drawn together into a central theme called the stem line hypothesis.[8] In
this construction, stem cells were defined as those cells in a tumor population
with a specific karyotype and as the principal progenitors of tumor growth.

Published 1983 by Elsevier Science Publishing Co., Inc.
Cancer: Etiology and Prevention, Ray G. Crispen, Editor

Cells with different karyotypes were considered to be the products of aberrant mitotic events, to be generally incapable of continued proliferation, and hence to be transient components of the tumor cell population. The stem line concept originated from studies of ascites cells, but was later extended to cover other tumor types and highly evolved in vitro cell populations.[9] Subsequent studies demonstrated that the original stem line hypothesis was an oversimplification. Improved cytogenetic technique led to the observation that karyotype deviations occurred within stem lines, and microspectrophotometric studies suggested that tumors may have multiple stem lines or no distinct stem lines. The published results from microspectrophotometric analyses are not easily interpretable and are sometimes at varience. Early studies suggested that chromosomally aneuploid cells also contained "aneuploid amounts" of DNA.[9] That is, if a cell population had an elevated level of variability in number of chromosomes per cell, it also had an elevated coefficient of variation (CV) for cellular DNA content. In contrast, a recent study using improved instruments and staining methods emphasized the relatively small variation in cell-to-cell DNA content in tumor cells.[10] Current discussions of chromosomal evolution in tumors refer to stem lines in indistinct terms and generally recognize that the available data are too incomplete to provide a precise definition.[11]

CHROMOSOME ANALYSIS AND FLOW CYTOMETRIC MEASUREMENTS OF DNA CONTENT IN TUMORIGENIC CELL POPULATIONS

The development of flow cytometry (FCM) permitted investigators to make DNA measurements of single cells at rates of several thousand cells per second. This capability provided a powerful new approach to the general problem of cell population analysis. The first FCM measurements of cell populations derived from tumors led to some unexpected results.[12] Although there was a broad range of number of chromosomes per cell, the intercellular variability in DNA content was as low as that of the euploid cells from which they were derived. An example of this phenomenon is illustrated in Fig. 1. Flow cytometric DNA measurements of human melanoma and HeLa cells are compared with diploid human WI-38 cells. The elevated dispersion of chromosome number per cell in the melanoma and HeLa cells is not reflected by an elevation in the CV of the G_1 peaks. In this case, the WI-38 cells have a CV of 4.87%, the human melanoma cells 4.76%, and the HeLa cells 3.16%. These original observations have been confirmed for numerous in vitro heteroploid cell lines[13] and for cells taken directly from human tumors.[14]

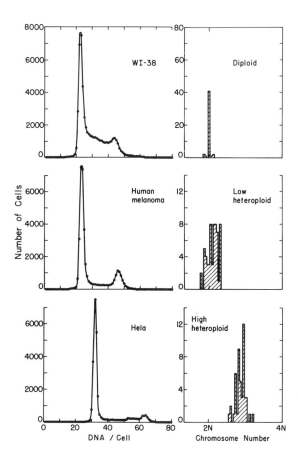

Fig. 1. Flow cytometric DNA distributions and chromosome number histograms of cultured diploid and heteroploid human cells.

Attempts to validate the original data included measurements of freshly cloned HeLa cells that had a narrower range of chromosome number per cell than the parental lines.[15] The rationale for the experiment was to determine if the low CV for DNA content in the parental cells could be further reduced by decreasing the dispersion in chromosome number per cell. The cloned HeLa cells had chromosome numbers of either 66 or 68 per cell, and the parental line had a dispersion of 62-74 per cell. The CVs for DNA content in the G_1 peaks were 3.75% and 3.52% respectively. This suggests, in an independent way, that within a heteroploid cell population, DNA content per cell is not always correlated with chromosome number per cell.

A second validation of the FCM measurements was made by inducing elevated dispersions of chromosome number per cell in heteroploid Chinese hamster cells.[16] Nondisjunction was induced in euploid and heteroploid cells by exposing them to low doses of Colcemid (0.06 μg/ml) for three hrs. In both cell types the cellular gain or loss of chromosomes was readily detected in the FCM spectra. The G_1 peaks were broadened by the presence of cells that had gained or lost chromosomes. The increased CVs were transient in both cases, returning to normal within 5 days after Colcemid reversal. This result supports the basic observation of DNA constancy in heteroploid cell populations and suggests that the mechanism that controls chromosome number dispersion is not mitotic nondisjunction.

Chromosome banding analyses were made on several of the lines previously measured for DNA content.[15] These provided useful information about specific chromosome complements that may ultimately help to resolve the paradox of constant DNA per cell in cells with chromosome number variability. Three HeLa lines were analyzed because they had broad distributions of chromosome number per cell, and because one of the three lines had a higher amount of DNA per cell than the other two. The two lines with identical DNA values of 1.5 times diploid human cells had similar chromosome number distributions, but the specific chromosome complements were markedly different. One line had about 40% abnormal chromosomes (rearranged as compared to normal human chromosomes), whereas in the other only 24% were abnormal. Another unexpected observation was the occurrence of large cell-to-cell differences in specific karyotype. Because many individual chromosomes had variable numbers of copies and because marker complements also varied in number from one cell to another, it was difficult to find two HeLa cells with identical karyotypes. This variability was as large among cells having the modal chromosome number as it was among nonmodal cells. The third HeLa line had twice the diploid human DNA content and had a higher number of chromosomes per cell than the other two lines (modal number of 83 as compared to 65 and 66 for the lower lines). Each of the lines contained a small number of identical HeLa marker chromosomes, suggesting that they had a common ancestry.

Because of the karyotype complexity of human heteroploid cells, a system originating from a relatively simple karyotype was selected for further studies. A heteroploid Chinese hamster cell line was cloned, and a series of these clones, selected on the basis of modal chromosome number, were karyotyped and measured for cellular DNA content.[16] The clones varied in modal chromosome number from a high of 39–40 to a low of 29–30, and each clone had a perimodal dispersion of at least 2 or 3 chromosomes. Some clones reverted rapidly to dispersions as great as the 10 chromsome dispersion of the parental line. The clones could not be distinguished from one another nor from the parental line on the basis of FCM DNA analyses. Chromosome analyses revealed similar characteristics as those found previously in the HeLa populations. Relative proportions of structurally altered chromosomes varied from one clone to another, individual chromosomes varied in number from one cell to another, and cells with identical numbers of chromosomes differed in specific chromosome content. In addition, there was an indication that the clones with high chromosome number contained more small chromsomes than the clones with low chromosome number.

Flow DNA measurements of isolated chromosomes from two of the clones described above are illustrated in Fig. 2. In each of the histograms in Fig. 2., the peak on the extreme left with the lowest intensity of fluoresence is composed of fluorescent beads used to standardize the flow karyotypes. The two peaks on the extreme right of each histogram represent chromosomes 1 and 2 of the Chinese hamster. The remaining peaks are composed of small and medium sized chromosomes that in some cases are normal, unaltered Chinese hamster chromosomes, while in others, they are structurally altered chromosomes formed during the evolution of the CHO-38 heteroploid line. The clone in the upper histogram (38-2) had a modal chromsome number of 36 with a range of 33–40 chromosomes per cell; the clone in the lower histogram (38-7) had a modal number of 32 with a range of 28–35. The histograms indicate that although the two clones share a number of chromsomes in common, some chromosomes are unique to only one clone. They also demonstrate the diversity of specific chromosome content between the two heteroploid clones. The fact that flow karyotypes are obtainable from these lines indicates that cell-to-cell chromosome diversity is primarily due to variable numbers of copies of individual chromosomes in each cell. If the cells contained a large number of structurally unique chromosomes, the flow karyotypes would not appear as a series of discreet peaks, but as broad curves or continuous distributions.

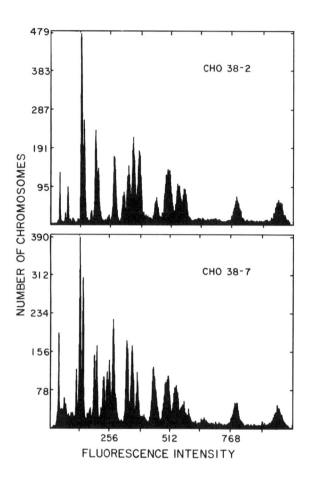

Fig. 2. Flow karyotypes of chromosomes isolated from heteroploid Chinese hamster clones 38-2 and 38-7. The clones have the same DNA content per cell, but clone 38-2 has a modal number of 36 while clone 38-7 has a modal chromosome number of 31. The profiles of isolated chromosomes show the diversity of specific chromosome content between the two clones.

DISCUSSION

All of the data reviewed or presented herein suggest that evolving tumori-genic cell populations maintain stringent control over cellular DNA content.

This process is expected and easily understood in euploid cells where mitotic division of daughter chromosomes ensures equal division and distribution of DNA. Similar distributions of chromatin probably occur during mitosis in heteroploid cells. This is indicated by the studies of induced nondisjunction discussed in this manuscript and by measurements that show that the DNA content in newly divided heteroploid cells is equal.[17] If this is the case, it is difficult to account for the variability in chromosome number and structure that characterizes these cells.

In order to explain the initial observations of DNA constancy in hetero-ploidy, a model was proposed that included variable sites for kinetochore and telomere expression.[12] According to this view, heteroploidy is maintained by aberrant packaging of chromosomes; cell-to-cell variability in specific chomosome content is the result of dividing the same amount of chromatin into different numbers of metaphase chromosomes. Although this model cannot be rigorously disproved at the present time, banding analysis of heteroploid cells has not provided critical support for it, and alternative explanations may be required.

Although the studies on induced nondisjunction are not inclusive, they suggest that this process alone is not responsible for the elevated dispersions of chromosome number and structure. Given the frequency of numerical chromo-some changes found in heteroploid cells, it is unlikely that the FCM analyses would not detect the resulting changes in DNA content per cell. If nondisjunc-tion is involved in the dispersions of chromosome number, then some type of compensatory exchange process must be invoked to explain the constancy of cellular DNA content. If a cell gains a large chromosome, it must lose a large chromosome or two small chromosomes at the same time in order to maintain a constant amount of DNA. There is little support in the literature for such a compensatory mechanism, and we conclude that a constant, relatively high level of compensatory nondisjunction is an unlikely origin of the elevated chromosome variability in evolving cell populations.

A more likely possibility is that evolving cells are directly or indirectly selected for favorable amounts of DNA. When a number of heteroploid lines were measured for cellular DNA content, they were found to cluster at multiple values of the haploid genome (2, 3, or 4C for G_1 peaks).[18] This phenomenon and cell-to-cell DNA constancy could be due to selective pressures. Cells with variant amounts of DNA are eliminated from the population because of growth disadvantages. The variability in specific chromosome content per cell could emerge from multipolar mitoses or unusual events such as compensatory nondisjunction. Because newly cloned lines of heteroploid cells vary in the extent of chromosome number dispersion, it is possible that the mitotic irregularities or other mechanisms that give rise to chromosome variability are under genetic control.[19]

Two independent studies[20, 21] have reached conclusions somewhat similar to those expressed in this paper. In these studies major emphasis was put on the number of chromosomes per cell or on variability of chromosome content in cells with equal numbers of chromosomes. In one of the studies,[20] it was concluded that the mitotic apparatus has "structural restrictions" that act as a control over chromosome number. Both reports conclude that cells with a constant number of chromosomes have a selective advantage over those with variant numbers, regardless of the specific chromosome content. Our data suggests that this advantage is coupled with specific amounts of DNA. It is possible that these earlier reports were studies of the same phenomenon, but that the investigators were attempting to express it in terms of chromosome number per cell. It is also possible that a constant amount of DNA per cell is coupled with some other nuclear phenomenon and is not the primary force in selection. Nuclear pore number or some other feature of nuclear topology could set restrictions that are manifested by constancy of cellular DNA content.

All of our studies suggest that stemlines should be defined on the basis of growth behavior and cellular DNA content. The specific chromosome complement appears to be of less importance. A more complete description of this phenomenon may be useful in defining the basic differences between tumorigenic and nontumorigenic cells.

SUMMARY

In 1959, Sajiro Makino defined stem cells as those cells in a malignant population that have identical karyotypes and as the principal progenitors of tumor growth. Cells with altered karyotypes, compared to stem cells, were considered to be the products of aberrant mitotic events, to be less competitive in growth rate, and hence to be minor and transient components of the tumor cell population. Although the original stem line concept has undergone a series of redefinitions and modifications, it continues to be a useful term in describing tumor progression. Recent studies of tumorigenic cell populations by flow cytometry and chromosome banding have shed new light on the essential characteristics of stem cells. These data suggest that stem line cells have lost the karyotype control found in euploid cells, but that control over the total ammount of cellular DNA is rather stringently maintained.

Selection for optimal amounts of DNA per cell appears to be an important aspect of cellular evolution in tumors that has not been recognized previously.

‑ACKNOWLEDGMENTS

This work was performed under the auspices of the United States Department of Energy. We wish to thank Sheila Palmer and Kathy Foster for assistance in manuscript preparation.

REFERENCES

1. Boveri, T. (1914) Zur Frage der Entwicklung maligner Tumoren, Gustav Fisher, Jena.

2. Koller, P.C. (1964) in Cellular Control Mechanisms and Cancer, Emmelotand, P. and Mulhock, O. eds., Elsevier, Amsterdam, pp. 174-189.

3. German, J. ed. (1974) Chromosomes and Cancer, John Wiley & Sons, New York pp. 1-756.

4. Sandberg, A.A. ed. (1980) The Chromsomes in Human Cancer and Leukemia, Elsevier, New York and Amsterdam, pp. 1-748.

5. Billing, J. (1927) J. Amer. Med. Assoc. 88, 396-418.

6. Kemp. T. (1930) Z. Zellforsch. Mikroskop. Anat. 11, 429-444.

7. Levine, M. (1930) J. Cancer Res. 14, 400-425.

8. Makino, S. (1952) Gann 43, 17-34.

9. Hsu, T.C. (1961) Int. Rev. Cytol. 12, 69-161.

10. Atkin, N.B. (1969) Acta. Cytol. 13, 270-273.

11. Nowell, P.C. (1976) Science, 194, 23-28.

12. Kraemer, P.M., Petersen, D.F., and Van Dilla, M.A. (1971) Science 174, 714-717.

13. Kraemer, P.M., Deaven, L.L., Crissman, H.A., and Van Dilla, M.A. (1972) in Advances in Cell and Molecular Biology, Vol. 2, Dupraw, E.J. ed., Academic Press, Inc., New York, pp. 47-108.

14. Barlogie, B., Gohde, W., and Drewinko, B. (1979) J. Histochem. Cytochem. 27, 505-507.

15. Deaven, L.L., Sanders, P.C., Grilly, J.L., Kraemer, P.M., and Petersen, D.F. (1975) in Mammalian Cells: Probes and Problems, Richmond, C.R., Petersen, D.F., Mullaney, P.F., and Anderson, E.C., eds, ERDA Symposium Series CONF-731007, National Technical Information Service, Springfield, Virginia, pp. 212-227.

70

16. Deaven, L.L., Cram, L.S., Wells, R.S., and Kraemer, P.M. (1981) in Genes, Chromosomes, and Neoplasia, Arrighi, F.E., Rao, P.N., and Stubblefield, E. eds., Raven Press, New York, pp. 419-449.

17. Stitch, H.S. and Steele, H.D. (1962) J. Nat. Can. Inst. 28, 1207-1217.

18. Deaven, L.L. and Petersen, D.F. (1974) in Methods in Cell Biology, Vol. 8, Prescott, D.M. ed., Academlic Press, Inc., New York, pp. 179-204.

19. Deaven, L.L. (1976) in The Automation of Uterine Cancer Cytology, Wied, G.L., Bahr, G.F., and Bartels, P.H., eds., Tutorials of Cytology, Chicago, pp. 304-310.

20. Terzi, M. (1972) J. Cell, Physiol., 80, 359-366.

21. Hughes, D.T. (1968) Nature 217, 518-523.

A MODEL FOR HUMAN CARCINOGENESIS: HEREDITARY CANCERS AND PREMALIGNANT LESIONS

SURESH H. MOOLGAVKAR, M.B.B.S., Ph.D.
Institute for Cancer Research, Fox Chase Cancer Center, 7701 Burholme
Avenue, Philadelphia, Pennsylvania 19111, USA

INTRODUCTION

   The recent spectacular advances in tumor virology lend some   support to
the proposition that activation of an oncogene is the final common pathway for
most cancers. On the other hand, the study of the dominantly inherited cancers
in man reveals the existence of another class of genes, distinct from oncogenes,
that is important in carcinogenesis. Unlike activated oncogenes, these genes
are recessive at the level of the cell: individuals who carry the gene have a
very high probability of developing a specific cancer; however, even though
every cell in the affected tissue carries the gene, only a few cells go on
to become malignant, suggesting that inheritance of the gene is not sufficient
and that another event is necessary. Second, these genes exert their effects
by a loss of their function rather than by activation[1]. Thus, in some cases
of hereditary retinoblastoma and Wilms' tumor, the gene site is deleted.

   What I would like to do in my talk today is to incorporate these two classes
of genes into a general model for carcinogenesis, and to discuss some of the
implications of this model.

THE MODEL

   The model described here is based on a genetic regulatory schema proposed
by Comings in 1973[2]. Specifically, he suggests that all cells contain genes
capable of coding for transforming factors that release the cell from normal
growth constraints. These oncogenes, supposed to be tissue specific, would
be temporarily expressed during embryogenesis and then turned off by diploid
pairs of regulatory genes, which, in effect, would be antioncogenes[1].
Malignant transformation of a cell would follow reactivation of the oncogenes.
Recent investigations on the model tumor viruses suggest various ways in which
this could happen. Chromosomal rearrangement could bring a host oncogene
adjacent to a "promoter" site or a viral "promoter" sequence could be inserted
next to an oncogene. Both these circumstances would lead to an abrogation
of normal cellular control of the oncogenes. Indeed, the latter mechanism
has been shown to be responsible for some virally induced avian tumors[3].
However, the body of epidemiologic and experimental data is consistent with

the notion that human tumors most commonly arise by mutations of the regulatory genes[4]. The possibility that some human tumors could arise by direct
activation of oncogenes must, however, be recognized. Candidates for such
tumors are the lymphomas and leukemias in which specific chromosomal rearrangements are a characterizing feature.

Thus, the model for carcinogenesis I am discussing today requires the
occurrence of two rare and irreversible events, namely mutations of each of
the two homologous antioncogenes (regulatory genes). There is evidence that,
at least in some tissues, mutations at one of several gene loci may be involved
in carcinogenesis. For example, in the colon as many as four distinct genes
may predispose to malignancy. Then, homozygous mutations at any one of these
loci would lead to malignancy. The direct evidence in support of this two
mutation model is sparse, and has recently been summarized[1]. However, this is
the only model that has been shown to be consistent with the main body of
epidemiologic and experimental data on carcinogenesis[4]. A crucial observation
is that when the kinetics of growth and differentiation of tissues are taken
into account, a two-stage model can generate all the age-specific incidence
curves observed in human populations[4,5].

GENETIC SUSCEPTIBILITY TO CANCER

There is now abundant evidence that there are single gene defects, both
dominant and recessive, that predispose to cancer. These mendelian conditions
are the strongest known risk factors for cancer in humans.

For cancers of many sites, pedigree data are consistent with the hypothesis
that a fraction of cases is due to the inheritance of an autosomal dominant
cancer gene. Thus 40% of all cases of retinoblastoma are estimated to be due
to inheritance of a dominant gene for retinoblastoma[6]. Dominant cancer genes
have been implicated in other childhood tumors as well, such as neuroblastoma
and Wilms' tumor. Familial polyposis coli is perhaps the best known example
of dominant inheritance of an adult tumor. The total number of dominant cancer
genes is not known, but approximately 30 are listed in McKusick's catalog of
human genes[7], and Knudson[8] has estimated that 100-200 such human cancer genes
exist.

Inheritance of a dominant cancer gene increases enormously the risk of
cancer. For example, the probability of retinoblastoma in the general population is approximately 1 in 30,000, whereas gene carriers develop on the average
3-4 tumors each. Thus, the risk to the individual cell (retinoblast) in gene
carriers is elevated some 100,000 fold. A similar computation for familial

polyposis coli shows that, at age 45, the risk of colon cancer in gene carriers is approximately 5000 times that in the general population. However, even though the gene confers a greatly elevated risk, the risk at the level of an individual <u>cell</u> is quite low: of the many millions of cells at risk only a few give rise to malignant tumors. Thus, inheritance of the gene is not sufficient for malignancy, and a second event must occur.

How do such autosomal dominant tumors fit into the two-stage model outlined above? An attractive hypothesis following from the model is that mutation of one of the regulatory genes has occurred in an ancestral germ cell and inherited by the gene carriers. Mutation of the regulatory gene on the homologous chromosome in a somatic cell would then lead to malignancy. Thus, although both mutations would be rare at the cellular level, gene carriers would have inherited one mutation, and there would be numerous cells in which a single event (the second mutation) would give rise to malignant transformation. Thus, with a high probability at least a few cells would undergo malignant change and pedigree analysis would be consistent with autosomal dominant inheritance with high penetrance. Thus, in this model, a gene that is recessive at the cellular level, is dominant on the population level (i.e., on pedigree analysis)[4].

The evidence in favor of this hypothesis comes mainly from the study of retinoblastoma and has recently been reviewed[1]. Briefly, as required by the model, the evidence suggests that the same genomic site is affected in both sporadic and hereditary cases of retinoblastoma. Further, there is one reported case of retinoblastoma in which the tumor cells show deletion of the same sites on homologous chromosomes[9].

The prototype of a recessive (on the population level) condition that predisposes to malignancy is xeroderma pigmentosum (XP). Afflicted individuals are remarkably sensitive to sunlight, the most lethal effect being skin cancers (basal cell and squamous cell carcinomas and melanomas). It is generally believed that this susceptibility to cancer is due to the defective repair of UV-induced DNA damage[10]. A recent report indicates that XP may predispose to chemical or spontaneous carcinogenesis at other sites than skin[11]. Within the context of the model, XP would predispose to cancer as a direct consequence of increased mutation rates, especially in the presence of UV light, of the regulatory genes.

Another recessive condition, Bloom's syndrome, is characterized by chromosomal fragility leading to increased frequency of sister chromatid and homologous chromosome exchanges[12], and elevated mutation rates[13]. Afflicted individuals are predisposed to cancer, especially leukemia. The predisposition to cancer may be attributable to the increase in mutation rates, but an intriguing possibility is that homozygosity could be brought about by mitotic recombination following mutation of one of the two homologous regulatory genes. Thus, Bloom's syndrome would preferentially increase the second mutation rate.

To summarize, according to the model, most human cancers are due to mutations at a pair of regulatory genes, thus abrogating cellular control of oncogenes. Mendelizing conditions that predispose to malignancy may be classified into two principal groups: 1) those conditions in which a non-functional antioncogene is inherited from a parent, such as hereditary retinoblastoma, familial polyposis coli, or BK mole (dysplastic nevus) syndrome (see table); 2) those conditions in which one or both mutation rates are increased, such as XP and Bloom's syndrome. In addition there are other recessive conditions predisposing to malignancy, such as Fanconi's anemia and ataxia telangiectasia, that do not fit neatly into the model. I do not wish to discuss these conditions today.

PREMALIGNANT LESIONS

In the model for carcinogenesis proposed here, cells that have sustained the first mutation may be thought of as initiated cells. It would clearly be of interest to identify and study such cells. Are there human lesions that could be considered to be premalignant in the sense that they are clones of such initiated cells? A study of cancers that occur in both a sporadic form and a form that is inherited in an autosomal dominant fashion provides leads to the identification of premalignant lesions and generates interesting and testable biologic hypotheses. In many of these cancers, gene carriers exhibit characteristic pathologic lesions in the tissue that is at high risk for cancer. These lesions may well represent identifiable clusters of initiated cells. These same lesions in non-gene carriers may then represent clones of initiated cells. Thus, for example, the abundance of polyps of the colon in familial polyposis coli suggests that adenomatous polyps represent clones of initiated cells in non-gene carriers. I must make it quite clear here that not all clones of initiated cells will be detectable as polyps: the polyps represent clones that have become large enough to be visible. A consequence of this is that many tumors of the colon would arise in pre-existing polyps; but at least some would not. The latter would presumably arise from clones of initiated cells that are too small to be visible.

As a consequence of the model, premalignant lesions would be clonal in sporadic cases and polyclonal in gene carriers[4]. Thus, for example, polyps in familial polyposis would be polyclonal, whereas those in sporadic cases would be clonal. However, in both cases, the malignant tumor arising from these lesions would be clonal. The reason that the model predicts this is as follows. In sporadic cases, the polyps would be due to the proliferation of a single cell that has sustained a rare event (the first mutation) and, thus, clonal. In contrast, all the cells in the colon of a gene carrier are initiated, and the polyps would be due to the improperly controlled proliferation of these cells, and, therefore, polyclonal. In both hereditary and sporadic cases, however, a second rare event would be necessary to produce malignancy, and therefore malignant tumors would be clonal. This prediction could be tested in affected females who are heterozygous at the X-chromosomal locus for the enzyme glucose-6-phosphate dehydrogenase. The prediction is that both alleles will be expressed in the premalignant lesions in hereditary cases, whereas only a single allele will be expressed in premalignant lesions in sporadic cases and in malignant lesions in both hereditary and sporadic cases[4]. Familial polyposis is used only as an example here. Clearly, the same argument can be made for any malignant tumor that occurs in both sporadic and autosomal dominant forms.

This prediction of the model has been partially fulfilled for one tumor type: sporadic neurofibromas are clonal, whereas the neurofibromas in von Recklinghausen's disease (neurofibromatosis) a dominantly inherited condition, are polyclonal[14]. The expectation is that the neurofibrosarcomas that arise from these lesions will be clonal. A partial list of tumors in which pre-malignant lesions may be identifiable is in the table.

CONCLUDING REMARKS

My discussion here of genetic factors in carcinogenesis has been limited to mendelian conditions, and has been conducted within the framework of a model for which there is some circumstantial evidence. The details of the model are largely speculative. However, they are consistant with the main body of data from experimental carcinogenesis and human epidemiology[4]. I have presented the model today, not as a description of reality, but as a working hypothesis to generate predictions that may be testable.

ACKNOWLEDGMENTS

This work was supported by USPHS grants CA-06927, CA-25588, CA-22780 and CA-30671 awarded by the National Institutes of Health, U.S.A.

TABLE 1

PUTATIVE PREMALIGNANT LESIONS AND THEIR CLONALITY

Premalignant Lesions		Malignant lesions, two-hit clonal, hereditary or non-hereditary
One-hit clonal, nonhereditary	One-hit multicellular, hereditary	
Sporadic adenomatous polyps	Polyps in familial polyposis	Carcinoma of colon[a]
Sporadic neurofibromas[a]	Neurofibromas in neurofibromatosis	Neurofibrosarcoma
?	C-cell hyperplasia of thyroid gland in MEA 2	Medullary carcinoma of thyroid gland[a]
?	Nodular renoblastema	Wilms' tumor
?	Neuroblastoma IV-S	Neuroblastoma
Lobular carcinoma in situ	Lobular carcinoma in situ	Carcinoma of the breast[a]
Superficially spreading melanoma, level I; lentigo maligna	B-K mole	Malignant melanoma

[a]Tumors in which clonality has been studied. The one reported case of carcinoma of the colon was said to have been of multicellular origin[15]. In this case, there were multiple metastases in the liver, and although each lesion exhibited a single Glc-6-PD allele, about half the lesions expressed one allele and half expressed the other. It was concluded from this finding that the primary tumor was multicellular. However, the case is an unusual one in that the patient died of her disease at 32 yr of age. In view of the young age at death, a polyposis syndrome cannot be ruled out. Multiple primary tumors in the colon could explain the expression of both alleles in the liver metastases. It is not clear from the paper whether this possibility was considered. Sporadic neurofibromas have been found to be clonal, whereas neurofibromas in von Recklinghausen's disease are multicellular[14]. Both carcinoma of the thyroid gland and pheochromocytomas in multiple endocrine adenomatosis type 2 (MEA 2) are clonal[16]. Carcinoma of the breast is also considered to be clonal. C-cell hyperplasia of the thyroid gland is likely to be the premalignant lesion in carcinoma of the thyroid gland[17]. A discussion of lobular carcinoma in situ as the possible premalignant lesion in breast cancer may be found in (18). It has recently been suggested that neuroblastoma IV-S consists of cells in the premalignant stage[19]. Differentiation of these cells could then lead to the spontaneous regression of tumor that is often seen in this condition.

REFERENCES

1. Knudson, A.G. (in press) in Proceedings of the XIII International Cancer Congress. American Elsevier.
2. Comings, D.E. (1973) Proc. Natl. Acad. Sci. USA, 70, 3324-3328.
3. Hayward, W.S., Neel, B.G. and Astrin, S.M. (1982) in Advances in Viral Oncology, Klein, G., ed., Raven Press, New York, pp.207-233.
4. Moolgavkar, S.H. and Knudson, A.G. (1981) JNCI, 66, 1037-1052.
5. Moolgavkar, S.H. and Venzon, D.J. (1979) Math. Biosci., 47, 55-77.
6. Knudson, A.G. (1971) Proc. Natl. Acad. Sci. USA, 68, 820-823.
7. McKusick, V.A. (1978) Mendelian inheritance in man: Catalogs of autosomal dominant, autosomal recessive, and X-linked phenotypes, 5th ed. Johns Hopkins Univ. Press, Baltimore.
8. Knudson, A.G. (1980) in Genes, chromosomes and neoplasia. Thirty-third annual symposium on fundamental cancer research: M.D. Anderson Hospital and Tumor Institute, Arrighi, F.E., Rao, N. and Stubblefield, E., eds., Raven Press, New York, 453-462.
9. Benedict, W.F., Murphree, A.L. and Banerjee, A. (1982) in Proc. Seventy-Third Annual Meeting of the American Association for Cancer Research (Abstract), 23, 40.
10. Cleaver, J.E. (1968) Nature, 218, 652-656.
11. Kraemer, K.H. (1980) in Carcinogenesis: Fundamental Mechanisms and Environ-mental Effects, Pullman, B., Ts'o, P.D.P. and Gelboin, H., eds. D. Reidel Publishing Company, Holland, pp.503-507.
12. Chaganti, R.S., Schonberg, S. and German, J. (1974) Proc. Natl. Acad. Sci. USA, 71, 4508-4512.
13. Warren, S.T., Schultz, R.A., Chang, C., Wade, M.H. and Trosko, J.E. (1981) Proc. Natl. Acad. Sci. USA, 78, 3133-3137.
14. Fialkow, P.J. (1977) in Genetics of Human Cancer, Mulvihill, J.J., Miller, R.W. and Fraumeni, J.F., eds., Raven Press, New York, pp.439-453.
15. Beutler, E., Collins, Z. and Irwin, L.E. (1976) N. Engl. J. Med., 276, 389-391.
16. Baylin, S.B., Gann, D.S. and Hsu, S.H. (1976) Science, 193, 321-323.
17. Jackson, C.E., Block, M.A., Greenawald, K.A. and Tashjian, A.H. (1979) Am. J. Hum. Genet., 31, 704-710.
18. Moolgavkar, S.H., Day, N.E. and Stevens, R.G. (1980) JNCI, 65, 559-569.
19. Knudson, A.G. and Meadows, A.T. (1980) N. Engl. J. Med., 302, 1254-1256.

GENETIC INSTABILITY AND TUMOR PROGRESSION

John T. Isaacs
Johns Hopkins Oncology Center and Department of Urology,
The Johns Hopkins University School of Medicine,
600 North Wolfe Street, Baltimore, Maryland, USA

INTRODUCTION

Much of the present inability to cure cancer patients is due to the fact that cancer cells often become resistant to initially effective treatments during therapy. The development of such resistance is due to the ability of cancer cells to change their basic biological properties from a sensitive to a resistant cancer cell phenotype during treatment. Such a change in cancer cell phenotype was originally defined by Foulds[1] as tumor progression and such progression has been repeatedly demonstrated in a variety of human as well as experimental animal cancers. While the phenomenon of tumor progression is a well-established principle of tumor biology, the exact mechanism responsible for these alterations of cancer cell phenotypes have not been completely resolved but must involve changes in the structure and/or regulation of the tumor genome. Regardless of the detailed mechanism, it is known that such a change in phenotype is both irreversible and inheritable[2]. This requires that some type of basic genetic change occurs in these cells. Genetic change is defined here as a heritable alteration of phenotype whether resulting from mutations, chromosomal alterations, or alterations in gene regulation. In order to experimentally study the nature of these genetic changes, the serially transplantable Dunning R-3327 rat prostatic adenocarcinoma system was used as a model. This system of tumors was used since it has been shown to be an appropriate animal model for human prostatic cancer, mimicking many of the important properties of the human disease[3], and because, within this system of cancers, spontaneous progression has occurred repeatedly.

Background on the Dunning R-3327 Tumor System. The history of the development of the various Dunning R-3327 rat prostatic tumor sublines used in the present study has been described in detail elsewhere[4]. In brief, the parent tumor from which cell the other sublines were derived, is the well-differentiated, slow-growing, androgen-sensitive H tumor. This H tumor, which arose spontaneously from the dorsal lobe of the prostate of a 22 month old male

Cancer: Etiology and Prevention, Ray G. Crispen, Editor

Copenhagen rat[5], is a heterogeneous tumor composed of clones of both androgen-dependent and -independent cancer cells[6]. By growing the H tumor in castrated male rats, it has been possible to clone _in vivo_ for only the slow-growing, well-differentiated, androgen-independent cancer cells. Using this method, the well-differentiated, slow-growing, androgen-insensitive HI-S subline was established[6].

Since 1975, the androgen-sensitive H tumor has been maintained at Johns Hopkins by continuous serial passage in intact male rats. While it has been possible to maintain the original characteristics of the H tumor over this period, there have evolved spontaneously, however, more aberrant sublines from the tumor at several subpassages. Subsequent serial passage of these individual sublines has allowed the development of 5 additional R-3327 tumors each with distinct biological characteristics and each more aberrant than the parent H tumor. The continuous serial passage of the androgen-insensitive HI-S tumor over the last 2 years likewise has resulted in the emergence of 3 new, more aberrant types of Dunning tumors. The present study, therefore, was undertaken to examine the mechanism(s) responsible for the progression of prostatic cancer wherein a cancer continuously evolves to an ever-increasingly aberrant phenotype using the H and HI-S tumor as prototypes.

RESULTS

Spontaneous Progression of the H Tumor. When 1.5×10^6 viable H tumor cells are injected s.c. into intact adult male rats, a tumor becomes palpable after 40 to 50 days. It requires 135 ± 16 (S.E.) days for such s.c. H tumor cell inoculations to produce 1 cu cm tumors. During the exponential phase of the H tumor growth in intact males, the tumor volume doubles with a constant 21 ± 6 day period. Histological examination of the H tumor during its exponential growth reveals a uniformly well-differentiated prostatic adenocarcinoma. The growth of the H tumor is androgen-sensitive as demonstrated by its response to castration. If a similar aliquot of 1.5×10^6 viable H tumor cells are inoculated into castrated male rats, a tumor does not become palpable until 90 to 100 days and does not reach the 1 cu cm size until 240 ± 25 days. In addition, if 1.5×10^6 viable cells are inoculated into intact male rats, the tumor is allowed to grow exponentially for 150 days, and then the rats are castrated, the tumor abruptly stops its exponential growth. For 50 to 60 days, the tumor does not increase in size.

DNA analysis of the H tumor, growing in intact males reveals that the DNA content per cell for the H tumor is identical with that of the normal adult dorsal prostate, which is the tissue of origin for the original spontaneous R-3327 tumor. Both H tumor and the normal dorsal prostatic cells have a diploid amount of DNA (Table 1). Chromosomal studies further revealed that the modal number of chromosomes for the H tumor is diploid at 42. Further analysis demonstrated that none of the cells from the H tumor which were karyotyped had any demonstrable chromosomal abnormalities[7].

Table 1
Comparative summary of biological characteristics of normal dorsal prostate and Dunning tumor sublines

R-3327 tumor sublines	Histology	Growth rate [tumor-doubling time (days)]	Androgen sensitivity	Metastatic potential[a]	DNA content/cell (pg/cell)	5α-Reductase activity[b]
Normal adult prostate	Well-differentiated	Static	Yes		8.7 ± 1.3^c	87.5 ± 8.5
H tumor	Well-differentiated	21 ± 6	Yes	Low	10.0 ± 2.1	17.0 ± 5.4
H tumor derived						
H-F	Moderately well-differentiated	5.4 ± 2.0	No	Low	8.9 ± 1.3	3.1 ± 0.4
AT-1	Anaplastic	2.5 ± 0.2	No	Low	15.5 ± 1.0	1.5 ± 0.3
MAT-LyLu	Anaplastic	1.5 ± 0.1	No	High	14.3 ± 1.2	1.4 ± 0.3
MAT-Lu	Anaplastic	2.7 ± 0.3	No	High	14.5 ± 1.5	1.1 ± 0.1
AT-2	Anaplastic	2.5 ± 0.2	No	Low to moderate	16.1 ± 2.5	2.1 ± 0.8
HI-S	Well-differentiated	24 ± 5	No	Low	9.5 ± 0.5	12.1 ± 3.0
HI-S tumor derived						
HI-M	Moderately well-differentiated	9.0 ± 0.8	No	Low	9.3 ± 1.3	3.3 ± 0.6
HI-F	Moderately well-differentiated	4.8 ± 1.8	No	Low	8.5 ± 1.9	1.5 ± 0.4
AT-3	Anaplastic	1.8 ± 0.2	No	High	13.8 ± 0.5	1.2 ± 0.1

[a] Low metastatic potential: <5% of s.c.-inoculated rats develop distant metastases; moderate; >5, <20%; high potential: >75% develop distant metastases.
[b] × 10^5 molecules of testosterone reduced per hr per cell.
[c] Mean ± S.E.

In order to maintain over the years the original characteristics of the H tumor (i.e., its androgen sensitivity and slow growth rate), it has been routinely necessary to constantly passage only the slowest-growing H tumor from each passage. If this is not done, tumors with increasing growth rates are eventually obtained. Recently, we have taken advantage of this fact to establish a new fast-growing subline from the parent slow-growing H tumor. By passage of the fastest-growing H tumor from an initial transplantation of the slow-growing H tumor and then by continuous selection of only the fastest-growing tumor produced for each subsequent passage, it has been possible to develop within 10 passages, a tumor which now has a doubling time of 5.4 ± 2 days as opposed to 21 days. This tumor, termed H-F, is histologically less well-differentiated than is the parent slow-growing H tumor, having less tumor stroma and smaller tumor acini. The H-F tumor, is, however, still a moderately well-differentiated tumor with no areas of anaplastic cells. Biochemically, the H-F is also less differentiated in that the level of 5α-reductase in this tumor is less than one-fifth that seen in the H tumor (Table 1). In addition to these histological and biochemical changes, the H-F is no longer androgen-sensitive; it grows equally well in intact or castrated male rats. This loss of androgen sensitivity occurred even though the tumor was always passaged in intact male rats.

Chromosomal analysis of H-F tumor cells revealed that this tumor has a diploid modal chromosomal number of 42 with a range of 34 to 45. Further analysis demonstrated that greater than 75% of cells from the H-F tumor which were karyotyped had marker chromosomes. All of these abnormal cells had lost the Y and one of the No. 1 chromosomes, and had a t(4;7) and t(1;2) translocation[7]. None of these types of chromosomal abnormalities were observed in karyotypes from the parent slow-growing H tumor, confirming that the progression of the H tumor to the less-differentiated fast-growing H-F tumor is associated with definitive chromosomal changes.

In contrast to progression of the slow-growing H tumor to the fast-growing H-F tumor which developed gradually over several passages, additional progressions have occurred within a single passage of the H tumor. At several distinct passages during the last 6 years, a few random H tumors growing in intact males began to grow at rates 8 to 10 times faster than normal. In these animals, the tumor volume doubling times increased from approximately 20 to less than 3 days. Histological examination of these unusually fast-growing tumors at a time when they are still less than 5 cu cm revealed heterogeneous tumors composed of distinct areas of well-differentiated glandular acini and areas of poorly-differentiated anaplastic cells. When such heterogeneous tumors were passaged, the subsequent tumors uniformly became palpable as early as 10 days after inoculation instead of the usual 40 to 50 day period for normal H tumors. These unusually fast-growing tumors often grew to the size of the host rat within 60 days. Histological examination of these unusually fast-growing tumors revealed uniformly anaplastic tumors with no indication of any areas of well-differentiated tumor cells. These fast-growing anaplastic tumors were thus termed AT tumors.

The first of these anaplastic tumors to be maintained in serial passage was termed the AT-1 tumor. Once developed, the AT-1 was completely androgen-insensitive with regard to its growth; it grew equally well in intact or castrated male hosts with a tumor volume doubling time of 2.5 ± 0.2 days. This is a growth rate 9-fold faster than the parent H tumor. In the earlier serial passages, the AT-1 tumor had a very low rate of distant metastases (<5%). Biochemically, as well as histologically, the AT-1 tumor was also much less differentiated than was the parent H tumor. The AT-1 tumor had no detectable levels of either high-affinity androgen-specific receptor or prostatic-specific acid phosphatase, and the levels of 5α-reductase were only about 10% of those seen for the H tumor (Table 1).

After 60 continuous serial passages in the Hopkins laboratories, the AT-1 tumor eventually became highly metastatic, spreading to both the lymph nodes and lungs in nearly 100% of all inoculated animals. This tumor was thus termed the MAT-LyLu tumor to denote its metastatic site specificity[8]. Continuous serial passage of the AT-1 tumor in Dr. W. D. W. Heston's laboratory at Washington University, St. Louis, Mo., also eventually led to a highly metastatic tumor; however, this tumor metastasizes almost exclusively to the lung and was thus termed the MAT-Lu tumor[9]. Unfortunately, the original AT-1 before it became highly metastatic was not karyotyped. Direct analysis of the DNA content per cell, determined by biochemical assay, did reveal, however, that the AT tumor before becoming highly metastatic was not diploid but polyploid (Table 1). Chromosomal analysis performed on the MAT-LyLu and MAT-Lu tumors demonstrated that both of these anaplastic tumors are hypotetraploid. For the MAT-LyLu tumor, the modal chromosomal number is 66 with a range of 51 to 71; in addition, there were numerous chromosomal markers including loss and gain of chromosomes and structural abnormalities. The consistent abnormalities were loss of the X chromosomes and 5 kinds of structural abnormalities which include a t(1;4) and t(4;X) translocation[7]. For the MAT-Lu tumor, the modal chromosomal number is 67 to 69 with a range of 61 to 72; again, there was both gain and loss of chromosomes and chromosomal structural abnormalities. The consistent abnormalities for the MAT-Lu tumor were the loss of a Y chromosome and 5 kinds of structural rearrangements including the t(4;7) translocation also seen in the HF tumor[7]. There is no common karyotypic abnormality characterizing the MAT-LyLu and MAT-Lu tumors, however, other than the facts that both tumors are hypotetraploid and both tumors are chromosomally distinct from the slow-growing H tumor.

During the last year, an additional anaplastic tumor spontaneously developed within one passage of the slow-growing H tumor. This anaplastic tumor too was completely androgen-insensitive, even though it was always passaged in intact male rats. This anaplastic tumor, termed AT-2 to distinguish it from the previous AT-1 tumor, like the latter tumor was fast-growing (doubling time, 2.2 ± 0.2 days) and in its early passage had a low metastatic potential (<5%). Chromosomal analysis of the AT tumor at its fifth passage demonstrated the tumor to be tetraploid with a modal chromosomal number of 84 and a range from 77 to 85. Karyotypes of cells from the fifth passage showed tetrasomy

(4 chromosomes) in almost all chromosomal groups, although deviation from tetrasomy (gain or loss) was observed in a few chromosomes; in addition, there were
2 unidentified minute chromosomes[7]. These results demonstrate that the H → AT-2
tumor progression, like the previously described H tumor progressions, was
clearly associated with definitive chromosomal changes. Further chromosomal
changes continued to develop with subsequent serial passage of the AT-2 tumor.
By its tenth passage, aneuploidization from tetraploidy (i.e., loss of chromosomes) and the development of structural abnormalities were observed in the
AT-2 tumor; the modal chromosomal number decreased to a value of 75 with a
range of 67 to 80.

Spontaneous Progression of the HI-S Tumor. The H tumor is heterogeneously
composed of both androgen-dependent and androgen-independent, slow-growing,
well-differentiated tumor cells. By serial passage of the H tumor in castrated
male rats, it has been possible to select in vivo for only the androgen-
insensitive, slow-growing clone of tumor cells. The tumor which such selection
produced is termed the HI-S tumor, and it is completely androgen-insensitive, as
demonstrated by its identical slow growth rate (doubling time, 24 ± 5 days) when
passaged in intact rats, castrated rats, or castrated rats treated with exogenous testosterone. In its slow growth rate, the HI-S tumor is essentially
identical with the parent H tumor. Following injection of 1.5 x 10^6 viable HI-S
tumor cells, 140 ± 20 days are required for the tumor to reach a size of 1 cu cm
regardless of the androgen status of the host. Histologically, the HI-S tumor
is also very similar to the H tumor, both being well-differentiated prostatic
adenocarcinomas. Biochemically, the HI-S tumor has 5α-reductase levels just
slightly lower than those of the H tumor (Table 1).

DNA analysis of the HI-S tumor growing in castrated males demonstrates that
the DNA content per cell for the HI-S tumor is identical with both the normal
adult dorsal prostate and the H tumor (Table 1). Unfortunately, chromosomal
analysis of the HI-S tumor in its earliest passage was not performed. Chromosomal analysis of the HI-S tumor from cells of the fifth serial passage,
however, revealed a diploid modal chromosomal number of 42 with a range of 33
to 42. Detailed chromosomal examination of the HI-S tumor at its fifth serial
passage reveals that, although 80% of the cells examined had a completely normal
diploid karyotype, approximately 20% of the examined cells had lost the Y
chromosome and had a t(4;7) translocation marker[7]. This t(4;7) translocation
marker was identical to that observed in the HF tumor. Histologically, biochemically, and by growth rate, the HI-S tumor at its fifth passage was very

similar to the first passage HI-S tumor. Upon continuous passage of the HI-S tumor, however, these parameters began to change. Between the fifth and seventh passages, the growth rate nearly doubled from a doubling time of over 20 days to one of only 9.0 ± 0.8 days. This 2-fold increase in growth rate was paralleled by decreases in 5α-reductase activities; 5α-reductase activity at the fifth and seventh passages were, respectively, 11.3 ± 2.0 versus $3.0 \pm 0.4 \times 10^5$ molecules of testosterone reduced per hr per cell. Histologically, the epithelial cells of the tumor acini of these latter passages are less well-differentiated, and they begin to pile up into the acinar lumen. The HI-S, after its seventh passage, was thus termed the HI-M tumor, first passage to denote its moderately fast (10 day doubling time) growth rate and its changed phenotype. Chromosomal analysis of the HI-M tumor demonstrated a modal number of 41 to 42 with a range of 37 to 84. The frequency of cells with abnormal karyotypes was increased to 50% in this tumor. Comparison of the karyotypes in these abnormal cells demonstrated the presence of at least 3 separate clones: one clone, accounting for 58% of the abnormal cells, had the $t(4;7)$ translocation and a ring No. 1 marker chromosome; the second clone, accounting for 25% of the abnormal clones, had the $t(4;7)$ and $t(1;2)$ translocation markers; and the third clone, accounting for 17% of the abnormal cells, had only the $t(4;7)$ translocation marker[7]. The $t(4;7)$ marker, seen in all the abnormal cells of the HI-M tumor, was also observed in all of the abnormal cells of the HI-S tumor (fifth passage), demonstrating the cellular continuity between these two tumors.

At the second serial passage of the HI-M tumor, 10 castrated male rats were inoculated with 1.5×10^6 viable HI-M tumor cells, and in all 10 rats a primary tumor grew. Nine of the 10 rats had tumors which doubled at a rate of 9.8 ± 0.9 days; however, one tumor grew with a doubling time of only 4.5 days. Passage of one of the 9 slower-growing second-passage HI-M tumors (doubling time, 9.2 days) into 5 castrated male rats produced third-passage tumors which grew with a doubling time of 8.8 ± 1.2 days. In contrast, passage of the one exceptionally fast-growing second-passage HI-M tumor (termed HI-F, first passage, to denote its increased growth rate) into 5 castrated males produced tumors, all of which had a fast doubling time of 4.8 ± 1.8 days. Serial passage of these fast-growing tumors established the HI-F tumor.

Histologically, the HI-F is less well-differentiated than is the HI-M tumor and possesses even lower 5α-reductase levels; 5α-reductase activities of HI-M and HI-F were, respectively, 3.1 ± 6.4 vs. $1.3 \pm 0.4 \times 10^5$ molecules of

testosterone reduced per hr per cell. There are, however, no areas of completely anaplastic tumor cells within the HI-F tumors. Chromosomal analysis revealed
that the HI-F tumor had a modal number in the diploid range. The frequency of
cells with abnormal karyotypes was increased in the HI-F tumor. One hundred
percent of all the cells karyotyped had the addition of a No. 4 chromosome and
had the t(4;7) translation markers, and 80% of the cells also had a ring No. 1
chromosome[7]. The morphology of the t(4;7) and ring No. 1 markers were completely identical with those of the major clone of the HI-M tumor, thus demonstrating
that the progression of the HI-M to HI-F tumors involved clonal selection.

At the eighth passage of the HI-F tumor, a single rat of 4 within the passage
developed a completely anaplastic tumor. This anaplastic tumor was serially
passaged and termed the AT-3 tumor. This AT-3, besides being anaplastic, is
completely androgen-insensitive and is even faster-growing than the HI-F tumor.
The doubling time for the AT-3 tumor is 1.8 ± 0.2 days regardless of the
androgen status of the host. Even in its earliest passage (first to fifth),
this AT-3 tumor has had a moderately high incidence of spontaneous metastases
(i.e., over 50% of rats inoculated developed axillary lymph node and lung
metastases). DNA analysis of the AT-3 tumor demonstrated that it had more than
the diploid amount of DNA per cell (Table 1). Chromosomal analysis further
revealed that the AT-3 tumor, at its third passage, has a modal number, 65, in
the hypotetraploid range. This deviation from tetraploidy involved the loss of
the Y chromosome and the gain of 5 kinds of structural chromosomal abnormalities
including a t(1;4) and t(4;X) translocation marker[7]. Thus, the progression of
the HI-F to the AT-3, like all previous progressions, was associated with
development of definitive chromosomal change.

DISCUSSION

A schematic summary of the development of the various Dunning sublines is
presented in Chart 1. Each of these sublines has a common direct lineage to
the parental H tumor. In addition, all of the sublines, except the HI-S,
spontaneously arose via progression. It is highly relevant that using the
Dunning R-3327 rat prostatic adenocarcinoma system of transplantable cancers as
a model, each time that progression occurred, concomitant chromosomal changes
could be detected. Unfortunately, the association of demonstrable chromosomal
changes and tumor progression does not in itself allow a decision as to the
mechanism for these phenotypic changes (i.e., genetic or epigenetic). Indeed,
these chromosomal changes may or may not be causally related to the phenotypic

changes involved in these tumor progressions. These chromosomal changes, however, do make it clear that the Dunning tumor cells, unlike normal prostatic cells, are genetically unstable (i.e., genetically changeable) under certain conditions. Numerous studies have demonstrated that normal mammalian tissues consist essentially of genetically homogeneous cell populations which upon cellular proliferation produce genetically identical progeny[10-12]. In direct contrast to this consistent genetic stability of normal cells, Dunning tumor cells can begin to produce novel tumor cell progeny that are genetically different from their parental cell precursors. That definitive genetic differences do exist between parental and progeny Dunning tumor cells when such genetic instability develops has been consistently demonstrated in the present study by comparison of the various karyotypes.

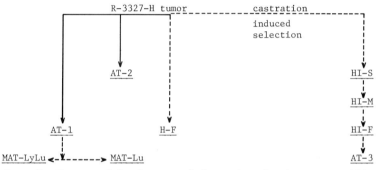

Chart 1. Summary of development of the various Dunning tumor sublines. ———, progression of tumor with a single passage; ----, progression of tumor which required multiple serial passages.

The observation that cancer cells are genetically more unstable than their normal cell counterpart raises the question of whether cancer cells are constantly genetically unstable or whether this genetic instability is a dormant characteristic, expressed only sporadically under certain conditions. It is possible, for example, that cancer cells are constantly genetically unstable (i.e., constantly giving rise to progeny cells with random chromosomal changes) but the effects of this instability are expressed only when the random chromosomal changes result in a specific rearrangement which confers to the new progeny cell a selective growth advantage (e.g., increased growth rate, etc.). In this explanation, the expression of genetic instability would be a stochastic event. How such random chromosomal changes could be constantly occurring among cancer cells is not entirely known. One possibility, however, is that one of the

earliest events in malignant transformation might involve activation of a gene
locus which increases the possibility of subsequent mitotic errors[13]. Indeed,
such genes have been demonstrated in Drosophila[14]. In addition, such genes have
been suggested in certain human families with "chromosomal breakage syndromes"
(e.g., Bloom's syndrome, Fanconi's anemia, ataxia telangiectasia, and xeroderma
pigmentosum) in which chromosomal breaks and rearrangements are increased as a
result of inherited defects[15-17]. In contrast to the possibility that cancer
cells are constantly genetically unstable, it is equally possible that cancer
cells are not constantly generating progeny cells with random chromosomal
changes but that the development of such genetic instability is actually an
inducible event caused by changes in the host microenvironmental conditions.
Exactly how this induction of genetic instability could occur is not completely
understood. It is known, however, that exposure of tissue culture cells to
medium deficient in single essential amino acids results in a decrease in
cellular proliferation with a specific inhibition of the cell cycle during the
S-phase. This inhibition also has been shown to induce the development of
genetic instability such that eventually, demonstrable chromosomal aberrations
occur[18]. The net results of this environmentally induced genetic instability
is that genetically novel progeny are produced from the original parent cell
precursors. Since one of the characteristic responses of initially sensitive
cancer cells to effective therapy is a substantial decrease in their cellular
proliferation, such effective therapy itself might induce genetic instability
in the originally sensitive cancer cells via a similar mechanism.

Regardless of whether the expression of the genetic instability of cancer
cells is a stochastic or inducible event, an important consequence of the expression of this genetic instability is that new clones of tumor cells are
capable of being added to the tumor population at any time. These additions,
when they occur, increase the heterogeneous nature of the initial tumor. For
example, in the progression of the Dunning HI-S to the HI-M tumor, 2 new clones
of tumor cells developed producing a heterogeneous tumor with at least 3 distinct but highly related tumor cell subpopulations. Once established, the
heterogeneous nature of a tumor can remain stable for years as long as all the
clones within a heterogeneous tumor have similar doubling times. This type of
stability can be seen with the H tumor which is a heterogeneous tumor composed
of both well-differentiated androgen-dependent and androgen-independent tumor
cells with identical slow growth rates. As long as there is no exogenous
selective pressure (i.e., androgen ablation) and no further expression of

genetic instability, this H tumor remains heterogeneous and highly stable as documented by its ability to be maintained in continuous passage for over 16 years.

In contrast to the relative stability of heterogeneous tumors composed of clones with identical doubling times, heterogeneous tumors having clones with differing growth rates are markedly unstable since eventually any clone(s) with a definitive growth advantage will selectively outgrow the other slower-growing clones initially present. This process, termed clonal selection, thus reduces the heterogeneous nature of tumors. Clonal selection has been consistently demonstrated in all of the progressions of the various Dunning sublines examined in the present study. In all of these progressions, a particular clone of cells within a heterogeneous tumor outgrew the other slower-growing clones producing a more homogeneous tumor. In this manner, the heterogeneous vs. homogeneous nature of a tumor, at any moment, is determined by the dynamic relationship between genetic instability increasing and clonal selection decreasing the number of tumor cell clones present within a tumor.

IN CONCLUSION:

The present study suggests that the process of genetic instability, which results in the addition of phenotypically new clones of cells to the tumor population, coupled with the process of clonal selection of these newly developed cells is at least one mechanism for the progression of prostatic cancer. Indeed, the idea that tumor progression involves such a coupled series of events has been proposed by Nowell[19] as a general model for all tumor progressions. Whether such a process is the only mechanism for tumor progression is not yet clear. In support of such a concept, however, there are a series of previous reports that, like the progression of the Dunning tumors, progression in other tumor systems is likewise associated with chromosomal changes and clonal selection. For example, both Mark[20], studying the mouse, and Mittelman[21], studying the rat, demonstrated that during the serial transplantation of Rous sarcoma virus-induced tumors there is a sequential change in the chromosomal makeup of the tumor which is associated with the progression of these tumors to a more malignant and less differentiated state. The studies of Mittelman[21] are particularly relevant since they demonstrate that the change in chromosomal number upon serial transplantation of rat sarcomas was typically associated with the progressive loss of differentiation, as determined both histologically and by decreased collagen production. In addition to these studies, Al-Saadi and Beierwaltes[22] have demonstrated that the serial transplantation of thyroid tumors in the rat is likewise associated with sequential chromosomal changes which are correlated with the progression of these tumors from a large degree of dependence on iodine deficiency and thyroidectomy for growth, to anaplastic, fast-growing, and metastatic tumors independent of hormonal modulation.

REFERENCES

1. Foulds, L. (1964) in Cellular Control Mechanisms and Cancer, Emmelot, P. and Muhlfork, O., eds., Elsevier, Amsterdam, pp. 242-258.
2. Medina, D. (1975) in Cancer: A Comprehensive Treatise, Vol. 3, F. F. Becker, ed., Plenum Press, pp. 99-120.
3. Isaacs, J. T., Heston, W. D. W., Weissman, R.M. and Coffey, D.S. (1978) Cancer Res., 38, 4353-4359.
4. Isaacs, J. T., Wake, N., Coffey, D.S. and Sandberg, A.A. (1982) Cancer Res., 42, 2353-2361.
5. Dunning, W. F. (1963) Natl. Cancer Inst. Monogr. 12, 351-369.
6. Isaacs, J.T. and Coffey, D.S. (1981) Cancer Res., 41, 5070-5075.
7. Wake, N., Isaacs, J.T. and Sandberg, A.A. (1982) Cancer Res., 42, 4131-4142.
8. Isaacs, J.T., Yu, G.W. and Coffey, D.S. (1981) Invest. Urol., 19, 20-25.
9. Lazan, D.W., Heston, W.D.W., Kadmon, D. and Fair, W.R. (1982) Cancer Res., 42, 1390-1394.
10. Ford, C.E., Hamerton, J.F. and Mole, R.H. (1958) J. Cell Comp. Physiol., 52 (Suppl. 1), 235-269.
11. Hauschka, T.S. (1961) Cancer Res., 21, 957-974.
12. Levan, A. (1959) in Genetics and Cancer, M. D. Anderson Hospital and Tumor Institute at Houston, Williams & Wilkins, Baltimore, pp. 152-182.
13. Cairns, J. (1975) Nature (London), 255, 197-200.
14. Green, M. M. (1980) Ann. Rev. Genet., 14, 109-128.
15. German, J. (1972) J. Prog. Med. Genet., 8, 61-101.
16. Cairns, J. (1981) Nature (London), 289, 353-356.
17. Feinberg, A.P. and Coffey, D.S. (1982) Cancer Res., 42, 3252-3254.
18. Freed, J.J. and Schatz, S.A. (1969) Cell Res., 55, 393-399.
19. Nowell, P.C. (1976) Science, 194, 23-28.
20. Mark, J. (1970) Hereditas, 65, 59-62.
21. Mittelman, F. (1972) Acta Pathol. Microbiol. Scand. Sect. A. Pathol., 80, 313-328.
22. Al-Saadi, A. and Beierwaltes, W.H. (1967) Cancer Res., 27, 1831-1842.

CHROMOSOME TRANSLOCATIONS, IMMUNOGLOBULIN GENES, AND NEOPLASIA

P. NOWELL[+], R. DALLA-FAVERA[++], J. FINAN[+], J. ERIKSON[+++], AND C. CROCE[+++]
[+]Department of Pathology and Laboratory Medicine, University of Pennsylvania
School of Medicine, Philadelphia, Pennsylvania 19104; [++]Laboratory of Tumor
Cell Biology, National Cancer Institute, Bethesda, Maryland 20205; [+++]The
Wistar Institute, 36th Street at Spruce, Philadelphia, Pennsylvania 19104.

INTRODUCTION

The widespread use of modern banding techniques has led, in recent years, to increasing recognition of chromosomal translocations which occur nonrandomly in a variety of human tumors, particularly leukemias and lymphomas[1,2]. Because all of the cells in a tumor typically have the same chromosome rearrangement, it is believed that these alterations confer a selective advantage on the neoplastic cells. Further, it has been suggested that these translocations indicate sites in the human genome where genes important in neoplastic development are located, although there is very little information concerning how gene function is altered and what the key gene products may be[3].

Several interesting possibilities have been indicated by the recent recognition that certain translocations in human lymphoid tumors involve chromosome segments where immunoglobulin (Ig) genes are located. The genes for human Ig heavy chains have been mapped to the terminal portion of the long arm of chromosome 14[4,5]. The genes for the kappa and lambda light chains have been mapped to the short arm of chromosome 2 (2p) and the long arm of chromosome 22 (22q), respectively[6,7,8].

At the same time, studies of chromosome changes in the Burkitt lymphoma have demonstrated that in approximately 90% of the cases the neoplastic cells have a characteristic translocation involving the terminal portions of 8q and 14q. In those few cases which do not have 8;14 translocation, there is in nearly every instance a translocation between 8q and 2p or between 8q and 22q[9,10].

In other lymphomas, translocations involving the terminal portion of 14q and another chromosome (often 11q or 18q) have also been observed to occur with non-random frequency[1,2,9]. Such translocations, producing 14q[+] marker chromosome, have also been reported in multiple myeloma and in chronic lymphocytic leukemia of both the B-cell and T-cell variety[11,12,13] as well as in the adult T-cell leukemia (ATL) endemic in Japan[14]. Although less common, translocations involving 2p and 22q also occur in human lymphoid neoplasms other than the Burkitt tumor[1,2,9,12].

Cancer: Etiology and Prevention, Ray G. Crispen, Editor

These observations, and similar findings in murine leukemias[3] have led to the suggestion by several workers[3,15] that chromosome translocations involving Ig gene segments might bring "promoter" sequences of these genes (transcriptionally active in a lymphoid cell) into juxtaposition with other DNA sequences (on chromosome 8 and elsewhere) that when thus activated might play an important role in cellular transformation and the development of neoplasia.

Additional support for such concepts has come from recent studies of both viral and human oncogenes and mechanisms for their activation. It now appears that there are DNA sequences in the human genome analogous to known retrovirus onc-genes, and that such sequences may be expressed in some human tumors and have the capacity, in transfection experiments, to transform other cells[16,17]. Furthermore, at least one mechanism by which such an onc-gene may be activated is the insertion of "promoter" DNA adjacent to it[18,19]. This "promoter-insertion" phenomenon for onc-gene activation has thus far been demonstrated only in the avian myelocytomatosis system, involving the myc oncogene[18], but it adds credence to the possibility that a similar promoter mechanism might be mediated by translocations in mammalian lymphoid cells that involve Ig genes.

In order to begin testing directly these concepts of human leukemogenesis, we have undertaken studies of several Burkitt tumor cell lines. Using techniques of mouse-human cell hybridization, we have been able to demonstrate that:

1. The breakpoint on chromosome 14 in the Burkitt tumor does involve the Ig heavy chain locus, with a portion of the locus translocated to chromosome 8[20].

2. The human analogue of the viral myc gene (c-myc) is located on the terminal portion of 8q and is translocated to chromosome 14, adjacent to Ig gene sequences, in the Burkitt tumor[21].

The details of these findings, and their possible implications, are discussed in the following sections.

Translocation of Ig genes in the Burkitt lymphoma

To obtain clones in which the human chromosomes involved in the 8;14 translocation in Burkitt lymphoma would segregate, we produced somatic cell hybrids between mouse myeloma cells and lymphocytes of the Daudi Burkitt lymphoma cell line. The resultant hybrid clones were then studied by isozyme and cytogenetic methods, including trypsin-Giemsa and G-11 banding, for the presence of the normal and translocated human 8 and 14 chromosomes[20]. We also analyzed the DNA derived from the parental Daudi and myeloma (NP3) cells and from the hybrid cells for the presence of the genes for the variable region

($V_{\underline{HIII}}$) of human heavy chains and for the µ and γ constant (C) regions by Southern blotting procedures[22]. As shown in Table 1, we detected the human µ and γ constant region genes in all hybrids containing either the normal chromosome 14 or the 14q⁺. Hybrids that did not contain either the normal or

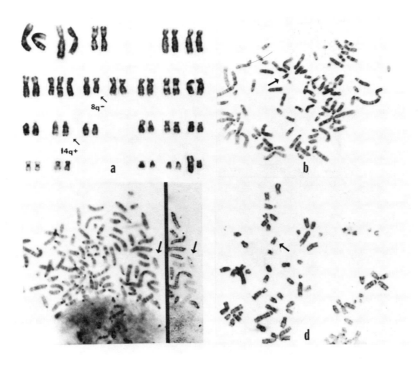

Fig. 1. (a) Karyotype of parental Daudi cell line with t8;14(q24;q32) (arrows) and small interstitial deletion in 15q. Trisomy 7 was present in a minority of the cells. (b) Trypsin-Giemsa banded metaphase from hybrid 3E5 Cl 3 containing normal 14 (arrow) and no 14q⁺. (c) Trypsin-Giemsa banded metaphase from hybrid 3F2 with 14q⁺ (arrow) and no normal 14. G-11 staining of the same metaphase (inset) indicates the human origin of 14q⁺. (d) Trypsin-Giemsa banded metaphase from hybrid 1E8 Cl 2 containing human 8q⁻ (arrow) and no 14 or 14q⁺[20].

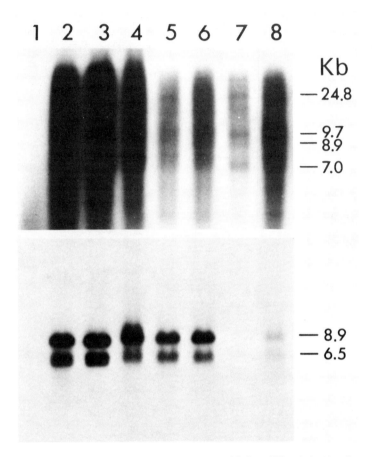

Fig. 2. Hybridization of HindIII-digested cellular DNA with the V_{HIII} probe (upper) and the same filter rehybridized with the γ cDNA probe (lower). In lane 1 is DNA from the mouse myeloma parent NP3, which shows no hybridization to either probe. Lane 2 is Daudi DNA, which hybridizes to both probes, as does DNA from 6M54VA, a simian virus 40 (SV40)-transformed human cell line, in lane 3. In lane 4 is the hybrid clone 3E5, which produces human μ chain. Lanes 5 and 6 are DNAs from two clones that are nucleoside phosphorylase positive. Lane 7 is DNA from the 1E8 Cl 2 clone, which is nucleoside phosphorylase negative and has the 8q⁻ chromosome. This DNA hybridizes to the variable region probe (upper) but not the (γ) constant region probe. In lane 8 is DNA from the 1D8 clone, which has the 14q⁺ chromosome but not the 8q⁻ chromosome. DNA from this clone hybridizes to both probes[20].

translocated chromosome 14, but did retain the 8q⁻ chromosome, had lost the genes for the μ and γ C regions.

The filters were then rehybridized with a probe specific for the human variable region gene (V_{HIII}). This human chromosome 14-specific probe has been used to demonstrate the synteny of the V_H and C_H genes in man by Rabbitts and his associates[23, 24]. As shown in Fig. 1 and Table 1, the two hybrids (1E8 Cl 2 and 2B8 Cl 22) that contained human chromosome 8q⁻ and had lost both the normal chromosome 14 and the 14q⁺ chromosome contained human V_{HIII} gene sequences. This result indicated that in the Daudi cells some of the variable region genes were translocated to chromosome 8. Because the 14q⁺ chromosome in clone 1D8, which lacked the 8q⁻ and the normal 14, had retained the V_{HIII} gene sequences (Fig. 2 and Table 1), we further concluded that the chromosomal breakpoint in the Daudi cells occurred in a region of chromosome 14 containing V_H genes.

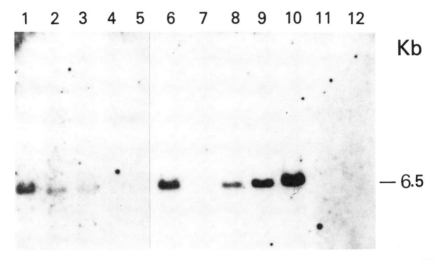

Fig. 3. Hybridization of the Xba I-digested cellular DNA with the μ cDNA probe, demonstrating the presence or absence of μ gene sequences in Daudi hybrids. Lanes 1 and 2 (clones 3E5 and 3A9) are DNAs from hybrid clones that produce μ chain. In lane 3 is DNA from clone 3F2, which is nucleoside phosphorylase positive. In lanes 4 and 5 are DNAs from two nucleoside phosphorylase-negative clones. In lanes 6-10 are human DNAs: lane 6 is Daudi; lane 7 is an IgA-expressing lymphoblastoid line; line 8 is an IgM-expressing lymphoblastoid line; and lanes 9 and 10 are two SV40-transformed human cell lines[36] (GM54VA and GM637). In lane 11 is DNA from NP3 and in lane 12 is DNA from a SV40-transformed mouse cell line, neither of which hybridizes to the human μ cDNA probe[20].

TABLE 1

HUMAN Ig GENES IN NP3-DAUDI CELL HYBRIDS

Cell line	Human chromosomes[a]				Human isozymes[b]		Expression of human μ chains	Human Ig genes		
	8	8q$^-$	14	14q$^+$	Glutathione reductase	Nucleoside phosphorylase		V_H	C_μ	$C\gamma$
Daudi	++	++	++	++	+	+	+	+	+	+
NP3	-	-	-	-	-	-	-	-	-	-
3E5 Cl 1	+	-	+	+	+	+	+	+	+	+
3E5 Cl 3	+	+	++	-	+	+	+	+	+	+
3F2	++	++	-	+	+	+	-	+	+	+
1D8	++	-	-	+	+	+	-	+	+	+
1E8 Cl 2	++	+	-	-	+	-	-	+	-	-
2B8 Cl 22	++	±	-	-	+	-	-	±	-	-

[a]Frequency of metaphases with relevant chromosome: - = none; ± = <10%; + = 10-30%; and ++ = >30%.
[b]Glutathione reductase is a marker for human chromosome 8; nucleoside phosphorylase is a marker for human chromosome 14[20].

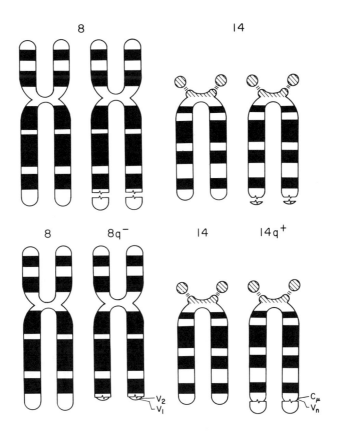

Fig. 4. Diagram of the (8;14) chromosome translocation in Daudi cells. (Upper) The breakpoint on chromosome 8 and 14; (lower) the t(8;14) reciprocal translocation. The figure also shows the postulated position of the genes for variable regions ($V_1 \rightarrow V_n$) and constant regions of Ig heavy chains on the involved chromosomes as indicated by our data[20].

Because the genes for the μ and γ C regions were all present in the hybrids 1D8 and 3F2, which contained the 14q$^+$ chromosome, and were not present in the hybrids containing only the 8q$^-$ (1B8 Cl 2 and 2B8 Cl 22) (Figs. 2 and 3, and Table 1), we also concluded that these heavy chain genes were proximal to the breakpoint observed in Daudi cells, and that the variable region genes are distal to the constant region genes on human chromosome 14 (Fig. 4).

The cellular DNA from the parental line was also cleaved with BamHI and, after agarose gel electrophoresis and Southern transfer, it was hybridized with μ-specific cDNA. As shown in Fig. 5, Daudi cells appeared to have the μ chains on both number 14 chromosomes rearranged. The results from the hybrids, in conjunction with the data in Table 1, indicated that the 14q$^+$ chromosome in these cells contained the BamHI μ chain-specific fragment (18.0 kb), whereas the normal chromosome 14 carried the smaller fragment (12.5 kb). Germline DNA gave a single band at 16.0 kb. We had previously shown that hybrids between Daudi cells and mouse myeloma cells secrete human IgM when the chromosomes carrying the active genes for light and heavy chains are present in the hybrids[25]. Therefore, we screened the hybrids described in Table 1 for the expression of secreted and cytoplasmic μ chains, and found that the presence of human cytoplasmic μ chains correlated with the presence of the normal chromosome 14 and not with the 14q$^+$ chromosome. There was no secretion of IgM

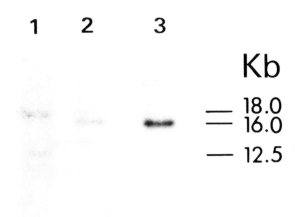

Fig. 5. Hybridization of BamHI-digested cellular DNA with the μ-specific cDNA probe. In lane 1 is Daudi DNA with two bands. In lane 2 is DNA from an adenovirus-transformed human cell line (FC Cl$_3$7)[37], and in lane 3 is GM54VA, a SV40-transformed fibroblastic human cell line[20]; both show a single band that does not comigrate with either of the Daudi bands.

because the hybrids did not produce light chains. These findings strongly suggested that in Daudi cells the μ chain genes on both number 14 chromosomes had undergone rearrangement, but that only the rearranged gene on the normal chromosome 14 was expressed.

Recently, these studies have been extended to the P3HR-1 Burkitt tumor line[26]. Using similar techniques, we demonstrated that in this cell line, which also has the 8;14 translocation, the breakpoint on chromosome 14 is between C_μ and V_H with V_H genes again translocated to the 8q⁻ chromosome, but none remaining on the 14q⁺ (Fig. 6). Thus, the breakpoint on chromosome 14 may differ in different Burkitt tumors, but in both instances, Daudi and P3HR-1, expression of Ig heavy chains was coded for by the non-translocated chromosome 14[20,26].

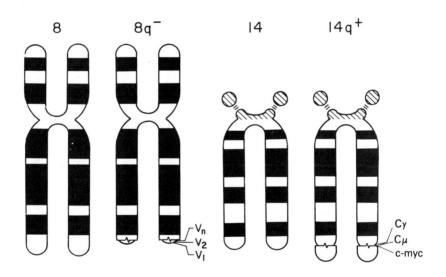

Fig. 6. Diagram of the t(8;14) chromosome translocation in P3HR-1 cells. The C_μ and C_γ genes are proximal to the breakpoint on chromosome 14, while the V_H gene translocates to the 8q⁻ chromosome. The human c-myc gene on the broken chromosome 8 translocates the heavy chain locus[26].

These various findings with the Daudi cell line and derived hybrids, as well as from additional Burkitt lymphoma cell lines (P3HR-1, CA46, JD38IV) (see below), were consistent with the hypothesis that the 8;14 chromosome translocation in the Burkitt tumor involved the Ig heavy chain locus, and that expression of malignancy might result from activation of a gene located on the long arm of chromosome 8, brought into association with the translocated V_H genes on the $8q^-$ chromosome or with retained Ig sequences proximal to the breakpoint on the $14q^+$ chromosome.

The possibility that the critical gene on chromosome 8 might be the human analogue of the viral oncogene of avian myelocytomatosis (c-myc) was suggested by parallel studies which indicated the location of c-myc on human chromosome 8[21]. The details of this work follow.

TABLE 2

PRESENCE OF THE HUMAN C-MYC HOMOLOGUE IN A PANEL OF RODENT X HUMAN HYBRID CLONES

Hybrids	\multicolumn{23}{c}{Human Chromosomes}	Human c-myc
	1	2	3	4	5	6	7	8	9	10	11	12	13	14	15	16	17	18	19	20	21	22	X	
DSK1B2A5 Cl2			■				■							■	■		■		■	■			■	+
DSK1B2A5 Cl20					■															■	■	■	■	−
Nu 9						■																		−
PAFxBalbIV Cl5	■						■						■					■						+
GMxLM Cl3			■											■										−
GMxLM Cl4														■										+
GMxLM Cl5												■		■										+
GMxLM Cl6											■	■												−
706B6-40 Cl17								■																+
77-B10 Cl5	■				■							■		■		■				■			■	+
77-B10 Cl8		■										■		■				■		■			■	+
77-B10 Cl25		■						■				■								■			■	−
77-B10 Cl26	■							■				■								■			■	+
77-B10 Cl28		■																		■			■	−
77-B10 Cl30								■				■								■			■	−
77-B10 Cl31	■							■				■		■				■					■	+

A black square indicates that the hybrid clone named in the left column contains the chromosome named in the upper row. An empty square indicates that the hybrid clone has lost the human chromosome indicated in the upper row[21].

Human c-myc onc-gene on the region of chromosome 8 translocated in Burkitt lymphoma cells

This study was also carried out with mouse-human hybrids as well as with a hybrid between Chinese hamster and human cells that had retained only human chromosome 8. The human c-myc probe used for Southern blotting studies was a recombinant pBR322 plasmid (clone pMC41RC) which contains the entire 3' c-myc exon[27]. Initial studies with human and mouse cellular DNA, using this probe, indicated that it was possible to distinguish between the human and the mouse

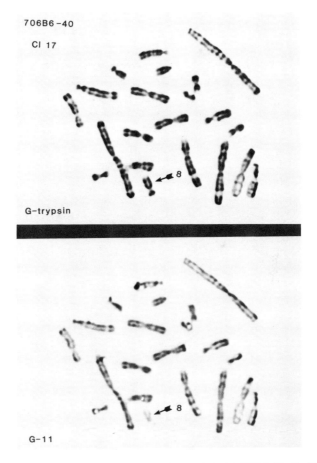

Fig. 7. Metaphase of Chinese hamster x human hybrid 706B6-40 Cl 17, which has retained human chromosome 8 and no other human chromosome, stained by the trypsin-Giemsa method (upper) and the G-11 method (lower)[26].

c-myc DNA sequences. Following digestion with ScT-1, the human c-myc DNA migrates as a 2.8 kb band while the mouse homologue migrates as a 17.0 kb band.

We then studied the segregation of the human-specific 2.8 kb band in a panel
of mouse-human hybrids to establish the chromosomal location of the human c-myc
homologue. Table 2 shows the results of the analysis of a panel of hybrid
clones that were studied for the expression of isozyme markers assigned to each
of the human chromosomes and for the presence of the human c-myc homologue.
Only human chromosome 8 segregated concordantly with the presence of the human
c-myc gene.

To confirm this indication that the human c-myc gene was located on chromosome 8, we also studied a somatic cell hybrid between Chinese hamster and human
cells that had retained only human chromosome 8 (Fig. 7). This hybrid
(706B6-40 Cl 17) also contained the human c-myc homologue (Table 2).

For regional mapping of the c-myc gene, mouse-human hybrids were utilized
from both the Daudi and the P3HR-1 Burkitt lymphoma cell lines. As indicated
in Table 3, hybrids M44 Cl 2S5 and M44 Cl 2S9, from the P3HR-1 line and re-
taining only the human $14q^+$ chromosome[21,26] also retained the human c-myc gene.
Hybrid 3F1, from the Daudi line, which had the $14q^+$ chromosome and neither the
normal nor the $8q^-$ chromosome, also contained the human c-myc gene (Table 3).
These results indicated that the human c-myc gene was located on region q24→qter
of human chromosome 8, the segment translocated to the $14q^+$ chromosome. Furthermore, since the human c-myc gene was present on the $14q^+$ chromosome of both
the Daudi and P3HR1 cell lines, we concluded that it must be distal to the
breakpoint on human chromosome 8 in both of these tumors. Interestingly, no

TABLE III

PRESENCE OF THE HUMAN C-MYC HOMOLOGUE IN HYBRIDS WITH THE BURKITT LYMPHOMA $14q^+$
CHROMOSOME

Hybrids	Isozymes[a]		Chromosomes				Human c-myc
	NP	GSR	8	$8q^-$	14	$14q^+$	
M44 Cl 2S5	+	-	-	-	-	+	+
M44 Cl 2S9	+	-	-	-	-	+	+
3F1	+	-	-	-	-	+	+

[a]NP = nucleoside phosphorylase; GSR = glutathione reductase.[21]

obvious rearrangement of the 3' exon of the human c-myc DNA segment was detected in its new location on the 14q$^+$ chromosome of these two cell lines.

The results of this study thus not only further supported the involvement of an Ig gene locus in a consistently observed translocation in a human lymphoid tumor, but also provided a possible candidate, the human c-myc gene, for an "oncogene" which might be activated by its new association with promoter regions of the Ig gene following translocation.

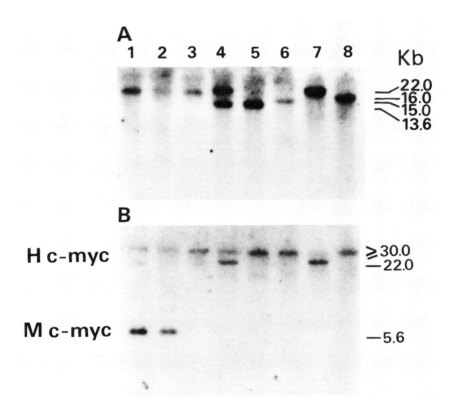

Fig. 8. Southern blotting analysis of BamHI-digested DNA derived from different Burkitt lymphoma cell lines. Lanes 1 and 2: two independent somatic cell hybrids between mouse myeloma cells and P3HR-1 Burkitt lymphoma cells. Lane 3: P3HR-1 Burkitt cell line. Lanes 4-7: Burkitt lymphomas CA46, AD876, EW36, and JD38-IV cell lines, respectively. Lane 8: PAF, an SV40-transformed human fibroblastic cell line. Panel A was hybridized with a C_μ probe. The probe was washed and the filter rehybridized to the human c-myc probe (panel B).[28]

This hypothesis has been strengthened by our recent evidence that the human c-myc gene translocation lies in close proximity to the human heavy chain locus in a number of Burkitt lymphomas with the 8;14 chromosome translocation. We have digested the DNA of five different Burkitt lymphoma cell lines with BamHI, a restriction enzyme that cuts outside the human μ gene[20] and the c-myc gene[28]. After agarose gel electrophoresis and Southern transfer, we have hybridized the nitrocellulose filter first with the μ-specific probe (Fig. 8a) and then with the human c-myc cDNA probe (Fig. 8b). As shown in Fig. 8, the same 22 kb band hybridized with both the c-myc and the μ probes, indicating that these two genes are contained in the same restriction fragment in some (CA46 and JD38-IV) of the Burkitt lymphomas with the 8;14 chromosomal translocation. Fig. 6 describes the organization of the c-myc gene and of the heavy chain gene in the P3HR-1, CA46, and JD38-IV cell lines.

We have detected a similar rearrangement of the c-myc gene with the Ig heavy chain locus in mouse plasmacytoma cells carrying the 12;15 chromosome translocation[28]. Interestingly, expression of high levels of myc transcription was detected in mouse plasmacytomas[28].

Implications of translocation model of onc-gene activation
_____

The results of the studies just described are consistent with the view that one mechanism of human leukemogenesis in lymphoid cells might involve chromosomal translocations that bring segments of Ig genes adjacent to human oncogenes, leading to their activation. Similar results have now been reported from at least one other laboratory[29], also involving the Burkitt tumor.

Although the critical gene product involved in these leukemogenic phenomena has not been identified, presumably a human or mouse lymphocyte with such a chromosome translocation acquires a selective growth advantage as the result of oncogene activation, and its progeny expand as a neoplastic clone. It has been generally assumed that the translocations themselves are random events, with only those cytogenetic changes that confer a selective growth advantage becoming apparent, but it is interesting to speculate on whether the chromosome breakage itself may be non-random. It is possible that Ig gene sequences engaged in physiological rearrangements are unusually susceptible to breakage and thus, in developing lymphoid cells, become fragile "hot spots". Our data on the Daudi and P3HR-1 lines indicate that the translocated chromosome is not the one expressing gene function (this activity resides with the rearranged gene of the normal chromosome 14), but the critical translocation could take place during an abortive attempt at physiological rearrangement.

As one attempts to extend these translocation-activation concepts to human lymphoid tumors other than the Burkitt lymphoma, it will be necessary to suggest other candidates for the activated oncogene. Although translocations involving the terminal portion of 14q are present in a variety of lymphoid leukemias and lymphomas, it is rare for chromosome 8 to be the "donor" except in the Burkitt tumor (and leukemic equivalent)[1,2,9]. As noted above, translocations between 14q and either 11q or 18q appear to be the two most common findings in the non-Burkitt lymphoid neoplasms. Mapping of a number of the human analogues of known onc-genes (other than c-myc) to specific human chromosomes is currently under way in several laboratories, including ours. A summary of recent assignments is incorporated elsewhere in this volume[30]. Obviously, those human "oncogenes" identified through their homology with viral oncogenes will not constitute the entire spectrum of genes importantly involved in human leukemogenesis, but the tools are currently available for the analysis of both structure and function of these DNA sequences in human tumors, and so they represent a fruitful area for immediate study.

It is also interesting to speculate as to whether certain of the non-random translocations observed in non-lymphoid human leukemias might also involve Ig gene sequences and/or onc-genes. For instance, the Philadelphia (Ph) chromosome in chronic granulocytic leukemia typically involves a translocation between the long arms of chromosome 22 and chromosome 9. The breakpoint in chromosome 22 (q11) is consistent with possible involvement of the lambda light chain locus[6], as well as the c-sis onc-gene[31]. Similar translocations involving 22q are also present in some disorders which present de novo as acute leukemia, classified as myeloid, undifferentiated, or lymphoid[32,2]. Although translocations involving 2q are much less common and a 14q+ chromosome is extremely rare in non-lymphoid tumors[33,34], the wide occurrence of the Ph chromosome at least suggests the possibility that Ig gene involvement, and also onc-gene involvement, may play important roles in tumors arising at the hematopoietic stem cell level as well as in those already differentiated along a lymphoid pathway.

In addition to speculations concerning the types of tumors in which these genes may be significant, there are also considerations of the nature of the "activation" process when onc-genes are involved in such chromosome translocations. The limited data available suggests that the transforming ability for 3T3 cells on onc-genes may result in some instances from point mutations within the gene, producing an altered gene product, and in other instances from an increased production of a normal gene product (R. Weinberg and M. Barbacid, personal communication). The possibility that point mutations are involved, however, requires additional careful investigation to exclude differences due to genetic polymorphisms. It is also not yet clear whether the ability to transform 3T3 cells reflects the role of the oncogene in the pathogenesis of the original tumor. In any event, there may be variation not only in different types of tumors but even in different individual cases of the same neoplasm. The numerous Burkitt cell lines available for detailed study as described above may provide some indication of the spectrum of changes in oncogene structure and expression associated with tumorigenesis, at least for this one tumor and one gene (c-myc).

It must be recognized, however, that even the elucidation of these questions, and the characterization of oncogene products, may still leave us some distance from complete understanding of the full development of a clinical tumor. In this regard, it is interesting to recall the recent history of our thinking about the Burkitt lymphoma. Its geographical distribution initially suggested the possibility of horizontal transmission of a causative agent by an insect vector. It now seems likely that these geographical patterns reflect a poorly explained influence of various infectious diseases, particularly malaria, on the development of the tumor, perhaps through distortion of the patient's immune system. Subsequently, the association of the Epstein-Barr virus (EBV) with the Burkitt tumor led to speculation as to its etiologic role. Again, our thinking has been modified since it has become apparent that EBV is frequently absent in non-African Burkitt tumors, appears not to integrate at consistent sites within the host-cell genome, and does not have direct damaging effect on host chromosomes. It now seems likely that EBV acts to "freeze" the infected B-cells in an actively proliferating state (analogous to its role in maintaining proliferation of normal B-cells in tissue culture)[35], and thus increases the probability that when a carcinogenic even occurs in a lymphocyte (the 8;14 translocation?), that cell will be actively proliferating and hence expand as a lymphoma. Subsequent progression of the tumor may be further promoted by additional genetic and cytogenetic changes within the neoplastic clone.

The specific translocation events that we have been discussing may thus represent only one essential step in a sequence necessary to produce the clinical disease. This does not reduce the significance of the findings, and the need to further elucidate the specific genes and gene products involved. It simply indicates the complexity of carcinogenesis, and the probability that we will need to dissect carefully a series of events if reasonably complete understanding is to be attained of the factors and mechanisms involved in the development of any human cancer.

ACKNOWLEDGMENTS

Dr. Croce is supported by grants CA-10815, CA-23568, GM-20700 CA-16685, CA-21124, CA-20741, CA-7712 and RR-04430 from the National Institutes of Health.

REFERENCES

1. Rowley, J. (1980a) Cancer Genet. Cytogenet., 2, 175.
2. Mitelman, F. and Levan, G. (1981) Hereditas, 95, 79.
3. Klein, G. (1981) Nature, 294, 313.
4. Croce, C.M., Shander, M., Martinis, J., Cicurel, L., D'Ancona, G.G., Dolby, T.W. and Koprowski, H. (1979) Proc. Natl. Acad. Sci., 76, 3416.
5. Kirsch, I.R., Morton, C.C., Nakahara, K. and Leder, P. (1982) Science, 216, 301.
6. Erikson, J., Martinis, J. and Croce, C.M. (1981) Nature, 294, 173.
7. McBride, O.W., Hieter, P.A., Hollis, G.F., Swan, D., Otey, M.C. and Leder, P. (1982) J. Exp. Med., 155, 1680.
8. Malcolm, S., Barton, P., Murphy, C., Ferguson-Smith, M.A., Bentley, D.L. and Rabbitts, T.H. (1982) Proc. Natl. Acad. Sci., 79, 4957.
9. Sandberg, A. (1981) Hum. Pathol., 12, 531.
10. Bernheim, A., Berger, R. and Lenoir, G. (1981) Cancer Genet. Cytogenet., 3, 307.
11. Gahrton, G. and Robert, K.-H. (1982) Cancer Genet. Cytogenet., 6, 171.
12. Nowell, P., Shankey, T., Finan, J., Guerry, D. and Besa, E. (1981) Blood, 57, 444.
13. Finan, J., Daniele, R., Rowlands, D. and Nowell, P. (1978) Virchow Archiv B Cell Pathol., 29, 121.
14. Ueshima, Y., Fukuhara, S., Hattori, T., Uchiyama, T., Takatsuki, K. and Uchino, H. (1981) Blood, 58, 420.
15. Cairns, J. (1981) Nature, 289, 353.
16. Murray, M.J., Shilo, B.Z., Shih, C., Corning, D., Hsu, H.W. and Weinberg, R.A. (1981) Cell, 25, 355.
17. Shih, C., Padhy, L.C., Murray, M. and Weinberg, R.A. (1981) Nature, 290, 261.
18. Hayward, W.S., Neel, B.G. and Astrin, S.M. (1981) Nature, 290, 475.
19. Oskarsson, M., McClements, W.E., Blair, D.G., Maizel, J.V. and Vaude Woude, G.F. (1980) Science, 207, 1222.
20. Erikson, J., Finan, J., Nowell, P.C. and Croce, C.M. (1982) Proc. Natl. Acad. Sci., 79, 5611.
21. Dalla-Favera, R., Bregni, M., Erikson, J., Patterson, D., Gallo, R.C. and Croce, C.M. (1982b) Proc. Natl. Acad. Sci., in press.
22. Southern, E. (1975) J. Mol. Biol., 98, 503.
23. Matthyssens, G. and Rabbitts, T. (1980) Proc. Natl. Acad. Sci., 77, 6561.
24. Robart, M.J., Rabbitts, T.H., Goodfellow, P.N., Solomon, E., Chambers, S., Spurr, N. and Povey, S. (1981) Ann. Hum. Genet., 45, 331.
25. Erikson, J. and Croce, C.M. (1982) Eur. J. Immunol., 12, 697.
26. Erikson, J., ar-Rushdi, A., Drwinga, H., Nowell, P. and Croce, C.M. (1983) Proc. Natl. Acad. Sci., in press.
27. Dalla-Favera, R., Wong-Staal, F., and Gallo, R.C. (1982a) Nature, 299, 61.
28. Marcu, K., Harris, L., Stanton, L., Erikson, J., Watt, R. and Croce, C.M. (1982) Proc. Natl. Acad. Sci., in press.

COMPLEMENT PHENOTYPES FOR PREDICTION OF RISK AND PROGNOSIS FOR
ACUTE LYMPHOCYTIC LEUKEMIA (ALL)

Bruce Budowle[†], James Dearth[†], Jeffry Roseman[‡],
Rodney Gott[‡] and William Crist[†],
Departments of Pediatrics[†] and Epidemiology[‡],
University of Alabama in Birmingham, Birmingham, AL, USA.

INTRODUCTION

A basic question for health scientists is why some
individuals contract a particular disease. There is evidence that
many diseases occur only in genetically susceptible individuals.
Genetic differences among individuals of a population and between
populations have become of interest in the past few years for
studies of etiology, pathogenesis and prognosis of disease.

The use of genetic markers is one method of determining if
genetic susceptibility is involved. Alleles or alternative forms
of a gene can occur in a population. A gene is said to be
polymorphic if the frequency of at least two alleles are both
greater than 1% in the population. Genetic markers are the
protein products encoded for by the alleles of polymorphic loci.

Two types of studies have been used to examine the
relationship between genetic markers and diseases: population
association, which is presented in this paper, and linkage
studies. Association studies evaluate the independence between
the presence of a particular disease and risk factors (in this
case the frequencies of genetic markers) in the population. This
is accomplished by phenotyping sufficiently large patient and
control samples for a particular polymorphic genetic marker(s).

© 1983 Elsevier Science Publishing Co., Inc.
Cancer: Etiology and Prevention, Ray G. Crispen, Editor

In association studies none of the subjects in either group can be related to each other. If the marker is associated with a particular disease, it will occur at a different frequency in the diseased sample than the control sample. For example, Aird et al[1] were first to demonstrate an increase in the erythrocyte antigen A of the ABO blood group and the presence of gastric carcinoma and duodenal ulcers. Since then a multitude of studies have found associations of genetic markers with diseases, the strongest being HLA-B27 and ankylosing spondylitis[2,3]. People carrying HLA-B27 have a 90 fold increased risk for developing ankylosing spondylitis. One of the most convincing reports of a genetic marker which may be causally involved in the pathogenesis of a disease is that of alpha-1 antitrypsin (Pi) and emphysema[4]. The S and Z alleles of the Pi locus produce functionally deficient gene products that do not inactivate elastase and, therefore, allow the destruction of elastin in the lungs resulting in emphysema.

There are several important considerations in association studies. First, the cases studied must be as homogeneous as possible. Any heterogeneity among cases can reduce the likelihood of finding a significant association. For example, if a gene product leads to susceptibility to non-T, non-B cell ALL, the inclusion of other forms of leukemia could obscure or mask the association. Also, if the disease has a high mortality rate, a sample of newly-diagnosed cases along with cases months or years from diagnosis can lead to associations which reflect genes which influence survival, not occurrence. For example, if those patients carrying the Human Lymphocyte Antigen (HLA) A2 are more likely to live longer after the onset of leukemia than those without A2, a sample of all cases being seen at a clinic will show an increase in A2 frequency over controls which may have nothing to do with leukemia susceptibility. Secondly, the frequencies of alleles of genetic markers vary among racial and ethnic groups. If certain racial or ethnic groups are more likely to develop the cancer in question, then it is possible to find genetic associations which simply reflect racial or ethnic differences. For example, melanoma is much more common in those of Celtic ancestry[5,6]. In the U.S., a sample of white melanoma cases would presumably have a much higher proportion of those with Celtic ancestry than would controls from the same region. If persons with Celtic ancestry have a higher proportion of HLA-DR4 and/or properdin factor B (Bf)S than those without such ancestry and if one found an increase in HLA DR4[5,6] and/or BfS[7] among melanoma cases, it could be that the increase was secondary to ethnic selection and not to linkage disequilibrium with a "melanoma susceptibility gene(s)". One way to control for this possibility is to match cases and controls for race and/or ethnic group. It is not necessary to match on gender for genetic markers encoded by genes of the major histocompatibility complex (MHC) since there are no known differences in allelic frequencies by gender.

The association of a given genetic marker and a disease may be due to either a causal relationship between the marker gene product and the disease (such as Pi and emphysema) or due to linkage disequilibrium of the marker with a disease

susceptibility gene(s).   Linkage refers to the proximity of gene
loci on a chromosome. The closer two gene loci lie on a
particular area of chromosome, the more closely linked they are
and, therefore, the less likely a crossover (an exchange of
chromosomal material between maternal and paternal chromosomes
during meiosis) will occur between the two loci. Closely linked
genes are usually transmitted as a single unit from one
generation to another.   There are at least three explanations
why a linkage disequilibrium (the occurrence of two or more
linked loci (a haplotype) appearing together in a population at a
frequency different than what would be expected by the product of
their independent occurrence) can occur. 1)There can be some
selective advantage conferred upon individuals carrying a
particular haplotype. 2) The haplotype may have arisen relatively
recently and has not yet reached random equilibrium. 3) A
"founder effect" which postulates that as a result of migration,
a foreign gene haplotype is introduced into a population [8].

True linkage of a genetic marker with a disease can be proven
only by linkage analysis of families of more than one generation
and not through population association studies. It is not in the
scope of this paper to discuss linkage analyses, and therefore,
it was only mentioned briefly.

In man, disease association studies have focused on the
genetic markers in the MHC on chromosome 6. The MHC contains a
diverse group of associated loci (HLA encoding genes, complement
component genes, immune response genes) that control a variety of
biological functions such as immune responsiveness, immune
surveillance, susceptibility and/or protection to disease and,

possibly, morphogenesis. Of the MHC loci, HLA has been associated with several malignant diseases which are reviewed elsewhere[9-12].

Since there is evidence for a genetic influence in ALL, we will use it as an example of a genetic marker-cancer association study. Lilly[13-16] was the first to show that certain antigens of the H-2 complex (lying within the MHC of the mouse) confer susceptibility to Gross and Friend virus leukemogenesis. Bearing in mind the remarkable structural and biochemical homology of the MHC in mouse and man[10,11], it seemed likely that the H-2 counterpart in man, HLA, would also be associated with leukemia susceptibility. This appears to be the case. Several studies have found significantly increased frequencies of HLA-A2[17-19] and B12[20] in ALL and a decreased frequency of A9[17] with ALL in Caucasians. In addition, longer survival was observed for patients carrying the A9 antigen[17,18,21,22] or the haplotypes A2/B12 and A2/B40[20]. Furthermore, ALL has been shown to occur with increased frequency with several genetic disorders, such as Down's syndrome[23], Bloom's syndrome[24], Fanconi's anemia[25] and ataxia telangiectasia[26].

Although HLA has been very useful, it lacks certain advantages of other MHC genetic markers such as properdin factor B (Bf) and the complement component C4. Bf[27,28] and C4[29-31] are both genetically controlled polymorphisms in man which lie within the MHC probably between HLA-B and -D/DR loci[32,33]. Bf has two commonly occuring alleles - BfF and BfS - and two rarer alleles - BfF1 and BfS1. C4 is encoded for by two tightly linked loci called C4A and C4B[29], each carrying 7 alleles (A0 - A6) and 5 alleles (B0 - B4), respectively, which makes C4 one of the most polymorphic markers described. Bf and C4 have been associated with diseases previously shown to be associated with HLA[7,35-38]. Both markers can be phenotyped from plasma samples. The ease of assay - agarose gel electrophoresis - which can be set up in any laboratory, the low cost, readily available sources of defined antisera and the ability to store samples make these markers ideal for large sample studies.

However, the most important aspect of Bf and C4 in studying malignant diseases is their potential role in immune response and host defense. Both markers occupy crucial steps as C3 convertases in the alternate (Bf) and classical (C4) complement pathways. They are involved in virus inactivation. A viral etiology has been demonstrated for leukemia in several animal species such as the cat[39-42], cattle[43-46], gibbons[47], rodents[48] and fowls[49]. A viral etilogy has been suggested for several human cancers, including some types of leukemia[50]. There is also evidence that two animal viruses, Bovine Leukemia virus[51-53] and Feline Leukemia virus[39,54], may cause ALL in man. Oldstone and Lampert[55] and Cooper and Welsh[56] have suggested that enveloped viruses are susceptible to lytic damage by the complement system, while non-enveloped viruses interact with antibodies and the early reacting complement components Cl, C2, and/or C4 resulting in virus neutralization. Viruses can be inactivated by serum containing C4 and/or Bf but not serum devoid of both factors. In addition, peptide fragments of C4 can alter the inflammatory response[57] and C4 may participate in cell-cell interactions[58]. Furthermore, Teisberg et al[59] have reported that there are non-functional variants of C4, such as C4A6, and there are reports that there is a high frequency of a null phenotype for C4 in several populations[29-31]. Therefore, certain allelic products of Bf and C4 may be efficient as C3 convertases, at altering the immune response, and at bacterial and virus inactivation. These biological characteristics of Bf and C4 coupled with their ease of assay make these markers ideal for disease association and linkage studies, especially for preliminary investigations.

CASE-CONTROL STUDY OF BF AND ALL IN WHITES

MATERIALS AND METHODS

The association of Bf with ALL has been reported previously by these investigators[36]. Serum samples from 164 Caucasian ALL patients obtained through the Pediatric Oncology Group were subjected to agarose gel electrophoresis for 90 minutes and subsequently immunofixed with Bf antisera[60]. The patients were obtained from throughout the United States, so a composite of 545 controls from various regions of North America was used[7,27,65,66]. Of the 164 patients, the most recent 90 were immune phenotyped[61-63]. The relative risks were estimated using Woolf's odds ratio method[64]. The significance of the associations was determined using the chi-square statistic. A p value of 0.05 was considered significant.

RESULTS

Bf phenotypes for patient and control samples are summarized in Table 1. The frequency of the BfF allele is increased and the BfS allele is decreased among ALL patients compared with controls. In fact, 73.1% of the ALL patients carry at least one BfF allele compared with 42.9% of the controls. This increase of the BfF allele is significantly associated with ALL (p<0.0001) and results in a relative risk of 3.6. There is no significant decrease of the BfS allele among the ALL patients compared with controls. However, those homozygous for BfS (BfSS patients) are at a significantly low risk (p<0.0001; relative risk = 0.3) for developing ALL. Although not significant, possibly due to small numbers, Bf SS homozygotes were 2.5 times more likely to have a non-B/T cell type than patients of other Bf phenotypes; in contrast those patients with the pre-B phenotype were 2.5 times more likely to be Bf FF homozygotes.

Table 1. Comparison of Bf Phenotypes Between ALL Patients and Controls

	No.	FF	FS	SS	FS1	F1S	SS1	FF1	F1S1
ALL	164	15	103	42	1	1	1	1	0
	(%)	9.1	62.8	25.6	0.6	0.6	0.6	0.6	0
Controls	545	41	186	291	3	6	13	4	1
	(%)	7.5	34.1	53.4	0.6	1.1	2.4	0.7	0.2

In addition, we reported[67] that BfFF homozygotes were more likely to have a white blood cell count greater than 50,000/mm2 at diagnosis (p<0.025) and more likely to be older (p<0.002). Furthermore, BfFF patients were 1.7 times more likely to relapse while BfSS patients were 1.9 times more likely to remain relapse-free after 12 months.

DISCUSSION

The data suggest that a gene(s) for susceptibility and/or protection is associated with Bf. There are two ways to interpret the data. 1) Despite the increase of the BfF allele, it is not a likely cause of the disease, since 26.8% of the patients did not carry the allele. Moreover, there is no evidence that any of the Bf allelic products are functionally different. This suggests that an ALL susceptibility gene(s) may be in linkage disequilibrium with BfF. 2) Etiologic heterogeneity may account for some patients lacking the BfF allele. Heterogeneity can obscure potential associations and, therefore, one needs to better define, both clinically and genetically, the various diseases.

Also, the Bf and ALL data suggest that BfFF homozygous patients have a poorer prognosis (high white blood cell count at diagnosis, older age, and pre-B immune phenotype) and do not respond as well to therapy (greater chance of relapse) than patients carrying other phenotypes. In contrast, BfSS patients have a better chance of maintaining a disease-free state.

Although informative, there is a problem using Bf alone as a disease association marker in Caucasian studies. Due to the low frequency of the BfF1 and BfS1 alleles in Caucasian populations, the Bf system is virtually a two allele system. Therefore, a change in the frequency of one allele automatically results in the reciprocal effect of the other allele. Since relative risk according to Woolf[64] is a measure of an association between phenotypes and considers only one antigen at a time[69], it is difficult to discern which allele, BfF or BfS, is associated with susceptibility or protection, respectively, to ALL and which is changing in response to the other. Therefore, Bf should be used only as an initial screening marker to determine if an association does exist.

C4 is an extremely polymorphic genetic marker that can encode for 420 possible haplotypes[30,31]. This polymorphic nature resolves the problem encountered with Bf. We are presently investigating C4 as a marker to possibly resolve the genetic versus environmental hypotheses for ALL susceptibility in Black Americans.

FUTURE APPROACHES AND CONCLUSIONS

The Bf data does show that genetic markers can be used for risk, prognosis and survival prediction for ALL, albeit weak. However, one must not forget that Bf, C4 and HLA comprise approximately one half dozen genes on a small segment of one chromosome. There are more than 100,000 genes on 23 different chromosomes making up the human genome, and to assume that only genes found in the MHC region are associated with malignant diseases would be naive. There are several reports demonstrating such associations; these include ABO and gastric carcinoma[1], Gm and melanoma[71] and Pi and hepatocellular carcinoma[72].

We have shown that the risk of whites carrying at least one BfF allele developing ALL is 3.6. This risk, as is the case with most disease association studies, is not high and, therefore, is not of much prognostic and/or prophylactic value. It is possible that the risk of developing a disease in those individuals carrying a particular genetic marker can be increased by better defining the disease and/or by increasing the resolution of the associated genetic marker. By subcategorization of a disease such as ALL into those of high and low white blood cell count at diagnosis, immune phenotype, age at onset, etc., one may obtain a more definitive association.

In addition to further defining the various diseases, superior resolution techniques for the detection of genetic polymorphisms are needed. Antibodies can only recognize external differences of a molecule; internal differences go unnoticed. By subjecting proteins to conventional electrophoresis (CE) followed by immunofixation, charge differences (internal and external) are also used to identify genetic polymorphisms previously undetected. Therefore, well-established genetic systems, such as ABO, Rh, Kidd, Duffy, MNS, etc., need to be electrophoretically investigated to identify possible previously undetected allelic products.

However, CE is not the best available resolving electrophoretic technique. Isoelectric focusing (IEF) utilizes carrier ampholytes to establish a pH gradient in a polyacrylamide or agarose gel. Each protein is electrically neutral at a particular pH called its isoelectric point (pI) and will migrate electrophoretically in a gel with appropriate ampholytes until it reaches a pH equal to its pI. With the recent advances of ultrathin layer gels[73,74] and more efficient cooling devices[74] resolutions of less than 0.01 pH units between protein moeities can be obtained. Moreover, silver staining procedures[75] with the sensitivity of radiolabeling have been developed which allows for the detection of nanogram quantities of protein. These advances have enabled investigators to detect common allelic products (or subtypes) for the biologically important proteins phosphoglucomutase[76], group specific component[77], transferrin[78] and Pi[79] not previously observed using CE. Therefore, it is conceivable that additional allelic forms will be found for genetic marker systems previously used for disease association studies. It is also possible that only one of the subtypes may be associated with a particular disease, and this would aid in the defining of the pathogenesis and/or prognosis of the disease.

In conclusion, genetic association studies have provided evidence that people can be genetically predisposed to disease. Once an individual comes in contact with an environmental insult(s) that can interact with his particular disease susceptibility gene(s), he may develop that disease. Moreover, there are additional genes that can interact with susceptibility genes and/or other environmental factors to modify the development of a diseae, the severity of disease and the response to various therapies[80]. The identification of these susceptible individuals and their prognosis would be of great prophylactic and economic value. Studies to better define disease heterogeniety and genetic polymorphisms, as well as the potential causal role of markers such as Bf and C4 should be vigorously pursued.

REFERENCES

1. Aird, I., Bental, H.,and Roberts, J. (1953) Br.Med. J. 1,799-801.
2. Brewerton, D.,Caffrey, M., Hart, F., James, D., Nichols, A., and Sturrock, R. (1973) Lancet 1, 904-907.
3. Schlosstein, L., Terasaki, P., Bluestone, R., and Pearson, C. (1973) N. Engl. J. Med. 228, 704-706.
4. Arnaud, P. and Allen, R. (1981) in Electrophoresis '81, Allen, R. and Arnaud, P., ed., Walter de Gruyter, Berlin, pp. 495-504.
5. Acton, R., Balch, C., Budowle, B., Go. R., Roseman, J., Soong, S-J, and Barger, B.(1982) in Melanoma Antigens and Antibodies, Reisfeld, R. and Ferrone, S., ed., Plenum Publishing Corporation, New York, pp. 1-21.
6. Acton, R., Balch, C., Barger, B., Budowle, B., Go. R., Soong, S-J, and Roseman, J. (1982) in Melanoma-1, Constanzi, J., ed., Martinus Nijhoff Publishers, The Hague. (In press.)
7. Budowle, B., Barger, B., Balch, C., Go. R., Roseman, J. and Acton, R. (1982) Cancer Genetics and Cytogenetics 5, 247-251.
8. Schaller, J. and Omenn, G. (1976) J. Pediatr. 88,913-925.
9. Acton, R. and Barger, B. (1981) in Pediatric Oncology, Vol. 1, Humphrey, G., Dehner, L., Grindley, G., and Acton, R., ed., Martinus Nijhoff Publishers, The Hague, pp. 47-77.
10. Svejgaard, A., Platz, P., Ryder, L., Nielsen, L., and Thomsen, M. (1975) Transplant. Rev. 22, 3-43.
11. Svejgaard, A. and Ryder, L., (1978) Birth Defects 16:27-46.
12. Terasaki, P. and McClelland, J. (1964) Nature 204, 998-1000.
13. Lilly, F. and Pincus, T. (1973) Adv. Cancer Res. 17:231-277.
14. Lilly, F. (1966) Genetics 53:529-539.
15. Lilly, F. (1970) J. Nat. Cancer Inst. 45,163-170.
16. Lilly, F. (1971) Transplant. Proc. 3, 1239-1241.
17. Sanderson, A., Mahour, G., Jaffe, N. and Dos, L. (1973) Transplantation 16, 672-673.
18. Rogentine, G., Trapani, R., Yankee, R., and Henderson, E. (1973) Tissue Antigens 3, 470-476.
19. Albert, E., Nisperus, B., and Thomas, F. (1977) Leukemia Research 1, 261-269.
20. DeBruyere, M., Cornu, G., Heremans-Bracke, T., Malchaire, J., and Sokal, G. (1980) Brit. J. Hematology 44(3), 243-251.
21. Lawler, S., Klouda, P., Smith, P., Till, M., and Hardesty, R. (1974) Brit. Med. J. 1,547-548.
22. Klouda, P., Lawler, J., Till, M. and Hardesty, R. (1974) Tissue Antigens 4,262-265.
23. Miller, R. (1970) Ann. N. Y. Acad. Sci. 171,637-644.
24. German, J., Bloom, D. and Pasarge, E. (1977) Clin. Genet. 12(3), 162-168.
25. O'Gorman Hughes, D. (1974) Med. J. Aust. 1, 519-526.

26. Hecht, F., McCaw, B. and Koler, R. (1973) N. Engl. J. Med. 289, 286-291.
27. Alper, C., Boenisch, T., and Watson, L. (1972) J. Exp. Med. 135, 68-79.
28. Budowle, B., Go., R., Barger, B. and Acton, R. (1981) J. Immunogenetics 8, 519-521.
29. Awdeh, Z. and Alper, C. (1980) Proc. Nat. Acad. Sci. 77, 3576-3580.
30. Budowle, B., Go., R., Roseman, J., Barger, B. and Acton, R., (1982) in Electrophoresis 1982, Stathakos, D., ed., Walter de Gruyter, Berlin, (In press).
31. Budowle, B., Roseman, J., Go, R., Louv, W., Barger, B. and Acton, R. (1982) Electrophroesis (Submitted).
32. Rittner, C., Grosse-Wilde, H. and Albert, E. (1976) Hum. Geret. 35, 79-82.
33. Bruun-Petersen, G., Lamm, L., Sorensen, I., Buskjaer, L., and Mortensen, J. (1981) Hum. Genet. 58, 260-267.
34. O'Neill, G., Yang, S., and Dupont, B. (1978) Proc. Nat. Acad. Sci. 75, 5165-5169.
35. Rittner, C. and Bertrams, J. (1981) Hum. Geret. 56,235-247.
36. Budowle, B., Acton, R., Barger, B., Go, R., Crist, W., Go, R., Humphrey, G., Ragub, A., Roper, M., Vietti, T., and Dearth, J. (1982) Cancer 50, (In press).
37. Budowle, B., Reitnauer, P., Barger, B., Go, R., Roseman, J. and Acton, R. (1982) Diabetologia 22, 483-485.
38. Budowle, B., Roseman, J., Louv, W., Go, R., Barger, B., and Acton, R. (In preparation).
39. Malone, G., Roseman, T., Crist, W. and Acton, R. (1982) in Pediatric Oncology, Humphrey, G., Dehner, L. Gromdley, G. and Acton, R., ed., Martinus Nighoff Publishers. The Hague (In press).
40. Cutter, S. (1976) Vet. Clin. N. Amer. 6, 367-378.
41. Hardy, W., Old, L., Hess, P., Essex, M. and Cutter, S. (1973) Nature 244, 266-269.
42. Jarret, W., Jarret, O., and Mackey, L. (1973) JNCI 51, 833-841.
43. Piper, C., Abt, D., and Ferrer, J. (1975) Cancer Res. 35(10), 2714-2716.
44. Dutcher, R., Larkin, E. and Marshak, R. (1975) J Nat. Can Inst. 33, 1055-1064.
45. Kettman, R., Portelle, D., Mammerick, SM., Cleuter, Y., Dekegel, D., Galou, M., Chysdael, J., Burney, A. and Chantrene, H. (1976) Proc. Nat. Acad. Sci. 73, 1014-1018.
46. Ferrer, J., Abt, D., Bhatt, D. and Marshak, R. (1974) Cancer Res. 34, 893-900.
47. Kawakami, T., Huff, S., Buckley, P., Dungworth, D., Snyder, S. and Gilden, R. (1972) Nature 225, 170-171.
48. Ioachim, H. (1970) Cancer Res. 30, 2661-2664.
49. Jarrett, W., Crawford, E., Martin, W. and Davie, F. (1964) Nature 202, 567-569.
50. Allen, D. and Cole, P. (1972) N. Engl. J. Med. 286, 70-82.
51. Donham, K., Berg, J. and Sawin, R. (1980) Amer. J. Epidemiology 112(1), 80-92.
52. Gupta, P. and Ferrer, J. (1982) Science 215, 405-407.

53. Ferrer, J., Kenyon, S. and Gupta, P. (1981) Science 213, 1014-1016.
54. Levy, S. (1974) N. Engl. J. Med. 290(9), 513-514.
55. Oldstone, M. and Lampert, P. (1979) Springer Semin. Immunopathol. 2, 261-283.
56. Cooper, N. and Welsh, R. (1979) Springer Semin. Immunopathol. 2, 285-310.
57. Porter, R. and Reid, K. (1979) Adv. Prot. Chem. 33,1-71.
58. Ferrone, S., Pellegrino, M. and Cooper, N. (1976) Science 193, 53-55.
59. Teisberg, P., Olaisen, B., Nordhagen, R., Thorsby, E., and Gedde-Dahl, T. (1980) Immunobiology 158, 91-95.
60. Alper, C. and Johnson, A. (1969) Vox Sang. 17, 445-452.
61. Vogler, L., Crist, W., Bockman, D., Pearl, E., Lawton, A., and Cooper, M. (1977) N. Engl. J. Med. 298, 872-878.
62. Cooper, M., Lawton, A. and Bockman, D. (1971) Lancet 2, 791-794.
63. Weiner, M., Branco, C. and Nussenzweig, V. (1973) Blood 42, 939-946.
64. Woolf, B. (1955) Ann. Hum. Genet. 19, 251-253.
65. Dornan, J., Allan, P., Noel, E., Larsen, B. and Farid, N. (1980) Diabetes 29, 423-427.
66. Walsh, L., Ehrlich, R., Falk, K., Cox, D. and Simpson, N. (1980) Amer. J. Hum. Genet. 32(b), 135A.
67. Budowle, B., Acton, R., Barger, B., Blackstock, R., Crist, W., Go, R., Humphrey, G., Ragab, A., Roper, M. Vietti, T. and Dearth, J. (1981) Blood 58(5), 136A.
68. Budowle, B. Louv, W., Roseman, J., Go, LR., Barger, B. and Acton, R. (1982) Immunogenetics (Submitted).
69. Curie-Cohen, M.(1981) Tissue Antigens 17, 136-148.
70. Ramot, B. and Macgrath, I. (1982) Brit. J. Hematology, 52, 183-189.
71. Walter, H., Brachtel, R. and Hilling, M. (1979) Hum. Genet. 49, 71-81.
72. Fargion, S., Klasen, E., Lalatta, F., Sangalli, G., Tommasini, M. and Fiorelli, G. (1981) Clinical Genetics 19, 134-139.
73. Radola, B. (1979) in Electrophoresis 1979, Radola, B., ed., Walter de Gruyter, Berlin, pp. 79-94.
74. Allen, R. (1980) Electrophoresis 1, 32-37.
75. Merril, C., Goldman, D., Sedman, S. and Ebert, M. (1981) Sciences 211, 1437-1438.
76. Sutton, J. and Burgess, R. (1978) Vox. Sang. 34, 97-103.
77. Kueppers, F. and Harpel, B. (1979) Hum. Hered. 29, 242-249.
78. Kuhnl, P. and Spielmann, W. (1979) Hum. Genet. 40, 193-198.
79. Genz,T., Martin, J. and Cleve, H. (1977) Hum. Genet. 38, 325-332.
80. Lappe, M. (1979) Birth Defects 15(2), 33-45.

GENES THAT CONTROL NATURAL KILLER CELL FUNCTION IN MAN AND MOUSE

JOHN C. RODER AND RONALD C. MCGARRY
Department of Microbiology and Immunology, Queen's University, Kingston,
Ontario, Canada   K7L 3N6

INTRODUCTION

Natural killer (NK) cells play an important role in rejection of transplantable tumors in mice[1,2]. Since NK cells exist in the unstimulated host at high frequency (0.6-2.4% of all lymphocytes[3]) and do not require a lengthy period of preactivation, one can hypothesize that NK cells provide a first line of defence against a newly arising malignancy or its metastases. Other potential effector cells such as T cells, activated macrophages or K cells participating in antibody-dependent cell-mediated cytotoxicity (ADCC), if they are important at all, would only be effective after a specific priming or activation period requiring days or weeks. It is not unreasonable to assume that under the selective pressure of such a lethal condition as malignancy, several independent defence mechanisms may have evolved. We have placed the NK cell as the foremost, but not necessarily the only, barrier to tumor development.

The mechanism by which the NK cell recognizes and destroys the developing tumor has been discussed elsewhere[1]. It is, however, instructive to consider some recent work by Collins, Patek, and Cohn[4] which shows a correlation between the tumorigenic potential of cloned, chemically transformed cell lines and their susceptibility to NK-mediated lysis in vitro. N cells, from a cloned fetal fibroblast line which does not grow in agarose, were not tumorigenic in vivo (in normal mice or lethally irradiated mice thymectomized as adults and reconstituted with fetal liver (ATxFL mice) and were not lysed by NK cells in vitro. When these cells were transformed by methylcholanthrene (MCA) they grew in agarose and after cloning could grow as tumors in ATxFL mice[5] which were NK deficient[4] but not in normal mice. This same mutation, N $\longrightarrow$ I, also made the cells susceptible to NK-mediated cytolysis in vitro. Cell lines derived from these I tumors were capable of growth in normal mice. This I $\longrightarrow$ C mutation, or selection, was accompanied by a loss of NK sensitivity, so that the tumor could escape NK surveillance and grow in normal mice.

It appears that NK cells may play some role in limiting tumor growth and are particularly efficient at preventing blood-borne metastasis to

Cancer: Etiology and Prevention, Ray G. Crispen, Editor

distant sites. It was important therefore to determine if NK function was subject to genetic abnormalities and if these defects lead to greater tumor suceptibility in both man and experimental animals.

MATERIALS AND METHODS

Lymphocyte preparations, fractionations, cytolytic assays, conjugate assays, cell lines, patients, normal donors, mice, reagents, immuno-fluorescence and other techniques are described in detail in the papers referenced in the Fig. and Table descriptions.

RESULTS

H-2 Linked Genes Control Target-Effector Recognition

The removal of adherent cells on nylon wool columns leaves a population of non-adherent lymphocytes which bind selectively to various NK-sensitive target cells as previously shown[3]. Most of the lymphocytes lyse the targets to which they are attached[6] and express a variety of NK markers including asialo-GM1, FcR for monoclonal IgG2b, Ly5 and Qa4[7]. Therefore the target binding lymphocytes are presumed to represent the NK population.

As shown in Table 1, the Fl progeny of high responder strains mated with low responder strains exhibited the cytolytic and target binding characteristics of the high reactive parent. In contrast a hybrid between two low responders (A/Sn and A.SW) maintained low levels of lysis and target cell binding. A backcross between C57Bl/6 and C57Bl/6 x DBA/2 Fl mice revealed that the level of responsiveness in conjugate activity and cytolysis was at least partially controlled by genes linked to the H-2 complex. Hence spleen cells from individually tested, heterozygous backcross progeny which were typed as $H-2^{d/b}$, had greater numbers of con-jugates than homozygous $H-2^{b/b}$ progeny. A similar H-2 linkage of cytolysis is shown in the same backcross and confirms the work of others[8,9,10]. These results suggest that the initial stage of target-effector interaction is regulated by dominant genes some or all of which may be linked to the H-2 region of chromosome 17. These genes would appear to control the size of the NK population expressing the putative recognition receptor. Whether these genes directly code for the recognition receptor or regulate some other aspect of cell differentiation cannot be ascertained at present.

Non H-2 Linked Genes Control Post Recognition Events in the NK Cytolytic Pathway

Since target cell recognition is only the first step in a complex series of events leading to target cell lysis we began a search for muta-

TABLE 1

GENETIC CONTROL OF TARGET-EFFECTOR BINDING

Strain	Responder phenotype	% lysis	% Conjugates
A) Dominance			
CBA	high	50 ± 5	20 ± 3
A/Sn	low	21 ± 3	6 ± 1
CBA x A/Sn F_1	high x low	40 ± 4	20 ± 2
C57Bl/6	intermediate	38 ± 2	12 ± 1.5
C57Bl/6 x A/Sn F_1	intermediate x low	52 ± 4	20 ± 2
A.SW	low	13 ± 3	7 ± 2
A.SW x A/Sn	low x low	12 ± 4	5 ± 2
B) H-2 Linkage			
C57Bl/6^b		38 ± 4	12 ± 1
C57Bl/6^b x DBA/2^d F_1		52 ± 3	19 ± 2
(C57Bl/6 x DBA/2) F_1 x C57Bl/6 - H-2$^{b/b}$		60 ± 4	22 ± 2
(C57Bl/6 x DBA/2 F_1 x C57Bl/6 - H-2$^{b/b}$		39 ± 2	12 ± 1.5 (p < .005)

Spleens were pooled from 6 age-matched mice per group and passed over nylon wool columns. Lymphocytes were assayed for frequency of target-binding cells (conjugates) and lysis of ^{51}Cr labelled YAC cells at a 50/1 E/T ratio (values represent the mean ± s.e. of triplicate samples). Twenty offspring were tested individually in the backcross experiment and differed significantly at the p < .005 level. The data in this Table is summarized from Roder and Kiessling[5].

tions which might affect discrete steps in the lytic pathway subsequent to target effector binding. As shown in Fig. 1 the recessive beige mutation (bg) in C57Bl/6 mice led to a marked impairment of NK cell mediated lysis. The heterozygous littermate controls (+/bg) responded as well as the wild type (+/+). With the exception of antibody dependent, cell-mediated cytotoxicity (ADCC) against tumor cells, all other forms of cell-mediated immune function in homozygous beige mice were normal as summarized in Table 2, thereby indicating that the NK defect may be selective. Since beige mice had a normal frequency of conjugate forming cells[11] it is inferred that the NK defect may lie within the lytic machinery of the cell rather than at the level of population size or recognition receptors.

A similar defect has recently been discovered in the human analog of the beige mutation, namely the Chediak-Higashi syndrome[12]. Eight patients carrying the autosomal recessive CH gene were examined and found to have a profound defect in their ability to spontaneously lyse various tumor cells by antibody dependent or independent mechanisms[12,13]. As shown in Fig. 1

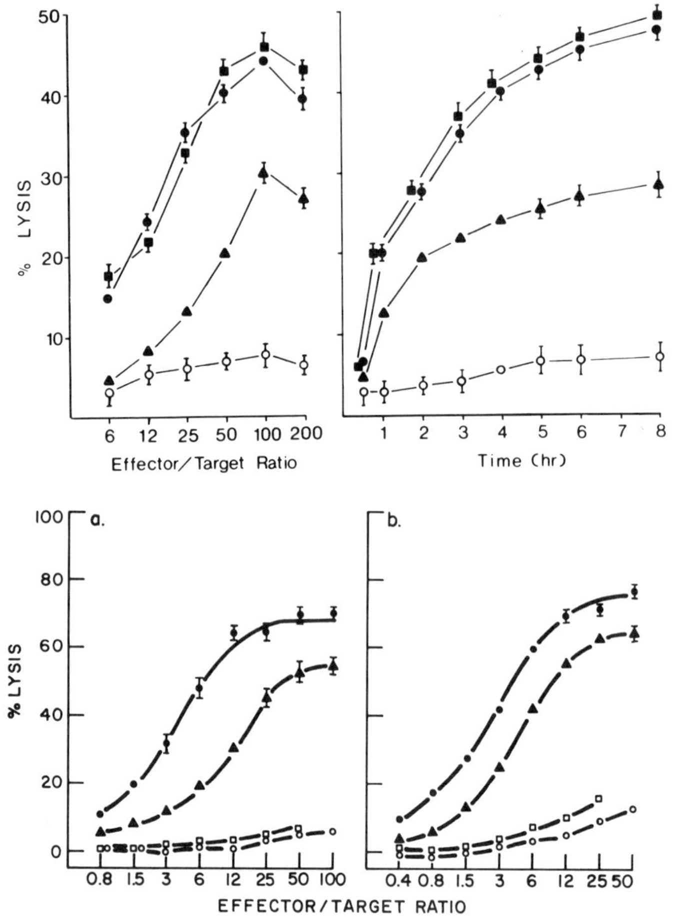

Fig. 1. Upper: Spleen cells were passed over nylon wool columns and incubated with ^{51}Cr labelled YAC tumor cells at various effector-to-target ratios in a 4-hr assay (left panel) or for various periods of time at a 100/1 effector/target ratio (right panel). ▲, A SN; ○, C57Bl/6, bg /bg ; ●, +/bg littermates; ■, age-matched +/+ controls. Lower: Peripheral blood lymphocytes from Chediak-Higashi patients (○, □) on age and sex matched normal controls (●, ▲) were tested in a 4 hr cytolytic assay against K562 cells (left panel) or an NK-insensitive cell line (P815) pre-coated with rabbit anti-P815 antibody. Values represent the mean % specific lysis ± s.e. in quadruplicate wells.

TABLE 2

IMMUNE FUNCTION IN BEIGE MICE AND CHEDIAK-HIGASHI HUMANS

Function	bg/bg mice	CH patients
NK cytolysis	low	low
Frequency of NK target-binding cells	normal	normal
ADCC vs tumor cells	low	low
ADCC vs erythrocytes	normal	normal
CTL-MLC	normal	normal
- in vivo alloimmune	normal	ND
- lectin induced	normal	normal
Skin graft rejection	normal	normal
Delayed type hypersensitivity	normal	normal
T cell - mitogens	normal	normal
B cell - mitogens	normal	normal
- lg production	normal	normal
Activated macrophage cytolysis	normal	normal
Promonocyte cytolysis - spontaneous	normal	normal
- ADCC	normal	ND
NK interferon boost	yes[†]	yes[†]
Interferon production	normal	ND
cGMP restoration of NK function	no	yes*
Lysosomal enzyme function	low	low

* In only two out of six patients.

[†] Does not approach level of untreated or IF boosted normal cells.

cytolysis of K562 cells by CH peripheral blood lymphocytes was depressed 100-fold, in terms of lytic units compared to age and sex matched normals. In addition, lysis of tumor cells precoated with an optimum dose of rabbit antibody was also severely depressed which is understandable since this form of antibody-dependent cellular cytotoxicity (ADCC) is mediated by NK cells. The selectivity of the antibody-independent NK cell defect is summarized in Table 2. Lymphocytes were blocked in their ability to spontaneously lyse tumor cells whereas spontaneous cytolysis of tumour cells by monocytes was normal. Cytostasis by neutrophils from CH patients against K562 cells was also normal as was lectin generated killing by this cell type. The population of T killer cells, as measured by lectin dependent cytolysis was normal in 5 out of 6 patients tested[13]. Others have previously observed normal mixed-lymphocyte culture (MLC) generated cytotoxic lymphocytes (CTL) in three CH patients and T cell mediated immunity in general, was previously shown to be normal in these and other CH patients as judged by skin testing and proliferative responses to T dependent mitogens. Percoll enriched NK cells from CH patients were completely normal in their ability to bind K562 tumor cells and, in addition, the frequency of cells bearing the NK specific marker, HNK-1, was normal in CH patients as detected by analysis on the fluorescence activated cell sorter[14] (Table 3). It was interesting to note that the HNK-1[+], NK cells from CH patients had a single giant granule instead of the 6-12 small granules found in HNK-1[+] cells from normal donors. The number of cells bearing other NK markers such as OKM1 and the large granular lymphocyte (LGL) morphology, was also normal in CH patients. These results suggest that NK cells are present in CH patients but do not function. Although the biochemical nature of the NK defect is unknown, recent success in restoring NK function to normal levels with cyclic GMP in some but not all CH patients, suggests that faulty cyclic nucleotide metabolism may be involved[15].

TABLE 3

NK CELL FREQUENCY IN CHEDIAK-HIGASHI PATIENTS

Donor	Unfractionated %HNK-1	Percoll enriched				Lytic Units/10[6]
		%OKM1	%HNK-1	%LGL	%Conjugates	
CH (n=8)	16.4 ± 2	53 ± 3	60 ± 4	50 ± 4	40 ± 3	294 ± 25
Normals (n=23)	14.3 ± 5	52 ± 6	57 ± 2	49 ± 3	41 ± 4	10 ± 5

Peripheral blood mononuclear cells were depleted of monocytes by plastic adherence and fractionated on Percoll density gradients to enrich NK cells[16] and then stained with the indicated monoclonal antibodies by indirect immunofluorescence. Large granular lymphocytes (LGL) were counted in cytocentrifuge preparations stained with Giemsa. Some cells were tested for binding to K562 target cells (conjugates) and also lysis of the same cells labelled with [51]Cr. Lytic units were calculated at 20% lysis. Values represent the mean ± s.e. of individually tested donors. This data is summarized from Abo et al[14] and Roder et al[17].

DISCUSSION

In the mouse there is a wealth of information on various genes directly involved in NK function. H-2 linked genes on chromosome 17 control the frequency of NK cells capable of recognizing tumor cells, as determined in a target-effector binding assay (Table 1) and functional cytolytic assays[8,9,10]. Fine mapping studies of segregating backcross populations as well as studies of congenic resistant and H-2 recombinant mice have shown that a locus within, or very near, the H-2D region affects NK activity against EL-4 and YAC-1 lymphoma targets[8,10]. The effect of the H-2D associated locus is most pronounced when certain non-H-2 genes are present[8,18]. A separate H-2 linked loci probably lies outside the H-2 region[9] as discussed previously[1]. Apparently at least two different H-2 linked loci on chromosome 17, as probably several other non-H-2 linked genes as well, are involved in the control of NK activity. Antibody-dependent, cell-mediated cytotoxicity (ADCC) activity against tumor cells was also shown to be H-2 linked, but it is important to note that the major histocompatability complex only accounts for a portion of the total NK and ADCC activity.

A separate gene, beige, (bg), on chromosome 13 was found to be intimately involved in a post-recognition event in the lytic cycle (Fig. 1). Hence NK cells from beige mutant mice could recognize and bind to the tumor cell target but failed to deliver the lethal hit. This defect was predetermined at the level of bone marrow progenitors[19] and was selective for NK cells since immune and cytolytic functions mediated by other cell types were normal (Table 2). As predicted, homozygous, NK-deficient, bg/bg mice were more susceptible to the growth and dissemination of transplantable tumors than normal, heterozygous +/bg littermate controls[21,22]. A variety of other mutant genes had minimal suppressive effect on NK activity and many were neutral whereas lymphoproliferative (lpr), and the nude(nu) loci on chromosome 11 were enhancing (Table 4). With the exception of bg, however, none of these genes are selective for NK cells and other immune functions are also altered within the immunological network. For example, motheaten (me) on chromosome 6 was the only mutation with NK activity suppressed to the same degree as exhibited by the beige gene[23]. However, motheaten mice are generally immunodepressed and also deficient in their ability to induce graft vs host disease, develop cytolytic T lymphocytes, and mount specific antibody responses. The advantage of a selective model, such as beige, is that it can be used to test the hypothesis that NK cells play a role in host surveillance against tumors or virus infected cells. However, there is one report showing that beige mice have a 2-3 fold decrease in alloimmune CTL against P815 tumor cells[24] whereas others report slightly decreased or normal H-2 restricted CTL against virus infected targets[25], alloimmune CTL generated *in vivo* or *in vitro*[29], skin graft rejection across H-2 barriers[20], and rejection of regressing MSV induced tumors (a T cell dependent phenomenon)[26]. It is difficult to rule out a

TABLE 4

THE EFFECT OF POINT MUTATIONS ON NK FUNCTION

Gene Name	Symbol	Chrom.	Strains	NK fnct.[a]	Trans.[b]	Select.[c]	Pleiotropy	Ref.
A) SUPPRESSIVE								
beige	bg	13	B6,C3H,SB	↓↓	yes	yes	giant granules ↑ secretion ↓	11,23,19,20
motheaten	me	6	C3H	↓↓	yes	no	GvH↓,CTL↓ Ab↓ immunodeficient	23
hairless	hr	14	SJL, HRS	rar[d]	ND[f]	no	GvH↓,DTH↓, Ab↓ immunodeficient	23
obese	ob	6	B6	↓	ND	no	Gr↓,Ab↓, insulin↑ corticosteroids↑	23
dominant spotting	w^v	5	WBB6 F1	↓	ND	ND	macrocytic anemia	23
steel	sl^d	10	WCB6 F1	↓	ND	ND	macrocytic anemia	23
microphthalmia	mi	6	B6	↓	yes	ND	osteopetrosis	30
reduced pigmentation	rp	7	B10	↓	ND	ND	lysomal enzymes in kidney ↑	27
pallid	pa	2	B6	↓	ND	ND	lysosomal enzymes	27
satin	sa	13	3H1 F1	↓	ND	ND	lysosomal enzymes	31
B) NEUTRAL								
pale ears	ep	19	B6	?	ND	ND	lysosomal enzymes ↑	23,27
pearl	pe	13	B6	↕	ND	ND	lysosomal enzymes ↑	23
ruby eye	ru-2	7	B6	↕	ND	ND	lysosomal enzymes ↑	23
sepia	sea	1	B6	↕	ND	ND	normal lysosomal enzymes	27
diabetes	db	4	BK	↕	ND	no	GR↓, CTL↓ obesity, hyperglycemia	23
yellow	A^Y	2	B6	↕	ND	ND	obesity, insulin ↑ adrenal hypertrophy	23

TABLE 4 (cont'd)

Gene Name	Symbol	Chrom.	Strains	NK fnct.[a]	Trans.[b]	Select.[c]	Pleiotropy	Ref.
X-linked immunodeficiency	Xid	X		↔	ND	no	B cell defect	32
LPS response	Lps	14	C3H	↔	ND	no	macrophage defect	33
Dominant hemimelia	Dh	1		↔	ND	ND	absence of spleen	32
C) ENHANCING								
nude	nu	11	B6,C3H,AKR	↑	ND	no	CTL , Ab , lack thymus and hair	34,35,23
lymphoproliferative	lps	?	NKR, B6	var[e]	ND	ND	hypergammaglobulinemia	23,36,37
D) COMBINATIONS								
nu + bg			B6,C3H	↑	ND	ND		23, 38
sa + bg			3H1 Fl	↓↓	ND	ND		31

[a] Natural killer cell function as measured in a 4 hr ^{51}Cr release assay.

[b] Defective or elevated NK activity can be adoptively transferred with bone marrow to phenotypically heterozygous littermates.

[c] The NK defect is selective for NK cells and no other cell type within the immunological system or host defense network is affected.

[d] Var, variable: reduced NK lysis if hr gene on SJL/J background but no effect if gene on HRS/J background.[23]

[e] Enhanced NK lysis if lpr gene on MLR/MP background but no effect if gene on C57Bl/6 background strain.[23]

[f] Abbreviations: Ab, specific antibody response following immunization; CTL, generation of cytolytic T lymphocytes; DTH, delayed type hypersensitivity; GR, allograft rejection; GvH, ability of lymphocytes to induce graft-versus-host disease; ND, not done; ?, unknown or conflicting data from different labs.

small (2 fold) T cell deficiency in beige mice but in view of a 10-100 fold defect in NK function, the model remains predominantly one of NK deficiency.

It is not possible to deduce one common mechanism of action for all the genes controlling NK cells since some will be involved at various steps in the cytolytic pathway, whereas others may control NK differentiation, although to date there have been no genes identified in this latter category. In one study of 5 pigment mutations[27], four were found to have suppressed NK cytolysis and these same four (bg, pa, ep, rp) also exhibited elevated kidney lysosomal enzyme levels whereas the fifth mutation (sea) had no effect on NK and also displayed normal kidney lysosomal enzyme activity. Since elevated kidney levels of lysosomal enzymes result from a block in secretion[28] these observations provided some support for the hypothesis that NK cells secrete a toxin, possible derived from lysosomes, which kills the target cells[29]. However, Clark et al has reported that two additional pigment mutants with elevated kidney lysosomal enzymes (pe, ru-2) have normal NK function which suggests that the pathway for lysosomal enzyme secretion and NK toxin secretion may overlap to some extent, but also have unique steps subject to different genetic control.

The genetic control of human NK cells is less well understood than in mouse. The beige mouse has been used for over 15 years as a model for the Chediak-Higashi (CH) syndrome in man. Both species exhibit abnormal leukocyte granulation and pigmentation whereas immune responsiveness (other than NK function) is intact. We reasoned that if the defective NK gene in the beige mouse was closely linked or identical with the gene controlling leukocyte granulation then CH patients should also have abnormal NK function. The data suggest that NK and ADCC activity against tumor cells is markedly impaired in patients with the CH syndrome (Fig. 1). Preliminary family studies are compatible with a recessive mode of inheritance. As summarized in Table 2, the CH gene is selective for NK cells within the immune system whereas other cellular functions, mediated by T cells, B cells, monocytes and granulocytes, are relatively normal. We believe NK cells are present in normal frequency (Table 3). They recognize and bind to the tumor cell target but may fail to deliver the lethal hit with normal efficiency. Thus far we have not been successful in universally restoring their function and we do not yet know if there is a connection between abnormal granule morphology and defective NK cytolysis. Since the NK deficiency in CH patients precedes the development of the accelerated phase, it is imperative to define more precisely the nature of the 'lymphoma' which arises. This model could provide evidence that NK cells are involved in surveillance against some forms of spontaneous tumor development in humans.

Other genes in the human have also been implicated in the control of NK function. Santoli et al[39] and Trinchieri et al[40], building on earlier work by Petranyi et al[41,42], attempted to correlate NK and ADCC activity in normal donors with the HLA-A3, B7 and a significant association between high activity and HLA-B12 was also reported. Formal proof of the NK-HLA association is lacking, however, since data showing a direct segregation of NK with HLA haplotypes in family studies has not been reported. It is of interest to note, as pointed out by Petranyi et al[41], that high multiple sclerosis incidence and low NK activity is associated with HLA-B7, whereas a low incidence of multiple sclerosis and high NK activity is associated with HLA-B12.

Several immunodeficiency disorders of proven or presumptive genetic origin have also been studied for NK function, as shown in Table 5. For example 10 out of 12 males with X-linked lymphoproliferative syndrome were found by Sullivan et al[43] to have impaired NK activity in a 4-h, ^{51}Cr - release assay against K562 when compared to 10 phenotypically normal XLP carriers (P < 0.001) or 33 normals. The magnitude of the deficiency was in the order of 10-fold in terms of lytic units. NK activity in affected males was enhanced slightly, but not restored, by interferon treatment. Chronic EB virus infection in males with XLP frequently (40%) leads to a lymphoproliferative disorder in which malignant cells contain the EB viral genome[43]. Since EB virus-infected cells have enhanced NK susceptibility[44], Sullivan et al[43] reasoned that the NK deficiency in XLP could conceivably predispose the patient to development of the lymphoreticular malignancy much as we have argued that NK deficiency in CH patients could lead to the 'lymphoma-like' lymphoproliferative disorder occurring in the accelerated phase [45]. It is not likely that interferon will be of much use in restoring NK function in vivo in either CH or XLP patients due to the marginal effects in vitro. In contrast, several interesting patients have been described with a combined NK deficiency and defective immune interferon production[46,47] which were completely restored in NK activity after five daily intramuscular injections of 10^5 U kg^{-1} interferon[48]. The same treatment did not restore or even improve NK activity in a CH patient.

Of the classical immunodeficiencies, only severe combined immuno-deficiency exhibited severely impaired NK activity, as shown in studies by Koren et al[49], and summarized in Table 5. In some disorders, such as IgA deficiency, ataxia telangiectasia and the Wiskott-Aldrich syndrome, some patients were low and others were normal, depending on the investigation and the assay employed. In general patients with X-linked agamma-globulinemia, common variable immunodeficiency hyper-IgM immunodeficiency, hypogammaglobulinemia and immunodeficiency thymoma were relatively normal with respect to NK function.

TABLE 5

POSSIBLE GENES AND GENETIC DISORDERS EFFECTING NK FUNCTION

Disorder	Inheritance	n	NK Activity	Ref.
CH syndrome	autosom. rec.	6	low	45
Chronic-granulomatous disease of childhood	autosom. rec. or X-linked	1	normal	54
Downe's syndrome	trisomy 21	4	normal	54
Agammaglobulinemia	X-linked	10	normal	46,49, 56
Common variable immunodeficiency	unknown	46	normal	49,46, 57,56
Hyper-IgM immunodeficiency	unknown	1	normal	49
Immunodeficiency-thymoma	unknown	1	normal	56
Ataxia-telangiectasia	autosom. rec.	7	variable	46,57
Wiskott-Aldrich	X-linked	6	variable	46,57
Hypogammaglobulinemia	unknown	1	normal	46
IgA deficiency	unknown	8	variable	46,57
Lymphoproliferative	X-linked	12	low	43
Severe combined immunodeficiency	autosom. rec.	5	low	49,46

n=Total number of patients tested. NK activity was assessed in ^{51}Cr-release assays against K562 or Chang tumor cells. Variable = some patients low, some normal. Some of this variation could be due to the pooling of data from different authors using different assays to assess NK function.

Another genetic disorder which might be thought to influence human NK activity, a priori, is Downe's syndrome (trisomy 21). Chromosome 21 is thought to contain a gene(s) coding for the interferon receptor[50] and hence cells, lymphocytes and fibroblasts from Downe's patients are much more sensitive to the action of interferon[51,52], due to the gene-dosage effect associated with an extra chromosome[53]. Interferon action increased logarithmically as the number of chromosome 21s increased linearly[53]. Since NK activity is influenced by interferon we expected Downe's lymphocytes to have altered NK activity, but as shown earlier[54] it was within the normal range. In addition, Downe's lymphocytes were not boosted more in NK activity than normal cells, whether measured early (1-6h) or late (18h) in the cytolytic assay after boosting. This experiment was repeated independently by Matheson et al[55] with similar results. The data suggest indirectly that there is more than one kind of interferon receptor and the NK-interferon receptor gene is not present on chromosome 21. The conventional interferon receptor on fibroblasts and lymphocytes modulates the anti-viral, anti-growth and immunosuppressive (blastogenesis) functions of interferon whereas a separate receptor may modulate enhancement of NK activity.

CONCLUSIONS

In the mouse, H-2 linked genes control tumor cell recognition whereas non-H-2 linked genes on other chromosomes control various steps in the post binding cytolytic pathway of the NK cell. In the human it has been shown that NK function is profoundly impaired in each of 8 CH patients examined. Preliminary evidence suggests that the NK population develops normally but fails to deliver the lethal hit to the tumor cell targets during the cytolytic process. We hypothesize that the NK deficiency in both CH and XLP patients could conceivably predispose the patient to develop the lymphoproliferative malignancies which characterize the terminal stages of these genetic disorders. HLA-linked genes and genes presumably involved in severe combined immunodeficiency may also lead to altered NK activity. The CH- and XLP-linked NK deficiency cannot be markedly improved by interferon in contrast to the dramatic restoration of NK function in patients with defective-immune-interferon-production. Due to the selective nature of the defect, the CH syndrome should allow a more precise understanding of the NK cytolytic mechanism and the in vivo role of NK cells in the human. Now that the various NK controlling genes have been identified in both man and mouse, future studies will be aimed at identifying the gene products.

REFERENCES

1. Roder, J.C., Karre, K., and Kiessling, R. (1981) Prog. Allergy 28, 66-159.

2. Roder, J.C. and Haliotis, T. (1980) Immunol. Today 1,96-100.

138

3. Roder, J.C. and Kiessling, R. (1978) Scand. J. Immunol. 8,135-144.

4. Collins, J.L., Patek, P.Q., and Cohn, M. (1981) J. Exp. Med. 153, 89-106.

5. Patek, P.Q., Collins, J.L., and Cohn, M. (1978) Nature (London) 276, 510.

6. Roder, J.C., Kiessling, R., Biberfeld, P., and Anderson, B. (1978) J. Immunol. 121, 2509-2517.

7. Beaumont, T.J., Roder, J.C., Elliott, B.E., Kerbel, R.S., Dennis, J.W., Kasai, M., and Okumura, K. (1982) Scand. J. Immunol. 16, 123-133.

8. Klein, G., Klein, G., Kiessling, R., and Karre, K. (1978) Immunogenetics 6, 651.

9. Petranyi, G., Kiessling, R., Povey, S., Klein, G., Herzenberg, L., and Wigzell, H. (1976) Immunogenetics 3, 15.

10. Harmon, R.C., Clarke, E., O'Toole, C., and Wicker, L. (1977) Immunogenetics 4, 601.

11. Roder, J.C. and Duwe, A.K. (1979) Nature 278, 451.

12. Roder, J.C., Haliotis, T., Klein, M., Korec, S., Jett, J., Ortaldo, J., Herberman, R.B., Katz, P., and Fauci, A.S. (1980) Nature 284, 553.

13. Roder, J.C., Haliotis, T., Laing, L., Kozbor, D., Rubin, P., Pross, H., Boxer, L., White, J., Fauci, A.S., Mostowski, H., and Matheson, D. (1982) Immunol. 46, 555-560.

14. Abo, T., Roder, J.C., Abo, W., Cooper, M.D., and Balch, C.M. (1982) J. Clin. Invest. 70, 193-197.

15. Katz, P., Roder, J.C., Zaytoun, A., Herberman, R.B., and Fauci, A.S. (1982) J. Immunol. 129, 297-302.

16. Timonen, T. and Saksela, E. (1980) J. Immunol. Meth. 36, 285.

17. Roder, J.C., Todd, R.F., Rubin, P., Haliotis, T., Helfand, S.L., Werkmeister, J., Pross, H.F., Boxer, L.A., Schlossman, S.F., and Fauci, A.S. (1982) Clin. Exp. Immunol. (in press).

18. Clark, E.A., Russell, P.H., Egghart, M., and Horton, M.A. (1979) Int. J. Cancer 24, 688-699.

19. Roder, J.C. (1979) J. Immunol. 123, 2168-2173.

20. Roder, J.C.,Lohmann-Matthes, M.L., Domzig, W., and Wigzell, H. (1979) J. Immunol. 123,2174-2181.

21. Karre, K., Klein, G.O., Kiessling, R., Klein, G., and Roder, J.C. (1980) Nature 284, 624-628.

22. Talmadge, J.E., Meyers, A.M., Prieur, D.J., and Starkey, S.R. (1980) Nature 284, 622-624.

23. Clark, E.A., Shultz, L.D., and Pollock, S.B. (1981) Immunogenetics 12, 601-613.

24. Saxena, R., Saxena, Q., and Adler, W.H. (1982) Nature 295, 240-241.

25. McKinnon, K.P., Hale, A.H., and Ruebush, M.J. (1981) Inf. Immunity 32, 204-210.

26. Karre, K. (1981) Ph.D. thesis, Dept. of Tumour Biology, Karolinska Institute, Stockholm, Sweden.

27. Orn, A., Hakansson, E.M., Gidlund, M., Ramstedt, U., Axberg, I., Wigzell, H., and Lundin, L.G. (1982) Scand. J. Immunol. 15, 305-310.

28. Brandt, E.J., Swank, R.T., and Novak, E.K. (1981) in Immunologic Defects in Laboratory Animals, Gershwin, M.E. and Merchant, B. ed., Plenum Press, New York, vol.1, chpt. 5, 99-117.

29. Roder, J.C., Argov, S., Klein, M., Petersson, C., Kiessling, R., Andersson, K., and Hansson, M. (1980) Immunol 40, 107-116.

30. Seaman, W.E., Gindhart, T.D., Greenspan, J.S., Blackman, M.A., and Talal, N. (1979) J. Immunol. 122, 2541-2547.

31. McGarry, R., Walker, R., and Roder, J.C. (manuscript in preparation).

32. Herberman, R.B. and Holden,H.T. (1978) Adv. Cancer Res. 27,305.

33. Roder, J.C., Lohmann-Matthes, M.L., Domzig, W., Kiessling, R., and Haller, O. (1979) Eur. J. Immunol. 9, 283.

34. Herberman, R.B., Nunn, M.E., and Lavrin, D.H. (1975) Int. J. Cancer 16, 216.

35. Kiessling, R., Klein, E., and Wigzell, H. (1975) Eur. J. Immunol. 5, 112.

36. Tai, A. and Warner, N.L. (1980) in Natural Cell-Mediated Immunity Against Tumors, Herberman, R.B. ed., Academic Press, New York, pp. 257-264.

37. Clark, E.A., Windsor, N.T., Sturge, J.C., and Stanton, T.H. (1980) in Natural Cell-Mediated Immunity Against Tumors, Herberman, R.B. ed. Academic Press, New York, pp. 417-429.

38. Karre, K., Klein, G.O., Kiessling, R., Klein, G., and Roder J.C. (1980) Int. J. Cancer 26, 789-797.

39. Santoli, D., Trinchieri, G., Zinijewski, C.M., and Koprowski, H. (1976) J. Immunol. 117, 765.

40. Trinchieri, G., Santoli, D., Zinijewski, C.M., and Koprowski, H. (1977) Transplant. Proc. 9, 881.

41. Petranyi, G., Benczur, M., Onody, C., and Hollan, S.R. (1974) Lancet 1, 736.

42. Petranyi, G., Ivanyi, P., and Hollan, S.R. (1974) Vox Sang 26, 470.

43. Sullivan, J.L., Byron, K.S., Brewster, F.F., and Purtilo, D. (1980) Science 210, 543.

44. Blazar, B., Patarroyo, M., Klein, E., and Klein, G. (1980) J. Exp. Med. 151, 614.

45. Roder, J.C., Haliotis, T., Klein, M., Korec, S., Jett, J., Ortaldo, J., Herberman, R.B., Katz, P., and Fauci, A.S. (1980) Nature 284, 553.

46. Lipinski, M., Virelizier, J.L., Tursz, T., and Griscelli, C. (1980) Eur. J. Immunol. 10, 246.

47. Virelizier, J.L., Lipinski, M., Tursz, T., and Griscelli, C. (1979) Lancet 2, 696.

48. Virelizier, J.L. and Griscelli, C. (1980) in Primary Immunodeficiencies, Seligmann, M. and Hitzig, W., eds., Elsevier/North Holland Biomedical Press, New York, p. 473.

49. Koren, H., Amos, B., and Buckley, R. (1978) J. Immunol. 120, 796.

50. Revel, M., Bash, D., and Ruddle, F.H. (1976) Nature 260, 139.

51. Cupples, C.G. and Tan, Y.H. (1977) Nature 1267, 165.

52. Tan, Y.H. (1976) Nature 260, 141.

53. Tan, Y.H. (1975) Nature 253, 280.

54. Roder, J.C., Laing, L., Haliotis, T., and Kozbor, D. (1982) in Human Cancer Immunology, Serron and Rosenfeld, eds., Elsevier/ North Holland Biomedical Press, New York, pp. 171-188.

55. Matheson, D.S., Green, B., and Tan, Y.H. (1981) Cell. Immunol. 65, 366.

56. Pross, H.F., Gupta, S., Good, R.A., and Baines, M. (1979) Cell. Immunol. 43, 160.

57. Nelson, D. (1980) in Primary Immunodeficiencies, Seligmann, M. and Hitzig, W., eds., Elsevier/North Holland Biomedical Press, Amsterdam, p. 141.

GENETIC REGULATION OF MAMMARY TUMOR CARCINOGENESIS IN MICE

PHYLLIS B. BLAIR, JOHN A. DANILOVS, AND CANDACE NEWBY
Department of Microbiology and Immunology, and the Cancer Research
Laboratory, University of California, Berkeley, California 94720, USA

INTRODUCTION

In the mouse, tumors of the mammary gland are a frequent result of neonatal infection with the mouse mammary tumor virus (MTV). Many strains of mice, such as the C3H, are naturally infected with MTV (of the MTV-S subtype), and the transfer of massive quantities of virus to the young through the milk of the infected mother insures the infection of each new generation. Because of this transmission without experimental manipulation, the resulting tumors, which often do not appear until the females are a year old, seem to be "spontaneous". Other strains of mice, such as the BALB/c, do not naturally carry the exogenous MTV, but can easily be infected with it, and will then transmit it to their offspring. However, some strains of mice are resistant to infection with MTV, and thus do not develop mammary tumors after neonatal exposure. Two well known examples of resistant strains are the C57BL and the I. These two strains are especially interesting because their hybrid is very susceptible to infection with MTV and develops mammary tumors in high incidence following neonatal infection.[1-5] From this, one can infer that the two strains possess different resistance mechanisms, and that the genetic control of each of these mechanisms is recessive in nature.

We present here a genetic analysis of the control mechanism existing in the C57BL strain. Our experimental results demonstrate that one major gene which is linked to the Major Histocompatibility Complex (MHC) on the 17th chromosome controls the inability of the C57BL mouse to support a productive virus infection, that, in backcross mice, the eventual development of mammary tumors is directly correlated with the presence of the susceptibility allele of this gene carried by the I strain, and that one or more modifier genes can enhance this productive infection and the subsequent development of tumors. In addition, we find that the major resistance gene linked to the MHC in the C57BL does not completely prevent virus infection and replication. Some of the females homozygous for the resistance gene (in the C57BL strain and in the backcross females) will late in life express MTV antigen in their milk,

Cancer: Etiology and Prevention, Ray G. Crispen, Editor

and a few will subsequently develop mammary tumors. In addition, it has been possible to develop inbred strains of mice carrying the MHC of the C57BL which are highly susceptible to MTV oncogenesis.

MATERIALS AND METHODS

Mice used were obtained from the colony of the Cancer Research Laboratory. Data presented in Tables 1-7 were obtained from 3 types of parous females: hybrid females resulting from matings of C57BL females with I males, first backcross females resulting from matings of hybrid females with C57BL males, and second backcross females resulting from matings of first backcross females with C57BL males. Data presented in Table 8 were obtained from virgin females of 6 recombinant inbred strains developed in this laboratory. Each of these strains is homozygous for the H-2^b haplotype of the MHC which is also carried by the C57BL strain. All females received MTV neonatally as a consequence of being foster-nursed on lactating MTV-infected females of the C3H strain.

Two bioassays were used in testing for the presence of infectious MTV in the experimental females.[1] Virus in blood was assayed by inoculation of fresh blood from the experimental females into young hybrid test females which were then subjected to hormonal stimulation to induce mammary gland growth and lactation; milk from each test mouse was tested for MTV antigen by immunodiffusion assay as evidence that infectious virus had been transmitted to them. Virus in milk was assayed by allowing susceptible test female babies (BALB/c) to suckle the experimental females during their first lactation; the test animals were subsequently mated, and their milk was sampled during the third lactation for MTV antigen by immunodiffusion assay to determine if infectious virus had been transmitted to them.

In a third assay procedure,[1] the experimental females were tested directly for evidence that they were productively infected with MTV by analysis of their milk for MTV antigen in immunodiffusion assay.

The two sensitive bioassays measure two different steps in the MTV infection process, first the infection of white blood cells, and subsequently the infection of the cells of the mammary gland. The less sensitive immuno-diffusion assay is a measure of massive replication of virus in the mammary gland.

The H-2 phenotypes of the first and second backcross females were determined by a facilitated hemaglutination technique, using rabbit anti-mouse IgG as the developing antiserum.[1]

RESULTS AND DISCUSSION

One major gene controlling resistance to MTV infection in C57BL mice

Previous studies[1-5] have demonstrated that the C57BL strain is highly
resistant to MTV infection whereas the (C57BL x I) hybrid is extremely
susceptible. To analyze the number of genes responsible for the recessive
resistance to MTV in the C57BL strain, we prepared backcross females by mating
(C57BL x I) hybrid females with C57BL males. The incidence of MTV infection
following neonatal introduction of the virus was analyzed by 3 assays. In
each case, the segregation pattern in the first backcross generation supports
a simple one-gene hypothesis for control of infection. As determined separately
for each of the 3 assays, almost exactly half of the backcross females
demonstrated the resistance trait of the C57BL (Table 1). Such a 50% ratio
is expected from the segregation of a single gene trait, and is significantly
different than the 25% or 75% expected from a two-gene segregation pattern.

TABLE 1

RESISTANCE TO EXPRESSION OF MTV IN FEMALES FROM THE BACKCROSS OF HYBRIDS TO
THE C57BL STRAIN*

Assay	Number Tested	Number Negative	Percent Negative
Bioassay of Blood	66	34	52%
Bioassay of Milk	76	40	53%
MTV Antigen in Milk[+]	115	57	50%

*The females were infected with MTV by neonatal fostering.
[+]Females were considered positive in this assay if MTV antigen was detectable
by immunodiffusion in their milk in lactations occurring during their first
7 months of life. The percentage given is based on the number tested at the
first lactation. Fewer mice were tested at subsequent lactations (due to
mortality or unsuccessful breeding and lactation), and adjustment of the
incidence to compensate for these losses decreases the percent negative to
46%.

H-2 linkage of the C57BL resistance gene

As just demonstrated, Mendelian segregation observed in the backcross
females for the resistance to MTV provides strong evidence for single-gene
control of the trait. This hypothesis can be independently verified by

demonstrating linkage to a known gene. Since the H-2[b] haplotype had previously been implicated in resistance to MTV-S induced mammary tumors,[6] the H-2 phenotype of some of the females tested in the 3 assays for MTV was also determined. A very close correlation was found between the inheritance, in the backcross females, of the H-2[b] haplotype from the hybrid and the resistance trait, or, conversely, the inheritance of the H-2[j] haplotype (originally from the I strain) of the hybrid and susceptibility to MTV infection (Table 2).

TABLE 2

LINKAGE, IN FIRST BACKCROSS FEMALES, OF THE GENE CONTROLLING MTV EXPRESSION WITH THE H-2 COMPLEX*

Expression of MTV		H-2 Phenotype of the Backcross Females[+]	
		H-2[j] H-2[b]	H-2[b] H-2[b]
Bioassay of Blood	+	22	0
	0	0	22
Bioassay of Milk	+	10	0
	0	1	15
MTV Antigen in Milk[x]	+	22	0
	0	1	21

*The females were infected with MTV by neonatal fostering.
[+]In the backcross females, one H-2[b] allele is inherited from the C57BL male parent. The hybrid mother contributes either the H-2[j] allele or a second H-2[b] allele.
[x]Females were considered positive in this assay if MTV antigen was detectable by immunodiffusion in their milk in lactations occurring during their first 7 months of life.

Verification of single gene segregation for resistance in a second backcross

After first backcross females had been typed for the presence of the H-2-linked resistance/susceptibility alleles, their offspring from a mating with C57BL males were collected and similarly typed. It was anticipated that, if

the one-gene hypothesis were correct, first backcross females negative for
the expression of MTV (and therefore homozygous resistant) would produce only
offspring similarly resistant and negative for MTV expression. In contrast,
first backcross females susceptible to MTV infection as measured by the assays
would be heterozygous, possessing one recessive resistance allele (from the
C57BL) and one dominant susceptibility allele (from the I), and should
contribute each allele to one-half of their off-spring. The results were as
anticipated (Table 3).

TABLE 3

EXPRESSION OF MTV IN FEMALES OF THE SECOND BACKCROSS TO THE C57BL CORRELATES
WITH THE STATUS OF THE FIRST BACKCROSS MOTHER*

Status of Mother	Status of Offspring	
	Positive	Negative
Negative for		
Bioassay of Blood	1	45
Bioassay of Milk	1	18
MTV Antigen in Milk[+]	3	39
Positive for		
Bioassay of Blood	18	18
Bioassay of Milk	9	5
MTV Antigen in Milk[+]	17	16

*The females were infected with MTV by neonatal fostering. Offspring of 8
negative and 12 positive mothers were tested in the assays.
[+]Females were considered positive in this assay if MTV antigen was detectable
by immunodiffusion in their milk in lactations occurring during their first
7 months of life.

Late expression of MTV in homozygous resistant females

First backcross females carrying the H-2-linked susceptibility allele of
the I strain demonstrated infectious MTV in their blood (tested in young
virgin females) and infectious MTV in their milk (tested during the first
lactation) as well as MTV antigen in their milk within the first 7 months of
life. Homozygous resistant females were negative for these expressions of
MTV at these times. Nevertheless, the resistance to MTV was not absolute, and

later in life a productive infection became detectable. Infectious virus could be detected in the blood, and MTV antigen could be detected in the milk (Table 4). One can infer from this delayed expression of MTV infection that a persistent though undetectable MTV infection exists in females of the MTV-resistant populations, and thus that the H-2 linked resistance gene of the C57BL strain (of the Crgl subline) appears to function by restricting pro-liferation of MTV at an early stage in the viral life cycle and may have no effect on the initial establishment of MTV infection.

TABLE 4

LATE EXPRESSION OF MTV IN RESISTANT $H-2^b$ $H-2^b$ FEMALES*

Assays	Number Positive / Number Tested	
	C57BL	First Backcross
Tests of Younger Females		
Bioassay of Blood[+]	1/10	0/34
MTV Antigen in Milk[x]	NT	1/11
Tests of Older Females		
Bioassay of Blood	6/19	14/31
MTV Antigen in Milk	9/35	13/42

*The females were exposed to MTV infection by neonatal fostering.
[+]The younger donors of blood for bioassay were 2 month old virgin females, whereas the older donors were 5-12 month old parous females.
[x]The younger donors of milk for detection of MTV antigen were 7 months of age or less, whereas the older donors were 8 months of age or older. NT = not tested.

A second gene affecting viral replication in susceptible females

Analysis of the time of first appearance of detectable MTV antigen (by immunodiffusion assay) in the milk of susceptible hybrid females and suscep-tible backcross females revealed a dramatic difference. At the first lactation, almost all of the hybrid females were positive for MTV antigen expression (Table 5). In contrast, only 29 of 115, or 25% of the backcross females were positive in this assay. This percentage is consistent with that expected if two genes are involved in the control of the trait. One of these we have already identified, the major susceptibility gene linked to the H-2 of the I strain (Table 2). There must be at least one more gene, segregating independently of the H-2, which enhances MTV expression such that sufficient antigen is produced even during the first lactation to allow its detection by the relatively insensitive immunodiffusion assay. Unfortunately, data which can unequivocally demonstrate that only a single second gene is involved are not available; first lactation milk samples were not tested in the second backcross, and linkage to another known gene of the mouse has not been found.

TABLE 5

EXPRESSION OF MTV ANTIGEN IN MILK OF HYBRID AND FIRST BACKCROSS FEMALES DURING THE FIRST LACTATION*

Type of Female	Number with MTV Antigen in First Lactation / Total	Percent
Hybrid	30/31	97%
First Backcross[+]	29/115	25%

*The females were infected with MTV by neonatal fostering.
[+]Although all the hybrid females are H-2^j H-2^b, only one-half of the backcross females are H-2^j H-2^b; the other half of the backcross females are H-2^{b}H-2^b and homozygous resistant for early expression of MTV antigen in milk.

Influence of the H-2-linked resistance/susceptibility gene on tumor development

As previously noted, although neonatally infected females of the C57BL or the I strains rarely develop mammary tumors, such tumors appear in a very high percentage of hybrid females after neonatal infection. In the backcross females studied here, tumor development was strongly associated with the presence of the I-introduced H-2-linked susceptibility gene; half of the backcross females carrying this gene developed mammary tumors within 15 months of age (Table 6). Mammary tumors were, however, not entirely restricted to these females. Approximately 10% of the homozygous resistant first and second backcross females also developed mammary tumors within 15 months; a similar low incidence has been reported in infected C57BL females.[4] In view of the fact that some of these resistant females do in later life express MTV (Table 4), the development of tumors in some of them is not surprising, and, indeed, all but one of the 14 tumors that occurred in homozygous resistant first and second backcross females occurred in individuals which expressed MTV antigen in their later lactations.

TABLE 6

INCIDENCE BY 15 MONTHS OF AGE OF MAMMARY TUMORS IN PAROUS FEMALES CARRYING THE
H-2-LINKED SUSCEPTIBILITY GENE FOR EARLY EXPRESSION OF MTV*

Type of Female	Number with Tumor/Total	Percent	Average Tumor Age
Hybrid	30/33	91%	8.6 months
First Backcross	40/80	50%	10.4 months
Second Backcross	8/17	47%	10.4 months

*The females were infected with MTV by neonatal fostering.

Other genes also affecting mammary tumor development

Examination of Table 6 reveals that at least one more gene than the H-2-
linked resistance/susceptibility gene must be important in the eventual
development of mammary tumors in infected mice. Although essentially all of
the hybrids developed mammary tumors, only half of the backcross females with
the H-2-linked susceptibility gene did so. This suggests that a second gene
is involved, and an immediate candidate is the one previously demonstrated to
enhance viral replication to detectable levels in immunodiffusion assay during
the first lactation (Table 5). However, this does not appear to be the only
factor involved; association of tumor development with first lactation
expression of MTV antigen is seen in the susceptible females (Table 7), but
it is not absolute. This suggests that multiple minor genes may be involved,
which cannot be separated on the basis of the data available.

TABLE 7

ASSOCIATION, IN SUSCEPTIBLE FEMALES OF THE FIRST BACKCROSS, OF EXPRESSION OF
MTV ANTIGEN IN THE FIRST LACTATION WITH DEVELOPMENT OF MAMMARY TUMORS*

Lactation	Number First Positive for MTV Antigen	Number Subsequently Developing Mammary Tumors	Percent
First	24	16[+]	67%
Second	15	8	53%
Third	13	3[+]	23%

*The females were infected with MTV by neonatal fostering.
[+]The difference in tumor incidence between these two groups is statistically
significant.

Differences in mammary tumor development in recombinant inbred strains

As part of another study, we have determined the mammary tumor incidence in female mice of 6 recombinant inbred strains which are homozygous for the $H-2^b$ MHC of the C57BL strain. One of these (B) was derived from an initial cross of BALB/c and C57BL mice, and the remaining 5 (ADP, ABS, AS, AD, and ADS) were derived from an initial cross of C57BL and I mice.[7] These mice were maintained as virgins and thus lacked the stimulating effect on mammary gland oncogenesis which multiple pregnancies and lactations provide. Nevertheless, two of the strains (AD and ADS) responded to the neonatal introduction of MTV with a significant incidence of tumor development (Table 8). We infer from this that a combination of modifier genes was established, during the inbreeding process by which the strains were brought to genetic homogeneity, which has made ineffective the resistance mechanism by which the $H-2^b$-linked recessive gene prevents the early expression of MTV.

TABLE 8

INCIDENCE BY 15 MONTHS OF AGE OF MAMMARY TUMORS IN 6 $H-2^b$ $H-2^b$ RECOMBINANT INBRED STRAINS OF MICE*

Strain	Number with Tumor/Total	Percent	Average Tumor Age (Months)
B	0/38	0	–
ADP	0/20	0	–
ABS	0/37	0	–
AS[+]	0/6	0	–
AD	5/8	63%	12.2
ADS	9/22	41%	11.3

*Females in this experiment were maintained as virgins. They were infected with MTV by neonatal fostering.
[+]Some of the AS females are only 14 months old at this time.

These observations on the susceptibility to oncogenesis of the $H-2^b$ homozygous recombinant inbred strains do not negate the demonstration that an MHC-linked recessive gene carried by the C57BL strain plays the dominant role in resistance to the expression of MTV infection and thus to its oncogenic

150

activity in that strain. The results do, however, provide a dramatic illustration of the important fact that the genetic background on which a gene is expressed can greatly alter the significance of its effect; the H-2^b linked gene is clearly of major importance in C57BL mice but of minimal if any importance in mice of the AD and ADS strains.

ACKNOWLEDGMENTS

These experimental studies were supported by research grants from the National Cancer Institute (CA-05388) and the American Cancer Society (IM-69), and by research funds of the University of California. J.A.D. and C.N. were supported by NIH training grant funds (CA-09041 and GM-07127) while these studies were being conducted; their current addresses are, respectively, Molecular Biology Institute, University of California, Los Angeles, California, and Department of Genetics, Stanford University, Stanford, California.

REFERENCES

1. Davilovs, J.A. (1978) The Genetics of Resistance to Mammary Tumor Virus Infection and Tumorigenesis in C57BL/Crgl Mice. Ph.D. Thesis, University of California, Berkeley.
2. Nandi, S. (1967) Proc. Natl. Acad. Sci. 58, 485-492.
3. Nandi, S. (1974) J. Natl. Cancer Inst. 52, 1797-1804.
4. Nandi, S., Handin, M., Robinson, A., Pitelka, D.R. and Webber, L.E. (1966) J. Natl. Cancer Inst. 36, 783-801.
5. Nandi, S., Haslam, S., and Helmich, C. (1972) J. Natl. Cancer Inst. 48, 1005-1012.
6. Muhlbock, O. and Dux, A. (1974) J. Natl. Cancer Inst. 53, 993-996.
7. Blair, P.B. (1980) in Natural Cell-Mediated Immunity Against Tumors, Herberman, R.B. ed., Academic Press, New York, pp. 401-409.

GENETIC CONTROL OF TRANSFORMATION AND TUMORIGENICITY
IN HUMAN CELL HYBRIDS

ERIC J. STANBRIDGE AND BERNARD E. WEISSMAN
Department of Microbiology, College of Medicine, University of California,
Irvine, California 92717

INTRODUCTION

The technique of somatic cell hybridization[1] has been extremely useful in studies of gene mapping[2] and control of expression of differentiated functions[3]. The technique has also been applied to the study of the genetic analysis of malignancy[4-9] but until recently the interpretations of these analyses have been quite controversial. By way of introduction to this controversy a brief history is presented. Early investigators in this field[4,10] isolated hybrid cells derived from the fusion of mouse cells of low malignant potential with those of high malignant potential. The intraspecific mouse cell hybrids derived from these fusions were as malignant as the highly malignant parent, thereby leading to the interpretation that malignancy behaves as a dominant trait. Similar conclusions were reached by others using polyoma-transformed mouse cells as the malignant parent[11]. However, Harris, Klein and their colleagues[5,12-14], based on an extensive series of experiments, came to the opposite conclusion. In their studies they showed that when highly malignant mouse cells were fused with normal mouse embryo cells or mouse cells of low malignant potential, the resulting hybrids were transiently suppressed in their ability to form tumors. Tumorigenic segregants appeared rapidly in these nontumorigenic populations. Analyses of the chromosome complements of the parental and hybrid cell populations indicated that the tumorigenic segregants had lost substantial numbers of chromosomes, including those originating from the normal parent. These findings have been confirmed by others[7,8,15,16] but there have been notable exceptions to this generalization[6,17]. The major drawback in all of these studies has been the chromosomal instability of intraspecific rodent hybrid cells where a significant proportion of the total chromosome complement is rapidly lost. This rapidity of chromosome loss, in addition to making the initial

premise of suppression of malignancy hard to evaluate, renders the identification of specific chromosome(s) which possibly control the expression
of the tumorigenic phenotype an extremely arduous task.

In another approach interspecific human-rodent hybrids have been used
in an attempt to identify the genetic elements regulating the control of
expression of the tumorigenic phenotype[6,9,18]. Here the situation is at
least as controversial as with intraspecific rodent cell hybrids--
different investigators working with the same cell combinations have again
reached opposite conclusions. Jonasson and Harris[18] found complete
suppression of tumorigenicity in hybrids formed between mouse A9 cells and
human fibroblasts whereas Kucherlapati and Shin found no such suppression
in their A9 x human fibroblast hybrids9. In another extensive study Croce
and colleagues[6,19] showed that when SV_{40} transformed human fibroblasts are
fused with normal mouse cells the tumorigenic phenotype continues to be
expressed until the integrated SV_{40} genome is lost by chromosome segregation. Once again, the general rule in the above studies is that chromosomes rapidly segregate from interspecific hybrids. However, other
investigators have found that the tumorigenic phenotype of SV_{40} transformed cells is suppressed following fusion with normal cells[20-22].

Recently we have developed an intraspecies human hybrid cell system
that eliminates the serious problem of chromosome instability[23,24]. In
the remainder of this article we present a brief description of this
system and discuss the possible nature of the genetic control of tumorigenic expression in human cell hybrids.

HUMAN CELL HYBRIDS

Although we have examined several combinations of malignant x normal
human cell fusions[24] we will restrict most of our remarks to the HeLa x
fibroblast and HeLa x keratinocyte hybrids that have been studied most
extensively. In our initial studies we fused the D98/AH-2 clone of HeLa[25]
with a series of different normal human fibroblasts. The hybrid clones
which arose in HAT selective medium[26] all had essentially the same morphology, which was intermediate between that of the HeLa and fibroblast
parental cells[23,27]. At a later stage hybrids derived from the fusion
between HeLa and keratinocytes were isolated and these hybrid cells all
had the morphology of epithelial-like cells[28].

TUMORIGENIC POTENTIAL OF THE HeLa/FIBROBLAST HYBRIDS

The primary objective of our early studies was to determine whether the tumorigenic phenotype of the malignant HeLa parent continued to be expressed in the HeLa/fibroblast hybrid cell or became suppressed due to the introduction of normal genetic material. The use of appropriately immunosuppressed animals was obviously necessary for these tumorigenicity assays. Mice immunosuppressed in a variety of ways were used and included (i) neonatally thymectomized and antithymocyte serum treated; (ii) adult thymectomized, whole body irradiated and bone marrow reconstituted (T^-B^+); and (iii) congenitally athymic nude mice. In all cases the same result was obtained: whereas 1×10^5 parental HeLa cells injected subcutaneously produced progressively growing tumors in 100% of animals no tumors were formed when as many as 1×10^8 hybrid cells were inoculated[23,29]. Thus it would appear that tumorigenic potential is initially completely suppressed in these hybrids. However, possible artifacts could include immunologic rejection of the hybrid cells by, for example, natural killer cell activity, a known complicating factor in nude mice in particular[30]. Also it might be possible that the human hybrid cells, like the rodent and interspecies human-rodent hybrids described previously, are chromosomally unstable and that the chromosomes responsible for malignant expression were rapidly lost from the hybrids in some non-random fashion. Both of these concerns were laid to rest when it was found that tumorigenic segregants arose from the nontumorigenic hybrids after prolonged times in culture. Extensive studies of the growth behavior of the hybrid cells in nude mice showed that immune rejection and natural killer cell cytotoxicity in particular[29] played no role in the control of the tumor growth.

The most valuable aspect of the human hybrid cell system was revealed when chromosome analyses were performed on the nontumorigenic hybrids and the tumorigenic segregants derived from them. It was found that immediately following fusion most (but not all) hybrid clones had lost a few - less than 5% - chromosomes based upon the calculated sum of the modes of the parental HeLa and fibroblast populations. Following this early minor loss the chromosomal compositions of the hybrids were extremely stable[31,32]. Detailed chromosome analysis of paired nontumorigenic and tumorigenic

HeLa/fibroblast hybrids showed that the tumorigenic segregant populations differed only slightly from their nontumorigenic counterparts with respect to chromosome number[32]. Furthermore, the loss of one copy of chromosomes 11 and 14, respectively, is correlated, with a high degree of statistical significance, with the reexpression of tumorigenicity. The chromosome stability of the hybrids provides us with the explanation why, in contrast to other hybrid cell systems, tumorigenic segregants appear only rarely in nontumorigenic human hybrid cell populations. The similarity in chromosomal makeup of the nontumorigenic and tumorigenic segregant hybrids also indicates that these paired populations are both genotypically and phenotypically very similar. This similarity therefore allows one to determine which phenotypic traits are specifically correlated with tumorigenic expression.

IN VITRO PHENOTYPIC CHARACTERISTICS OF HeLa/FIBROBLAST HYBRIDS

Two major factors prompted the comparative analysis of nontumorigenic hybrids and their tumorigenic segregants. In the first place, it is becoming increasingly clear from both epidemiological[33] and experimental[34,35] studies that the progression of a normal cell to a frankly neoplastic one involves multiple steps. We consider, as will be apparent from the description below, that the nontumorigenic hybrids behave as transformed cells in culture and are analogous to an intermediate step in the progression of a normal cell to a neoplastic state in naturally occuring cancers. Secondly, it has been shown that the process of neoplastic transformation is accompanied by a bewildering array of phenotypic changes in cultured cells. These changes include altered cellular morphology, loss of density-dependent inhibition of growth, reduced requirement for serum growth factors, enhanced proteolytic activity, altered metabolic rates, expression of new products and surface antigens, anchorage independence and alterations in cytoskeletal and membrane architecture (reviewed in ref. 36). In the majority of cases these "markers of malignancy" have been identified on the basis of comparisons between the neoplastic cells and their normal progenitors. We felt that it might be more useful to compare a tumorigenic cell with its transformed but nontumorigenic precursor in order to determine which phenotypic characteristics of the tumorigenic cells differ not only from the normal cells but also the transformed precursor and thereby specifically correlate with tumorigenic expression.

A summary of our findings is given in Table I. We will not dwell on the details of these findings, which have been published elsewhere[23,27,32,37-41]. However, it is clear that many of the phenotypic traits examined are expressed in both nontumorigenic and tumorigenic segregant hybrid populations. Thus the expression of these "tumor-specific" markers may be necessary but are not sufficient for full tumorigenic expression. Those phenotypic traits that distinguish tumorigenic HeLa/fibroblast hybrids from their nontumorigenic hybrid counterparts include morphology, fibronectin distribution and microfilament organization. All three phenotypic traits are completely reversible. Addition of low concentrations of dexamethasone or sodium butyrate to tumorigenic hybrid cells results in a phenotypic shift of these three traits to that corresponding to the nontumorigenic hybrids. Two tumor-associated markers have, however, been identified in HeLa/fibroblast hybrids. They are the expression of a 75 kilodalton phosphoprotein in the membranes of parental HeLa cells and tumorigenic segregant hybrid cells[40], and the expression of the α subunit of human chorionic gonadotropin in these tumorigenic cells[41]. Neither phenotype is expressed in normal parental cells or nontumorigenic hybrids. The functional significance of these findings is as yet unclear.

One phenotype we do wish to discuss briefly is that of anchorage independent growth of cells in soft agar or methyl cellulose. It has repeatedly been documented[42,43] that the ability of cells to grow in suspension in these milieus is correlated with tumorigenic expression. Although most of the studies have involved rodent cells the dogma that anchorage independent growth is synonymous with tumorigenicity has been extrapolated to other species, including human[44]. Our studies, which have been confirmed by others[16,45], indicate that this phenotype does not correlate specifically with tumorigenicity (although it may be a necessary alteration in the progression to malignancy since many malignant cells express this trait) since transformed nontumorigenic cells grow perfectly well in suspension in agarose or methyl cellulose. Thus, in human cells this phenotypic trait may represent an early alteration in the progression from normalcy to malignancy. In fact, we have recently shown[46] that normal human fibroblasts are capable of anchorage-independent growth in methyl cellulose under certain nutritional conditions. These findings illustrate the dangers of extrapolating from one mammalian system to another and

underscore the necessity of working with human cells in order to unravel
the complexities of the human cancer phenotypes.

TUMORIGENIC EXPRESSION - DOMINANT, RECESSIVE OR GENE DOSAGE CONTROL?

Our studies with HeLa/fibroblast hybrids in particular, described in
the preceding sections, clearly indicate that tumorigenicity is completely
and stably suppressed and that tumorigenic segregants appear when certain
specific chromosomes are lost from the hybrid cell. With this particular
combination of malignant x normal cell fusion tumorigenicity does not
behave as a dominant trait. We attempted to investigate the possibility
that chromosome (gene) dosage may play a role in the control of tumorigenic expression by taking nontumorigenic or tumorigenic segregant HeLa/
fibroblast (H/F) hybrids and fusing them with one more HeLa or fibroblast
parental cell. The results, given in Table 2, show that when tumorigenic
segregant H/F hybrids are fused with normal fibroblasts suppression of
tumorigenicity is reestablished. However, when nontumorigenic H/F hybrids
are fused with HeLa the resulting multiparental hybrid, containing 2
genomic copies of HeLa and one of normal fibroblast, remains nontumorigenic. Tumorigenic segregants appear rather rapidly in these populations
and their appearance is correlated with extensive chromosome loss. It
would seem, therefore, from this rather crude approach, that tumorigenic
expression in HeLa behaves as a recessive trait rather than being a gene
dosage phenomenon.

A most interesting result was observed when nontumorigenic H/F hybrids
were fused with normal fibroblasts. The vast majority of the triparental
hybrids were capable of only limited proliferation and then underwent a
"senescent" phase similar to that seen in normal fibroblasts in culture[47].
Thus, in this case the transformed phenotype seems to be under some form
of gene dosage control and normal growth properties are restored when the
combination of 1x HeLa with 2x normal fibroblast genomes is accomplished.

A quite different interpretation is found with other combinations of
malignant x normal cell fusions. Croce and colleagues[48] have shown that
when the human fibrosarcoma cell line HT1080 was fused with normal human
fibroblasts all of the hybrid clones recovered were highly tumorigenic.
On the basis of these findings they concluded that tumorigenicity behaves
as a dominant trait. We have also undertaken a rather extensive series of

experiments with this cell line and have arrived at somewhat different conclusions[49].

The HT1080 human fibrosarcoma cell line is predominantly pseudodiploid, with a tight mode of 46 chromosomes that includes two distinct marker chromosomes, involving chromosomes 5 and 11[50]. The cell line, however, has a propensity to accumulate subtetraploid cells and if the cells are propagated long enough this population will predominate. We selected both pseudodiploid and subtetraploid clones of HT1080 cells and fused them with normal fibroblasts. When the subtetraploid clones were used many hybrid colonies were generated. All clones, without exception, were highly tumorigenic in nude mice. However, when the pseudodiploid HT1080 clone was fused with normal fibroblasts a very different picture emerged. Many hybrid colonies appeared in the primary fusion plates. These colonies were isolated and transferred to other dishes where the majority underwent only a few population doublings and then ceased to proliferate. Thus, these hybrids appeared to express the growth control and limited proliferative lifespan of the normal parental fibroblast. From a number of different experiments three hybrid clones have been isolated that proliferate indefinitely in culture. These hybrid cells are completely nontumorigenic in nude mice. A tumorigenic segregant has been obtained from one of these hybrid clones[49].

Thus, at least in our hands, the tumorigenic potential and the transformed phenotype of HT1080 appears to be influenced by gene dosage. Hybrid cells containing 1x HT1080 and 1x fibroblast genomic complements behave like normal cells. Segregants that progressively express transformed and then tumorigenic characteristics have been isolated from these suppressed populations. Hybrid cells that contain 2x HT1080 and 1x fibroblast genomic complements are both transformed and tumorigenic.

Insofar as experiments with somatic cell hybrids can take us it is suggestive that chromosome or gene dosage may play a role in control of expression of the transformed and tumorigenic phenotypes of some, but not all human cancer cells. A similar role of chromosome dosage in the control of neoplastic expression has been described in rodent cell systems, both experimentally and in naturally occurring leukemias[51-53].

COMPLEMENTATION OF THE TUMORIGENIC PHENOTYPE

The fact that tumorigenic expression can be suppressed by introduction of normal genetic information would indicate that this phenotype behaves as a recessive trait or involves gene dosage effects rather than behaving as a dominant trait. This property allows one to attempt a complementation analysis of the genetic lesions determining this phenotype in a manner similar to that used in the study of other heritable recessive traits in somatic cells[54]. The rationale here would be the assumption that more than one chromosomal region is involved in the control of malignant expression and that alterations at any one of these chromosomal regions would result in a neoplastic cell. If this were the case then malignant cells obtained from a variety of neoplasms might have accrued damage at different chromosomal loci. Fusion between two such malignant cells might then result in a hybrid cell that is complemented for these defects and would now be nontumorigenic. We undertook a study where different carcinoma cells were fused together and were also fused with lymphoma, fibrosarcoma, and melanoma cells. All parental cell populations were highly tumorigenic in nude mice. It was found that when HeLa was fused with other carcinoma cells or with lymphoblastoid cells containing integrated Epstein-Barr virus (EBV) genetic material the resulting hybrids were also tumorigenic. However, when HeLa, or another carcinoma cell line, A549, was fused with pseudodiploid HT1080 fibrosarcoma cells, most of the hybrid clones isolated were nontumorigenic (Table 3). After varying periods of time in culture tumorigenic segregants could be recovered from these hybrid populations. When HeLa was fused with melanoma cells the hybrids isolated showed a full spectrum, ranging from nontumorigenic to highly tumorigenic. Interpretation of these latter results is difficult because, unlike other intraspecific human cell hybrids[31], the HeLa x melanoma hybrid cells rapidly segregated chromosomes.

The fact that fusions between different carcinoma cells, which are all of epithelial origin, result in no complementation and, therefore, continued tumorigenic expression, raises the intriguing possibility that a single common genetic locus governs the neoplastic expression of cancerous cells of similar somatic origin. It is also possible that lymphoblastoid cells may share this putative common genetic locus, although the presence of EBV in this case complicates matters since the control of neoplastic expression in hybrid cells derived from virally-transformed parental cells is quite complex[55,56]. Conversely, in cells of diverse somatic origin, e. g. HeLa or A549 lung carcinoma cells fused with fibrosarcoma cells, different genetic loci may control tumorigenic expression and can therefore be complemented, resulting in suppression of tumorigenicity.

The results described above, although preliminary, indicate that a family of genes, rather than a single common genetic locus may control neoplastic expression in human cells; possibly a distinct one for each somatic cell type. This situation is somewhat analogous to that seen with the different retroviral transforming genes which induce neoplastic transformation of different somatic cell types[57]. This analogy may become even more pertinent if the suspicion that retroviral transforming genes are actually acquired host cellular genes[58,59] is confirmed.

CANCER GENES AND CELL HYBRIDS - A RECONCILIATION OF GENETIC THEORIES

In the last 2 - 3 years there have been some very exciting breakthroughs and advances in our understanding of the molecular genetic basis of naturally occurring cancers. Two major findings contributed to this understanding - firstly, it was found that the individual transforming genes, or oncogenes, of "acute" transforming retroviruses are homologous to DNA sequences present in normal uninfected cells[60,61]. It appears, therefore, that at some time in the past recombination between nontransforming retroviruses and normal cellular genes occurred and, at least in some cases, these "recombinant" viruses now became highly oncogenic by virtue of their promoting an abnormally high level of expression of this acquired cellular gene in infected cells[62]. At least 13 distinct retrovirus transforming genes have now been identified[57].

The second major breakthrough was the transfer of biologically active eukaryotic DNA from one mammalian cell to another (termed transfection) and, in particular, the transfer of cellular transforming genes from human cells to mouse cells[63,64]. These latter studies have clearly established that DNA fragments obtained from human cancer cells and transfected into mouse 3T3 cells induce the neoplastic transformation of these rodent cells. Several of these transforming sequences have now been cloned and induce transformation at high frequencies when subsequently transfected into 3T3 cells[65,66]. It has also been shown that <u>normal</u> cellular DNA sequences will induce transformation of 3T3 cells, albeit at a significantly lower frequency than human cancer cell DNAs[67].

The demonstration that transfection of human cancer cell DNA into mouse 3T3 cells results in neoplastic transformation of the recipient cells has been interpreted as evidence that carcinogenesis in various neoplasms appears to involve dominant genetic alterations, either by mutations or gene arrangements[57]. Such an interpretation is obviously contrary to our observations on the control of tumorigenic expression in human cell hybrids. It is possible, of course, that certain neoplasms arise as a consequence of dominant mutations whereas others involve recessive mutations or gene dosage effects. In fact, DNA fragments from approximately 50 percent of chemically induced and spontaneously occurring neoplasms tested failed to induce efficient transformation of mouse 3T3 cells[57]. HeLa cell DNA was one of the cancer cell types that did not induce transformation. However, it has been recently reported that DNA from HT1080 fibrosarcoma cells efficiently transforms 3T3 cells[68]. In cell hybridization experiments we have established that control of tumorigenic expression of the HT1080 cell line is governed by gene dosage effects[49]. There are a number of possible explanations for the apparently contradictory results obtained from DNA transfection studies versus cell hybridization analyses. The transforming activity of normal cell DNAs suggests that these DNA sequences, which have undergone shearing prior to transfection, have been removed from flanking sequences that normally control the level of expression of these genes. The situation with cancer cell DNAs is different because the regulatory control of flanking sequences would presumably already have been lost by mutation or genetic rearrangement. In somatic cell hybrids, derived from the fusion between a malignant cell and a normal cell, the regulatory control of tumorigenic expression exerted by the normal cell DNA sequences presumably operates in a trans-acting fashion. However, in certain combinations, for example HT1080 fibrosarcoma x normal fibroblast hybrids, the trans-acting control of tumorigenic expression may be governed by gene dosage. In the case of human cancer cell DNA transfected into mouse 3T3 cells there may be an interspecies "barrier"

preventing control of expression of human DNA sequences by cis or trans
acting mouse DNA regulatory sequences. Alternatively, there may be
integration of multiple copies (perhaps only two are necessary) of the
human cancer DNA sequences thereby overcoming the "suppressor" control of
the cis or trans acting mouse DNA sequences by gene dosage effects.
Finally, there is the possibility of position effects where the human
cancer gene integrates into the mouse genome at positions where they come
under strong promoter control that neutralizes any cis or trans acting
regulatory control and promotes high level expression of the cancer gene.
Strong promoter effects have been noted in experimental systems where the
long terminal repeat (LTR) sequences of nontransforming retroviruses have
been ligated to normal cellular homologs of the viral transforming genes
and these recombinant molecules now have significant transforming
activity[69,70].

Further understanding of the nature of the control of human cancer gene
expression will come when it is possible to transfect and transform normal
human cells rather than aneuploid mouse 3T3 cells with human cancer cell
DNA.

CONCLUSION AND FUTURE PROSPECTS

This brief survey of our experiences with the use of somatic cell
hybrids in the analysis of malignancy in human cells illustrates some of
the advantageous features of the system in tackling this complex problem.
Human cell hybrids are chromosomally stable and thereby provide a system
whereby one may probe with confidence into the chromosomal control of
expression of transformation and tumorigenicity, secure in the knowledge
that mass populations of cells may be propagated and harvested for experimentation and yet still represent a homogeneous population. This is a
definite advantage over the more unstable intraspecific rodent and interspecific human-rodent systems previously described.

Using this system we have shown that: (i) transformed and tumorigenic phenotypes are under separate genetic control; (ii) nontumorigenic
and tumorigenic segregant hybrid cells have very similar phenotypes in
culture; (iii) tumor-specific antigens can be identified by comparing
paired NT and TS populations; (iv) reexpression of tumorigenicity is
correlated with the loss of specific chromosomes; (v) control of tumor

formation is due to differentiation-inducing signals; and (vi) differentiation-specific products have been identified.

One major disadvantage of this intraspecific human hybrid cell system is that identification of those chromosomes controlling the expression of the transformed and tumorigenic phenotypes is very difficult - there are usually 95-100 chromosomes per metaphase spread to analyse by banding techniques. Furthermore, identification of the parental origin of a given chromosome in a parental cell is well nigh impossible unless it is accompanied by some type of marker such as isoenzyme polymorphism or actual translocation of chromosome material. It would also appear that relatively few chromosomes, perhaps only 1 or 2, are involved in the control of tumorigenic expression. Therefore, fusion of a normal cell, containing 46 chromosomes, with a malignant cell in order to suppress tumorigenicity presumably involves considerable redundancy of transferred normal chromosomes.

Fortunately, recent technological advances now make it possible to transfer isolated chromosomes and even isolated genes into recipient cells. We are currently developing the technology whereby isolated, specific individual chromosomes may be transferred from a normal cell to a malignant cell and vice versa. Success in this approach will be followed, hopefully, by the cloning of the discrete DNA sequences responsible for the expression and suppression of tumorigenic potential. Such technology will greatly accelerate our quest for the identification of those regulatory elements governing the neoplastic behavior of human cells.

ACKNOWLEDGMENTS

These studies were supported by National Institute of Health grant CA-19401 and a gift from the Florence A. Clark Memorial Fund. Eric J. Stanbridge is the recipient of National Institute of Health Research Career Development Award CA-00271.

REFERENCES

1. Harris, H., and Watkins, J. F. (1965) Nature, 205, 640-646.
2. McKusick, V. A., and Ruddle, F. H. (1977) Science, 196, 390-405.
3. Davidson, R. L. (1974) "Somatic Cell Hybridization." Raven Press, New York.
4. Barski, G., and Cornefert, F. (1962) J. Natl. Cancer Inst. 28, 801-821.
5. Harris, H., Miller, O.J., Klein, G., Worst, P., and Tachibana, T. (1969) Nature, 223, 363-368.
6. Croce, C. M., Aden, D., and Koprowski, H. (1975) Proc. Natl. Acad. Sci. USA, 72, 1397-1400.
7. Stanbridge, E. J. (1976) Nature, 260, 17-20.
8. Sager, R., and Kovac, P. E. (1978) Somat. Cell Genet., 4, 375-392.
9. Kucherlapati, R., and Shin, S. (1979) Cell, 16, 639-648.
10. Scaletta, L. J., and Ephrussi, B. (1965) Nature, 205, 1169-1171.
11. Defendi, V., Ephrussi, B., Koprowski, H., and Yoshida, M. C. (1967) Proc. Natl. Acad. Sci. USA, 57, 299-305.
12. Harris, H. (1971) Proc. Royal Soc. B., 179, 1-20.
13. Wiener, F., Klein, G., and Harris, H. (1971) J. Cell Sci., 8, 681-692.
14. Wiener, F., Klein, G., and Harris, H. (1974) J. Cell Sci., 15, 177-183.
15. Kao, F., and Hartz, J. A. (1977) J. Natl. Cancer Inst., 59, 409-413.
16. Klinger, H. (1980) Cytogenet Cell Genet., 27, 256-266.
17. Aviles, D., Jami, J., Rousset, J., and Ritz, E. (1977) J. Natl. Cancer Inst., 58, 1391-1397.
18. Jonasson, J, and Harris, H. (1977) J. Cell Sci., 24, 255-263.
19. Croce, C. M., Aden, D., and Koprowski, H. (1975) Science, 190, 1200-1202.
20. Gee, C. J., and Harris, H. (1979) J. Cell Sci., 36, 223-240.
21. Howell, N., and Sager, R. (1982) Cytogenet. Cell Genet., (in press).
22. Weissman, B. E., and Stanbridge, E. J. (1982) (submitted for publication).
23. Stanbridge, E. J., and Wilkinson, J. (1978) Proc. Natl. Acad. Sci. USA, 75, 1466-1469.
24. Stanbridge, E. J., Der, C. J., Doersen, C.-J., Nishimi, R. Y., Peehl, D. M., Weissman, B. E., and Wilkinson, J. (1982) Science, 215, 252-259.
25. Szybalski, W. S., Szybalska, E. H., and Ragni, G. (1962) Cancer Inst. Monogr., 7, 75-88.
26. Littlefield, J. W. (1964) Science, 145, 709-710.
27. Der, C. J., and Stanbridge, E. J. (1978) Cell, 15, 1241-1251.
28. Peehl, D. M., and Stanbridge, E. J. (1981) Int. J. Cancer, 27, 625-635.
29. Stanbridge, E. J., and Ceredig, R. (1981) Cancer Res., 41, 573-580.
30. Kiessling, R., Klein, E., and Wigzell, H. (1975) Eur. J. Immunol., 5, 112-117.
31. Weissman, B. E., and Stanbridge, E. J. (1980) Cytogenet. Cell Genet., 28, 227-239.
32. Stanbridge, E. J., Flandermeyer, R. R., Daniels, D. W., Nelson-Rees, W. A. (1981) Som. Cell Genet., 7, 699-712.
33. Armitage, P. and Doll, R. (1954) Brit. J. Cancer, 8, 1-12.

164

34. Barrett, J. C., and Ts'o, P. O. (1978) Proc. Natl. Acad. Sci. USA, 75, 3761-3765.
35. Mondal, S., Brankow, D. W., and Heidelberger, C. (1976) Cancer Res., 36, 2254-2260.
36. Nicolson, G. L. (1976) Biochem. Biophys. Acta, 457, 57-108.
37. Der, C. J., and Stanbridge, E. J. (1980) Int. J. Cancer, 26, 451-459.
38. Stanbridge, E. J., and Wilkinson, J. (1980) Int. J. Cancer, 26, 1-8.
39. Der, C. J. and Stanbridge, E. J. (1981) J. Cell Sci., 52, 151-166.
40. Der, C. J. and Stanbridge, E. J. (1981) Cell, 26, 429-438.
41. Stanbridge, E. J., Rosen, S. W., and Sussman, H. H. (1982) Proc. Natl. Acad. Sci. USA, (in press).
42. Freedman, V. H. and Shin, S. (1974) Cell, 3, 355-359.
43. Shin, S., Freedman, V. J., Risser, R., and Pollack, R. (1975) Proc. Natl. Acad. Sci. USA, 72, 4435-4439.
44. Hamburger, A. W., and Salmon, S. E. (1977) Science, 197, 461-463.
45. Kahn, P., and Shin, S. (1979) J. Cell Biol., 82, 1-16.
46. Peehl, D. M., and Stanbridge, E. J. (1981) Proc. Natl. Acad. Sci., USA 78, 3053-3057.
47. Hayflick, L. and Moorhead, P. S. (1961) Exp. Cell Res., 25, 585-621.
48. Croce, C. M., Barrick, J., Linnenbach, A. and Koprowski, H. (1979) J. Cell Physiol., 99, 279-286.
49. Benedict, W. F., Weissman, B. E., Mark, C. and Stanbridge, E. J. (submitted for publication).
50. Rasheed, S., Nelson-Rees, W. A., Toth, E. M., Arnstein, P. and Gardner, M. B. (1974) Cancer, 33, 1027-1033.
51. Hitotsumachi, S., Rabinowitz, Z. and Sachs, L. (1971) Nature, 231, 511-514.
52. Benedict, W. F., Ruck, N., Mark, C. and Kouri, R. E. (1975) J. Natl. Cancer Inst., 54, 157-162.
53. Klein, G. (1981) Nature, 294, 313-318.
54. Littlefield, J. W. (1976) Variation, Senescence and Neoplasis in Cultured Somatic Cells. Harvard University Press, Cambridge, Mass., USA, pp. 1-163.
55. Koprowski, H. and Croce, C. M. (1977) Proc. Natl. Acad. Sci. USA, 74, 1142-1146.
56. Gee, C. J. and Harris, H. (1979) J. Cell Sci., 36, 223-240.
57. Cooper, G. M. (1982) Science, 217, 801-806.
58. Hanafusa, H., Halpern, C. C., Buchhagen, D. L. and Kawai, S. (1977) J. Expt. Med., 146, 1735-1747.
59. Oskarrson, M., McClements, W. L., Blair, D. G., Maizel, J. V. and Vande Woude, G. F. (1980) Science, 207, 1222-1224.
60. Der, C. J., Krontiris, T. G. and Cooper, G. M. (1982) Proc. Natl. Acad. Sci. USA, 79, 3637-3640.
61. Santos, E., Tronick, S. R., Aaronson, S. A., Pulciani, S. and Barbacid, M. (1982) Nature, 298, 343-347.
62. Collett, M. S., Brugge, J. S. and Erikson, R. L. (1978) Cell, 15, 1363-1369.
63. Shih, C., Shilo, B.-Z., Goldbarb, M. P., Dannenberg, A., and Weinberg, R. A. (1979) Proc. Natl. Acad. Sci. USA, 76, 5714-5718.

64. Cooper, G. M. and Neiman, P. E. (1980) Nature, 287, 656-659.
65. Shih, C. and Weinberg, R. A. (1982) Cell, 29, 161-169.
66. Goldbarb, M., Shimizu, K., Perucho, M. and Wigler, M. (1982) Nature, 296, 404-409.
67. Cooper, G. M., Okenquist, S. and Silverman, L. (1980) Nature, 284, 418-421.
68. Pulciani, S., Santos, E., Lauver, A. V., Long, L. K., Robbins, K. C., and Barbacid, M. (1982) Proc. Natl. Acad. Sci. USA, 79, 2845-2849.
69. Oskarsson, M. McClements, W. L., Blair, D. G., Maizel, J. V., and Vande Woude, G. (1980) Science, 207, 1222-1224.
70. DeFeo, D., Gonda, M. A., Young, H. A., Chang, E. H., Lowy, D. R., Scolknick, E. M. and Ellis, R. W. (1981) Proc. Natl. Acad Sci. USA, 78, 3328-3332.

TABLE I. SUMMARY OF IN VITRO PROPERTIES OF PARENTAL AND HYBRID HUMAN CELLS

In Vitro Phenotype	Parental Cells		Nontumorigenic HeLa/Fibroblast Hybrids	Tumorigenic HeLa/Fibroblast Segregants
	HeLa	Fibroblast		
Morphology	Epithelial	Fibroblastic	Intermediate	Epithelial*
Requirement for Serum Growth Factors	Reduced	High	Reduced	Reduced
Lectin Agglutination	+++	±	+++	+++
Anchorage Independent Growth	Yes	No	Yes	Yes
Fibronectin Expression	None	High	Reduced (short branched filaments)	Reduced (unbranched* stitch pattern)
Cytoskeleton: Microtubules Microfilaments	Organized Poorly organized	Organized Organized	Organized Organized	Organized Poorly organized*
Placental Alkaline Phosphatase	High	Low	High	High
Ganglioside Analysis	Simple	Complex	Relatively Complex	Relatively Complex
α-Human Chorionic Gonadotropin (α-hCG)	Present	Absent	Absent	Present
75K Membrane Phospho-protein	Present	Absent	Absent	Present

* Reversible properties – addition of dexamethasone or sodium butyrate induces a phenotypic shift to that of the nontumorigenic hybrid cells.

TABLE 2

TUMORIGENIC PROPERTIES OF TRIPARENTAL HeLa/FIBROBLAST HYBRIDS

Biparental Hybrid	Fusion Partners	Triparental Clone	Chromosome Mode (Range in Parentheses)	No. Tumors/No. Mice Inoculated
NT[a]-1	HeLa	C1	(89-131)	0/3
NT-2	HeLa	C3	136 (85-143)	0/4
		C5	131 (106-135)	0/4
		C6	105,128 (93-131)	0/4
NT-3	HeLa	C1	(140-150)	0/3
NT-4	HeLa	C5	118 (106-124)	0/3
		C5 (Scl. 2B)	103 (95-106)	3/3
		C5 (Scl. 10)	111 (101-114)	3/3
TS[b]-1	HDF[c]	C1	116,117 (100-125)	0/2
		C2	125,127 (108-128)	0/2
		C4	126,127 (89-134)	0/3
		C6	122,132 (113-143)	0/3
TS-2	HDF	C1	123 (88-128)	0/4
		C2	119 (111-124)	0/4
		C3	116 (106-121)	0/3
		C4	135 (104-185)	0/4
TS-3	HDF	C1	123 (112-137)	0/4
		C2	128 (114-134)	0/4
		C3	123 (109-132)	0/4
		C4	134 (114-144)	0/4
		C5	132 (118-136)	0/3
NT-5	HDF	12 clones	N.D.[d]	N.T.[e]

a = nontumorigenic HeLa/fibroblast hybrid.
b = tumorigenic segregant HeLa/fibroblast hybrid.
c = human diploid fibroblast.
d = not done.
e = not tested. The cells ceased proliferating in culture within
    10 population doublings.

TABLE 3

TUMORIGENIC POTENTIAL OF HYBRID CELLS DERIVED FROM THE FUSION
BETWEEN TWO MALIGNANT PARENTAL CELLS

Hybrid Cell Description	Chromosome Mode (Range)	No. Tumors No. Animals Inoculated
HeLa x A549 (Lung Carcinoma)		
Clone 1	121 (709-126)	4/4
Clone 3	114 (104-125)	4/4
HeLa x PET-1 (Metastatic Carcinoma)		
Clone 1	112 (105-116)	4/4
Clone 3	111 (100-114)	6/6
HeLa x Paxton (Teratocarcinoma)		
Clone 1	106 (72-108)	4/4
Clone 2	104 (97-115)	2/2
HeLa x HTD114 (Fibrosarcoma)		
Clone 1	107 (101-110)	0/7
Clone 2	102 (85-107)	1/9
A549 x HTD114 (Fibrosarcoma)		
Clone 1	107 (101-110)	0/7
Clone 2	102 (85-107)	1/9
HeLa x HS294 (Melanoma)		
Clone 1	110 (97-112)	2/7
Clone 5	102 (86-112)	3/3
Clone 6	111 (102-120)	0/2

NATURAL CELL-MEDIATED CYTOTOXICITY AGAINST TUMORS IN MICE

OSIAS STUTMAN AND EDMUND C. LATTIME
Cellular Immunology Section, Memorial Sloan-Kettering Cancer Center, 1275 York Avenue, New York, New York 10021, U.S.A.

INTRODUCTION

The idea of natural cell-mediated cytotoxicity (NCMC) being mediated by an heterogeneous system of effector cells[1], is derived from two types of observations: 1) Depending on the targets, assays and effector cell donors used, NCMC effector cells with different properties have been described, two of the prototypes being natural killer (NK)[2] and natural cytotoxic (NC)[1] cells and their variants[1,2]; and 2) A variety of effector cells, especially those induced in culture and probably polyclonally activated by xenogeneic serum or other mechanisms, can kill some of the NK-susceptible prototype targets, the best examples of those being promonocytes[3], anomalous killers (AK)[4] or the T-like killers[5,6] described in different laboratories. One may argue that the first case is the actual reflection of NCMC being a truly heterogeneous system, as we originally proposed[1,7-11], and extensively corroborated in other laboratories[5,12-16]. The second alternative is probably a spurious heterogeneity, since as we indicated in a recent review, "...not everything that kills YAC or K-562 in vitro is an NK cell..."[17].

The NCMC effector system has some unique properties that sets it aside from the conventional T,B or macrophage-mediated phenomena. These properties are: 1) Pre-existence at high levels in normal hosts with no need for priming, once the system develops in ontogeny; 2) shows no evidence of immunological memory, although it may show some "specificity" or "selectivity"; 3) the levels of activity are regulated by interferon (at least for the NK system); 4) the effector cells show no restriction for target killing related to the major histocompatibility complex; 5) have complex genetic influences which affect the levels and type of activity, different from those regulating conventional immune responses; and 6) is mediated by an heterogeneous population of effector lymphocytes of still undefined lineage. Although NK and NC cells in the mouse share most of the properties described above, they certainly have different genetic control and different regulatory mechanisms. In the present paper we will discuss some of these differences, as well as the questionable

Cancer: Etiology and Prevention, Ray G. Crispen, Editor

target preference of both systems[18,19] and their possible role as an anti-tumor surveillance mechanism[20].

SOME COMPARISONS BETWEEN NK AND NC CELLS

In the past we produced long listings comparing the properties of murine NC and NK cells[1,7,8,10,11,17], which we certainly are not going to repeat here. The picture that emerged from those listings was that although there were some clear differences between the two systems (especially in genetic control and surface antigenic markers; see refs. 1, 10, 21 & 22 for genetics of NC cells and ref. 23 for review on NK genetics; see refs. 1, 7-9, 11, 18 & 24 for surface markers on NC cells, as well as comparisons with NK cells; see ref. 2 for extensive review on murine NK markers), there were substantial similarities to warrant the proposition that NC and NK cells belonged to a family of effector cells mediating NCMC[1,7]. Several of our more recent studies are worth mentioning. For example, using a marker such as Qa5 which is present in resting or spontaneous NK cells, as well as in activated NK cells[5,25], but absent from NC cells[11], we could show that the NC activity detected in the long-term assays (18 to 24 hrs) was not due to an in vitro activated NK cell[24,26]. Conversely, the cytotoxicity detected in long-term assays when using NK-susceptibile targets and mice with genetically determined low NK activity, such as those carrying the beige mutation or other strains such as A/J, PL/J, I/St or SJL/J, is mediated exclusively by Qa5$^+$ NK cells[22,26]. Using velocity sedimentation at unit gravity we could also separate NC and NK, as well as other effector cells (K and macrophages) from murine peritoneal washings[27], based on differences in volume; a task which was not so easy with more overlap when comparable studies were done with spleen cells[8]. In addition, NK cells with different volume of size have also been described, depending on target used and stage of activation[14]. Thus, as is the case with NK cells[14], NC cells also show differences in size and/or volume depending on tissue source[8,27]. Concerning the genetics, we could define three genes which possibly control NC activity and which do not have detectable effects on NK activity[22], however, the three genes are probably located in a region of chromosome 17 distal to the D-end of H2[22], which has been shown to be an important region in the control of NK activity[23]. Finally, although the prototype NK and NC-susceptible targets are derived from tumors of different histologic types (lymphomas for the former and chemically-induced fibrosarcomas or "solid tumors" for the latter[1,2]), we could show that such different targets share "antigens" or "recognition structures" based on cold target competition studies[11,28,29].

Thus, NK-susceptible targets could block the killing of NC-susceptible targets[28] and NC targets could block the killing of NK-susceptible targets[11], by the appropriate effector cells.

The nature of the target structures being recognized by NK and NC cells is still undefined[1,2]. The blocking of NK or NC-mediated cytotoxicity by simple monosaccharides associated to the cell membrane[28,29] suggested the hypothesis that lectin-like receptors on the effector cells were recognizing appropriate concentrations or displays of sugars associated with cell surface glycoproteins or glycolipids[29], however, such is not the case since the monosaccharides appear to affect a post-recognition event related to lysis (our unpublished studies). However, it is still of interest and perhaps related to the "antigens" (as well as to surface receptor endocytosis[30]) that the NC-susceptible targets show a preference for D-mannose, not shown by the NK-susceptible targets[29].

On the other hand, since the emergence of the "large granular lymphocyte" (LGL) in human blood as the main NK effector cell in humans[31], there has been such a concentration of studies on these cells[32-34], that other possible NCMC effector cells are quite neglected, in spite of some possible human NC homologues when studying melanoma adherent targets[35], or the marked serological heterogeneity of the LGL population[34]. One additional point is that in all of the studies with LGL cells separated by Percoll fractionation, (see for one example ref. 32), it is apparent that while in some of the fractions there is excellent agreement between LGL numbers and cytotoxic activity, it is usual that the fraction above has too many LGL and too little cytotoxicity, while the fraction below has too much cytotoxicity for the number of LGL in that fraction. Thus, the present situation with the human studies with NK cells (i.e. LGL) is somewhat comparable to the early studies with the murine NK system, where the properties of the effector cell capable of killing YAC targets was considered the absolute paradigm that defined the system, ignoring the apparent heterogeneity of effector mechanisms and regulation (see ref. 36 for a good example of the dogmatic simplification of the earlier studies, which is worth comparing with reference 2, also analysing murine NK cells). In mice, although an LGL homologue has been described which indeed has NK-like activity[37], it is apparent that heterogeneity of effector cells based on effector cell type, surface markers and regulatory factors is well accepted. Table 1 summarizes some of the main properties of the different NCMC effector subsets, as well as the different terminologies proposed for such populations.

TABLE 1

TERMINOLOGY AND CHARACTERISTICS OF MURINE NATURAL CELL-MEDIATED CYTOTOXICITY

Nomenclature of references:

1,7,11	NK	–	–	NC	–	–
13	NK_L	–	–	NK_S	NK_C	–
15,16	NK_A	–	–	NK_B	NK_C	–
5	NK_I	NK_T	T_K	NK_M	–	–
4	–	–	–	–	AK	–
40,41	–	–	–	–	–	NK lines

Antigens:

Thy 1^-	Thy 1^+	Thy 1^+	Thy 1^-	Thy 1^+	Thy 1^+
Lyt 2^-	Lyt 2^-	Lyt 2^+	Lyt 2^-	Lyt 2?	Lyt 2^-
NK^+	NK?	NK?	NK^-	NK^+	NK?
Qa 5^+	Qa 5^+	Qa 5^-	Qa 5^-	Qa 5^+	Qa 5?
Ly 5^+	Ly 5^+	Ly 5^+	Ly 5^+	Ly 5?	Ly 5^+

Regulators:

IF	IL-2	IL-2	IL-2	IF	IL-2
			IL-3	IL-2	
				FCS	

Nomenclature: Shows the different nomenclatures for the NCMC effector cells and their appropriate references.

Antigens: Describes the surface antigens detected on the different subtypes. "NK" applies to the NK 1 and 2 antigens described in reference 42 and 43; the antigenic profiles of the different cell types are also described in the above cited references.

Regulators: See text. IF means interferon, FCS means fetal calf serum.

FACTORS THAT REGULATE NCMC ACTIVITY: INTERFERON AND INTERLEUKINS

   In addition to the overall genetic differences in NCMC reactivity described in the previous section, one established fact about NCMC is that its levels and activity are affected by soluble cellular products such as interferon[2,19,36] or interleukin-2 (IL-2)[5,38]. As a matter of fact, we included in one review[1] that the regulation by interferon was one of the properties of the NCMC system. However, we have recently found that the NC system seems less susceptible to regulation by interferon or interferon-inducers than the NK system[18], at schedules of administration and dosages which produced marked increase in NK activity either after in vivo or in vitro treatment[18]. Furthermore, in all instances in which boosting of cytotoxicity was observed after in vivo treatment with the interferon inducer poly-IC, when tested with otherwise NC-susceptible targets, all of the increased cytotoxic activity was due to a superimposed activated NK population, defined serologically by the presence of the Qa5 surface marker[18]. An interferon insensitive "NK-like" cell in bone marrow termed NK_M has been recently described[5], which we feel is comparable to the NC cells detected in spleen and marrow[1] (see also Table 1).

Table 2 shows that IL-2 can augment both NK and NC activity, when the spleen cells are preincubated for 24 hrs with the factor, and that interleukin-3 (IL-3)[39] augments only NC activity without affecting NK levels. Table 2 also shows that, based on expression of the Qa5 surface marker (which is present on NK[5,25] and absent from NC cells[11]) the IL-2 augmented cytotoxic activity is mediated by distinct populations of NK and NC cells, depending on the target used for testing. Similarly, the augmented activity induced by IL-3 is exclusively mediated by a Qa5⁻ cell population, i.e. by NC cells. These differences in regulation by "factors" is also depicted in Table 1.

TABLE 2

EFFECT OF PREINCUBATION (24 hr) WITH IL-2 OR IL-3 ON NC AND NK ACTIVITY AND EFFECT OF TREATMENT WITH ANTI-Qa5 AND C ON CYTOTOXIC ACTIVITY AGAINST WEHI 164 (NC TARGET) AND YAC.1 (NK TARGET)

| Treatment of cells | Anti-Qa5 + C | Type of target and % cytotoxicity at different E:T | | | | | |
| | | WEHI 164 | | | YAC 1 | | |
		100	50	25	100	50	25
Fresh	No	47	37	21	27	24	18
24 hr. inc.	No	46	29	26	9	9	3
IL-2	No	79*	63*	51*	47*	38*	15*
IL-3	No	62*	56*	45*	11	8	7
Fresh	Yes	47	33	24	8	3	1
24 hr inc.	Yes	48	33	27	4	4	1
IL-2	Yes	70*	53*	48*	9	5	4
IL-3	Yes	66*	55*	36	4	5	1

Spleen cells from C57BL/6 mice were incubated alone or with IL-2 or IL-3 preparations for 24 hrs, washed and used either directly or submitted to treatment with anti-Qa5 monoclonal and C before assay for cytotoxicity on ^{51}Cr labelled cells (18 hr assays, using the above indicated E:T ratios). WEHI 164 is an NC-susceptible target (see ref. 13). IL-3 was a kind gift from Dr. J.N. Ihle and was used at a concentration of 20 ED50/ml per $5x10^6$ spleen cells/ml; see ref. 39 for further details on IL-3. IL-2 was prepared in our laboratory as described in ref. 44 and used at a concentration of 20 U/ml per $5x10^6$ spleen cells. * = significant differences.

In summary, it is apparent that NC and NK cells are both regulated by the T cell product IL-2, but are differentially affected by interferon (which augments NK but not NC) and IL-3 (which augments NC but not NK).

SOLID TUMORS ARE SUSCEPTIBLE TO NC AND NK CELLS

The fact that most of the interferon or poly-IC boosted activity, when detectable, is mediated by a superimposed NK component, rather than by NC cells, when target cells derived from solid tumors are used (i.e. putatively susceptible to NC and not to NK lysis, as in the original descriptions of NC[7,8], indicates that solid tumors, even some that belong to the NC-susceptible category, are also susceptible to lysis by activated NK cells[18]. By screening a relatively low number of solid tumors (approximately 25 tumors in which chemically induced fibrosarcomas were predominant) we could obtain examples of almost all the possible permutations (see ref. 18, also our unpublished observations): 1) Solid tumors killed only by NC cells (with no detectable augmentation by poly-IC, but showing augmentation by IL-2 or IL-3); 2) Solid tumors killed by NC and NK cells (usually with the NK component only detectable after poly-IC boosting; the most common case being tumors killed by spontaneous resting NC cells and by an additional component of poly-IC boosted NK cells) and 3) Solid tumors killed only by NK cells, (in some cases even by spontaneous resting NK cells, although in most cases killing was observed only after poly-IC augmentation). To complete the above picture, a recent paper has described a lymphoma which is lysed by an NC-like cell type[16]; in addition to the lymphomas usually lysed by resting or augmented NK cells[2].

The corollary of these observations is that the frequently quoted statement equating NK cells to an anti-lymphoma system[2,36] and NC as an anti-solid tumor (i.e. non-lymphoid, and certainly not meaning that "non-solid" tumors are gaseous or liquid!; a poor terminology indeed, retained by custom and which certainly is informative in spite of being inaccurate) is probably inaccurate and reflects only the apparent properties of the limited number of target cells used in the studies.

In addition, the fact mentioned above that NK and NC-susceptible targets share "antigens" or recognition structures[11,28,29], should be taken into account. Thus, it is not surprising that studies in man concentrating only on the peripheral blood NK population which can be recognized as LGL, would show that both lymphoid as well as solid tumors are susceptible to lysis by such cells[32].

NCMC AND SURVEILLANCE

A popular interpretation is the NCMC effector cells may be operative as a possible in vivo anti-tumor surveillance devise in a "Burnetian" sense[19]. We have discussed this possibility in some detail[20], indicating that indeed NCMC has some unique properties which act on incipient tumors in situ, especially the lack of time-consuming priming or activation (which are properties of T cells or macrophages) as well as the capacity to handle small numbers of tumor cells in situ[20]. We even postulated that since there are regional differences in tissue distribution of NK and NC cells, as well as of resting versus boosted activity[1], one may consider that tumor development or growth of transplanted tumors may depend on local factors such as mobilization of NCMC effectors or activation of NCMC precursors. The tumors that did develop would be on the "weak spots" of the NCMC system[17,20]. These peculiar weak spots may even explain the well known regional differences in tumor growth or development, recently reviewed by Auerbach and Auerbach[45]. On the other hand, it may well be that NCMC activity against tumors is only a by-product of its real function as a more general early defense mechanism against bacterial or other parasitic invaders, as we proposed for immune surveillance some time ago[20,46]. Immune surveillance, mediated by any imaginable defense mechanism, will probably remain for a long time as part of our voluntaristic ideology of imagining that the organism must have a defense system against malignancy, even in the face of its lack of accurate predictions as an hypothesis.

ACKNOWLEDGMENTS

We would like to thank Mr. Gene Pecoraro and Mr. Michael Cuttito for their technical help, and Ms. Linda Stevenson for preparing the manuscript. We would also like to apologize for the biased bibliography, but do to page limits we could not expand it to include many of the appropriate references. The experimental part of our work was supported by NIH grants CA-08748, CA-15988 and American Cancer Society grant IM-188.

REFERENCES

1. Stutman, O., Lattime, E.C. and Figarella, E.F. (1981) Federation Proc. 40, 2699-2704.
2. Roder, J.C., Karre, K. and Kiessling, R. (1981) Prog. Allergy 28, 66-159.
3. Lohmann-Mattes , M.L., Domzig, W. and Roder, J. (1979) J. Immunol. 123, 1883-1886.
4. Karre, K. and Seeley, J.K. (1979) J. Immunol. 123, 1511-1518.
5. Minato, N., Reid, L. and Bloom, R.B. (1981) J. Exp. Med. 154, 750-762.
6. Burton, R.C., Chism, S.E. and Warner, N.L. (1978) Contemp. Topics Immunobiol. 8, 69-106.
7. Stutman, O., Paige, C.J. and FeoFigarella, E. (1978) J. Immunol. 121, 1819-1826.
8. Paige, C.J., FeoFigarella, E., Cuttito, M., Cahan, A. and Stutman, O. (1978) J. Immunol. 121, 1827-1835.
9. Stutman, O., FeoFigarella, E., Paige, C.J. and Lattime, E. (1980) in Natural Cell-Mediated Immunity Against Tumors, Herberman, R.B., ed., Academic Press, New York, pp 187-229.
10. Stutman, O. and Cuttito, M.J. (1981) Nature 290, 254-257.
11. Lattime, E.C., Pecoraro, G.A. and Stutman, O. (1981) J. Immunol. 126, 2011-2014.
12. Kumar, V., Luevano, E. and Bennett, M. (1979) J. Exp. Med. 150, 531-547.
13. Burton, R.C. (1980) in Natural Cell-mediated Immunity Against Tumors, Herberman, R.B., ed., Academic Press, New York, pp. 19-35.
14. Tai, A., Burton, R.C. and Warner, N.L. (1981) J. Immunol. 124, 1705-1711.

15. Burton, R.C., Bartlett, S.P., Kumar, V. and Winn, H.J. (1981) Transplant. Proc. 13, 783-786.
16. Lust, J.A., Kumar, V., Burton, R.C., Bartlett, S.P. and Bennett, M. (1981) J. Exp. Med. 154, 306-317.
17. Stutman, O. (1982) in Human Cancer Immunology, Vol.6: NK cells, Fundamental Aspects and Role in Cancer. Serrou, B., Rosenfeld, C. and Herberman, R.B. eds., Elsevier, Amsterdam, in press.
18. Lattime, E.C., Pecoraro, G.A., Cuttito, M. and Stutman, O. (1982) in NK Cells and Other Natural Effector Cells. Herberman, R.B., ed., Academic Press, New York, in press.
19. Herberman, R.B. and Ortaldo, J.R. (1981) Science 214, 24-30.
20. Stutman, O. (1981) in The Handbook of Cancer Immunology, Vol. 7., Waters, H., ed., Garland STPM, New York, pp. 1-25.
21. Stutman, O. and Cuttito, M.J. (1980) in Natural Cell-Mediated Immunity Against Tumors, Herberman, R.B., ed., Academic Press, New York, pp. 431-442.
22. Stutman, O. and Cuttito, M.J. (1982) in NK Cells and Other Natural Effector Cells, Herberman, R.B., ed., Academic Press, New York, in press.
23. Clark, E.A. and Harmon, R.C. (1980) Adv. Cancer Res. 31, 227-285.
24. Lattime, E.C., Ishizaka, S.T., Pecoraro, G., Koo, G., and Stutman, O. (1982) in NK Cells and Other Natural Effector Cells, Academic Press, New York, in press.
25. Chun, M., Pasanen, V., Hammerling, U., Hammerling, G.F. and Hoffman, M.K. (1979) J. Exp. Med. 150, 426-431.
26. Lattime, E.C., Pecoraro, G.A., Stutman, O. (1982) Int. J. Cancer, in press.
27. Lattime, E.C., Pelus, L.M. and Stutman, O. (1982) in NK Cells and Other Natural Effector Cells, Herberman, R.B., ed., Academic Press, New York, in press.
28. Stutman, O., Dien, P., Wisun, R., Pecoraro, G. and Lattime, E.C. (1980) in Natural Cell-Mediated Immunity to Tumors, Herberman, R.B., ed., Academic Press, New York, pp. 949-961.
29. Lattime, E.C., Pecoraro, G.A., Stutman, O. (1982) in NK Cells and Other Natural Effector Cells, Herberman, R.B., ed., Academic Press, New York, in press.
30. Goldstein, J.L., Anderson, R.B.W. and Brown, M.S. (1979) Nature 279, 679-685.
31. Saksela, E., Timonen, T., Ranki, A. and Hayry, P. (1979) Immunol. Rev. 44, 71-123.
32. Landazuri, M.O., Lopez-Botet, M., Timonen, T., Ortaldo, J. and Herberman, R.B. (1981) J. Immunol. 127, 1380-1383.
33. Timonen, T., Ortaldo, J.R. and Herberman, R.B. (1981) J. Exp. Med. 153, 569-582.
34. Ortaldo, J.R., Sharrow, S.O., Timonen, T. and Herberman, R.B. (1981) J. Immunol. 127, 2401-2409.
35. Saal, J., Riethmuller, G., Hadam, M., Rieber, E.P., and Fleiner, J.M. (1979) in Natural and Induced Cell-Mediated Cytotoxicity, Riethmuller, G., Wernet, P. and Cudkowicz, G., eds., Academic Press, New York, pp. 89-98.
36. Kiessling, R. and Wigzell, H. (1979) Immunol. Rev. 44, 165-208.
37. Luini, W., Boraschi, D., Alberti, S., Aleotti, A. and Tagliabue, A. (1981) Immunology 43, 663-668.
38. Henney, C.S., Kuribayashi, K., Kern, D.E. and Gillis, S. (1981) Nature 291, 335-338.
39. Ihle, J.N., Rebar, L., Keller, J. Lee, J.C. and Happel, A.J. (1982) Immunol. Rev. 63, 5-32.
40. Dennert, G., Yogeeswaran, G. and Yamagata, S. (1981) J. Exp. Med. 153, 545-556.
41. Nabel, G., Bucalo, L.R., Allard, J., Wigzell, H. and Cantor, H. (1981) J. Exp. Med. 153, 1582-1591.

42.Glimcher, L., Shen, F.W. and Cantor, H. (1977) J. Exp. Med. 145, 1-8.
43.Burton, R.C. and Winn, H.J. (1981) J. Immunol. 126, 1985-1989.
44.Miller, R.A. and Stutman, O. (1982) J. Immunol. 128, 2258-2264.
45.Auerbach,R and Auerbach, W. (1982) Science 215, 127-132.
46.Stutman, O. (1975) Adv. Cancer Res. 22, 261-422.

RECOGNITION SITE HETEROGENEITY IN THE HUMAN NATURAL
KILLER CELL POPULATION

PAMELA J. JENSEN, PH.D.[+] AND HILLEL S. KOREN, PH.D.[++]

[+]NCI-Frederick Cancer Research Facility, P.O. Box B, Frederick, Maryland,
USA; [++]Immunology Division, Duke University Medical Center, Durham,
North Carolina, USA.

INTRODUCTION

Natural killer (NK) cells can lyse a variety of tumor target cells,
but the recognition mechanisms leading to productive interaction of the
effector cells with different target cells are not clearly understood.
To investigate whether NK cell recognition sites are heterogeneous, we
have developed a cellular immunoadsorption technique. NK cells selectively bind to monolayers of NK-sensitive target cells, permitting us
to isolate nonadherent and adherent populations that are respectively
depleted of or enriched for NK activity. By using several target
cells in a quantitative analysis of the depletion of NK activity in the
nonadherent fraction, we obtained evidence for donor-dependent heterogeneity in NK cell recognition sites.

MATERIALS AND METHODS

Effector cells. Human peripheral blood lymphocytes (PBL) depleted
of cells that adhere to plastic[1], were prepared for all experiments.
Large granular lymphocytes (LGL)[2] were also used in some experiments.

Cell lines. HSB, K562, and MOLT4, three human tumor cell lines
grown in suspension culture, were used as NK target cells and/or for monolayer fractionation. SB, a relatively NK cell-resistant human line, was
used as the target cell in the antibody-dependent cellular cytotoxity
(ADCC) assays.

Published 1983 by Elsevier Science Publishing Co., Inc.
Cancer: Etiology and Prevention, Ray G. Crispen, Editor

Monolayer fractionation. PBL or LGL were incubated on K562 or HSB monolayers[3] that had been prepared on plates coated with poly-L-lysine. Nonadherent cells were removed by decanting,[3] and adherent cells were recovered by further incubation[4] of the plates in 5 mM ethylenediamenetetraacetic acid. Fractions were tested immediately after separation and/or after overnight incubation at 37°C.

Cytotoxicity assays. NK and ADCC activities were measured[1] in 2-3 hr ^{51}Cr-release assays, using 4 or more effector-cell-to-target-cell (EC:TC) ratios. For determination of ADCC, SB target cells were labeled with trinitrobenzenesulfonic acid (SB-TNP) and a rabbit hyper-immune anti-TNP serum was added to the assay.

RESULTS AND DISCUSSION

Cytotoxic activity of PBL nonadherent and adherent to target cell monolayers. When tested on the day of fractionation or after overnight

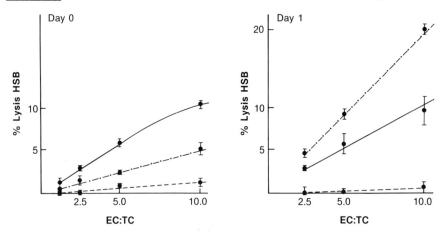

Figure 1. NK activity of nonadherent and adherent cells assayed on day 0 and day 1 after fractionation on HSB monolayers. PBL adherent (-·-) and nonadherent (---) to HSB monolayers were washed and assayed for NK activity immediately after separation (Day 0) or after incubation of the cells at 37°C for 16 hr (Day 1). Unfractionated control PBL (—) were also assayed concurrently. (From Jensen, P.J. and Koren, H.S., (1982) Immunobiol. 161, 494-506.)

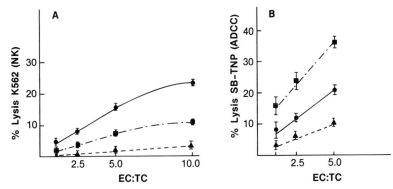

Figure 2. NK and ADCC activities of cells adherent and nonadherent to a K562 monolayer. PBL adherent (-·-) and nonadherent (---) to a K562 monolayer were washed and assayed immediately after separation, along with unfractionated PBL (——), for NK activity against K562 and ADCC activity against SB-TNP. (From Jensen, P.J. and Koren, H.S. (1982) Immunobiol. 161, 494-506.)

incubation, PBL nonadherent to HSB or K562 monolayers showed depleted NK activity [3,4] (Figs. 1 and 2A). In contrast, NK activity of the adherent cells measured on the day of fractionation[4] was intermediate between that of control, unfractionated PBL and that of nonadherent cells (Figs. 1 Day 0, and 2A). After overnight incubation, the cells adherent[4] to HSB monolayers consistently had greater NK activity than control PBL (Fig. 1 Day 1). This enhancement of NK activity was not routinely observed in fractions adherent to K562 monolayers after incubation; the reason for the difference in the two adherent fractions is presently unclear.

Since, in many cases, ADCC has been found to parallel NK activity, and the same cells may very well express both activities, we also examined ADCC levels in the monolayer-nonadherent and -adherent fractions. After fractionation on K562 or HSB monolayers, the nonadherent cells had depressed ADCC activity[5] (Fig. 2B). The cells adherent to either monolayer had levels of ADCC activity enriched relative to control PBL,

even when assayed on the day of fractionation[4] (Fig. 2B). These
data strongly suggest that NK cells selectively adhere to target monolayers and that this technique can be used to isolate NK cell-enriched
and NK cell-depleted populations.

NK activity of LGL adherent and nonadherent to target cell monolayers.
To investigate the possibility that other cell types might play a role in
the cellular interactions responsible for the enrichment and depletion of
NK cells after monolayer fractionation, we performed several experiments
with LGL, a population shown to be highly enriched for NK cells.[2] Fractionation of LGL on HSB or K562 monolayers yielded nonadherent and adherent
fractions that were respectively depleted of and enriched for NK activity
relative to control LGL. The results were very similar to those obtained
with whole PBL populations; therefore contaminating cell types probably
do not strongly influence the monolayer fractionation procedure.

Quantitative analysis of target monolayer adsorption. To examine
the question of NK cell recognition site heterogeneity, we quantitatively
analysed[3] the extent of depletion of NK activity in populations non-
adherent to K562 or HSB monolayers. Cytotoxic activity of control and
nonadherent populations as a function of EC:TC ratio was compared using
the slope ratio method. Slopes were always calculated in the linear
range of the curve with a weighted least squares linear regression
program. A comparison of the cytotoxic activity of the two populations
was generated with the following ratio:[3]

$$\text{slope ratio} = \frac{\text{slope of nonadherent PBL NK activity}}{\text{slope of control PBL NK activity}}$$

By comparing the ability of a single monolayer to deplete PBL
populations of NK activity against several different target cells, we
found two patterns of NK activity in the pool of seven donors tested.[6]
In one group, represented by donor HK in Table 1, K562 monolayers were

TABLE 1

RELATIVE DEPLETION OF NK ACTIVITY OF PBL AGAINST TUMOR TARGET CELLS

		K562 monolayer			HSB monolayer		
Target Cell:		K562	HSB	MOLT4	K562	HSB	MOLT4
			Slope ratios			Slope ratios	
PBL Donor	Expt. #						
HK	1	.26	.23	N.D.	.55	.40	N.D.
	2	.39	.35	.43	N.D.	N.D.	N.D.
	3	N.D.	N.D.	N.D.	.68	.33	.16
PJ	1	.23	.98	N.D.	.51	.17	N.D.
	2	.07	.85	N.D.	.41	.17	N.D.
	3	.33	1.05	.89	.53	.13	.17

Control PBL and PBL nonadherent to either HSB or K562 monolayers were
tested for NK activity against K562, HSB, and/or MOLT4 target cells at
four or more EC:TC ratios. The data from each target were expressed
as slope of activity of nonadherent PBL divided by slope of activity
of control PBL. N.D. = not determined.

able to deplete a PBL population of cytotoxic activity against K562,

HSB, and MOLT4 cells to an equivalent extent. In contrast, with the

other group of donors, represented by PJ in Table 1, fractions

nonadherent to K562 monolayers were much more depleted of anti-K562

activity than of anti-HSB or anti-MOLT4 activity. With either group of

donors when PBL nonadherent to HSB monolayers were tested, we found that

NK activity against HSB was depleted to a greater extent than NK

activity against K562 (Table 1). The donor-dependent differences in the

patterns of NK activity were stable during repeated experimentation over

the course of at least a year.

The findings described above from experiments that used only a

limited pool of donors and target cells suggest that the process of NK

cell recognition involves both heterogeneous and shared components.

K562 and HSB cells each appear to have at least one unique recognition site not found on the other, although they may share additional ones as well. NK effector cells also appear to be heterogeneous, with some cells recognizing either K562 or HSB cells and some recognizing both target cells. In addition, individual donors differ in their repertoire of NK cells. The biochemical nature of these heterogeneous recognition sites and the mechanism through which specific binding leads to cell lysis remain intriguing questions.

ACKNOWLEDGEMENTS

Research sponsored by Public Health Service grants CA23354 and CA09058-05 and in part by the National Cancer Institute, DHHS, under contract No. N01-CO-23909 with Litton Bionetics, Inc. The contents of this publication do not necessariy reflect the views or policies of the Department of Health and Human Services, nor does mention of trade names, commercial products, or organizations imply endorsement by the U.S. Government.

REFERENCES

1. Koren, H. and Williams, M. (1978) J. Immunol., 121, 1956-1960.
2. Timonen, T., Ortaldo, J.R. and Herberman, R.B. (1981) J. Exp. Med. 153, 569-582.
3. Jensen, P.J., Amos, D.B. and Koren, H.S. (1979) J. Immunol. 123, 1127-1132.
4. Jensen, P.J. and Koren, H.S. (1982) Immunobiol. 161, 494-506.
5. Jensen, P.J. and Koren, H.S. (1980) J. Immunol. 124, 395-398.
6. Jensen, P.J. and Koren, H.S. (1980) in Natural Cell-mediated Immunity Against Tumors, Ronald B. Herberman, ed., Academic Press, New York, pp. 883-892.

CHARACTERIZATION OF HUMAN NK CELLS BY USE OF MONOCLONAL ANTIBODIES

GERHARD WIEDERMANN[+], HELMUT RUMPOLD, GERHARD OBEXER, DIETRICH KRAFT[++] AND PETER MOSCHL[+++]

[+]Institute for Specific Prophylaxis and Tropical Medicine, University of Vienna, Kinderspitalgasse 15, A 1095 Vienna, Austria;[++]Institute of General and Experimental Pathology, University of Vienna, Währinger Straße 13, 1090 Vienna, Austria [+++]Second Department of Surgery, University of Vienna, Spitalgasse 23, 1090 Vienna, Austria

INTRODUCTION

Since the detection of the phenomenon of natural killing (NK) NK cells are increasingly considered as a surveillance mechanism of the body's defence against tumor cells and virus infected cells.[1] These cells present themselves as a functional entity. Recent studies indicate[2,3] that NK cells are included in a cell population of typical morphology, namely large lymphocytes with azurophilic granules (large granular lymphocytes, LGL). There is still not too much known, however, about their origin regarding T-B-cell or myelomonocytic lineage. In man low avidity E receptors and some other T cell associated antigens were found to be expressed on NK cells.[4-8] In other studies NK cells were unreactive with a monoclonal antibody (OKT3) recognizing an antigen common to all mature T cells;[9-11] they were marked, however, with OKM1 antibody which reacts with myelomonocytic and some E rosetting cells[9-11] and this contributed to the controversy about a possible myelomonocytic origin of NK cells. Recently, another monoclonal antibody, HNK-1, has been described,[12] which is considered to react selectively with NK cells.

In this study we investigated the expression of myelomonocytic as well as T cell associated antigens on human LGL by using various monoclonal antibodies.

MATERIAL AND METHODS

Monoclonal antibodies. Anti-Leu 1, -Leu 2a, -Leu 3a, -HLA-DR were purchased from Becton Dickinson (Sunnyvale, CA), anti-human Lyt-3 was obtained from New England Nuclear (Boston, MA) and OKM1 was acquired from Ortho Diagnostic Systems (Raritan, NJ). VEP8, VEP9, VEP13, either biotinylated or not, were those as described previously.[13,14] The characteristics of the used monoclonal antibodies are summarized in table 1.

TABLE 1

SUMMARY OF MONOCLONAL ANTIBODIES USED IN THIS STUDY

MoAb	IF-reactivity with (except LGL)	reference
VEP8	$76\pm5\%$ BM cells, > 95% PMNL, < 1% monocytes	13
VEP9	$68\pm6\%$ BM cells, > 95% PMNL, > 95% monocytes	13
VEP13	$6,8\pm4\%$ BM cells, > 95% PMNL	14
OKM1	20% periph. T (T_γ), > 95% PMNL, > 95% monocytes	15
anti-Leu 1	> 95% periph. T cells, 95 % thymocytes	16
anti-Leu 2a	20-40% PBL (T cytotoxic/suppressor subset) 80-90% thymocytes	17
anti-Leu 3a	40-60% PBL (T helper/inducer subset) 95% thymocytes	17
anti-human Lyt-3	> 99% peripheral T cells, > 99% thymocytes	18
anti-HLA-DR	B cells, monocytes / macroph., activ. T cells	19

MoAb = monoclonal antibody, BM = bone marrow, PMNL = polymorphonuclear-leucocytes. PBL = peripheral blood lymphocytes

Preparation of cells. Lymphocytes from human peripheral blood were prepared as discribed priviously by Rumpold et al.[20] Phagocytic cells were depleted by carbonyl iron and magnet treatment. LGL were enriched according to Timonen et al.[3] using Percoll gradient centrifugation.

Indirect membrane immunofluorescence (IMF) test. IMF tests were performed according to Schauenstein et al.[21] Fluorescein isothiocyanate (FITC) conjugated F(ab')$_2$ rabbit anti-mouse Ig reacting with IgG and IgM was used throughout the study. The commercially available antibodies were used according to the manufacturers instructions, VEP8 and VEP9 containing ascites were diluted 1:200. Purified VEP13 IgM or biotinylated VEP13 IgM antibodies were used 2 titer steps below the titer showing plateau fluorescence. For double staining cells were reacted with monoclonal antibody, subsequently with FITC-conjugated F(ab')$_2$ anti mouse Ig and thereafter with biotinylated monoclonal antibody and avidin-TRITC.

Cytotoxicity tests were performed as ^{51}Cr-release assays for 3 hours as reported previously.[20]

RESULTS

NK aktivity of PBL and LGL-enriched cell preparations

LGL enriched cell preparations were tested for spontaneous cytolytic activity against K562 targets. The LGL fractions (purity 75±15% LGL) showed a six to tenfold increase of cytotoxicity as compared to unfractionated lymphocytes (table 2).

TABLE 2

NK ACTIVITY OF PBL AND LGL PREPARATIONS ENRICHED BY PERCOLL^R GRADIENT CENTRIFUGATION AGAINST K562 TARGET CELLS

| E/T ratio | Cytotoxicity of | |
	PBL	LGL enriched prep.
40 : 1	43.8 ± 1.4	n.d.
20 : 1	36.8 ± 1.1	61.9 ± 1.4
10 : 1	27.6 ± 0.7	56.3 ± 2.5
5 : 1	17.9 ± 0.5	47.1 ± 1.9

spontaneous release 2.4 ± 0.4. Values are given as % ^{51}Cr release of triplicate samples (mean ± SD).

Phenotypes of LGL enriched cell preparations

Monoclonal antibodies reacting solely with myelomonocytic cells (VEP8 and VEP9) exhibited no reactivity with LGL enriched preparations (Table 3). Antibodies reacting with T cells or T-cell subsets showed the following pattern: only a low percentage of LGL was stained with the pan T cell marker anti-Leu 1 and the anti helper/inducer T cell antibody anti-Leu 3a, whereas a high number of cells was marked with anti-Leu 2a (59 ± 8 %) and anti-human Lyt-3 (55 ± 4%) which are directed against T suppressor/cytotoxic cells and the E receptor on lymphocytes, respectively. Monoclonal antibodies against antigens shared by myelomonocytic and lymphocytic cells exhibited strong reactivity in case of OKM1 (81 ± 11%), anti-HLA-DR, however, marked only 7 ± 3% of cells. VEP13 which in addition reacts with granulocytes stained a high number of LGL (75 ± 15%).

TABLE 3

REACTIVITY OF LGL ENRICHED CELL PREPARATIONS WITH VARIOUS MONOCLONAL ANTIBODIES
(NUMBER OF EXPERIMENTS IN PARENTHESES)

MoAb	reactivity by IMF %	MoAb	reactivity by IMF %
anti-Leu 1	13 ± 6 (3)	OKM1	81 ± 11 (7)
anti-Leu 2a	59 ± 8 (6)	HLA-DR	7 ± 3 (3)
anti-Leu 3a	4 ± 5 (3)	VEP8	< 1 (6)
anti-human Lyt-3	55 ± 4 (4)	VEP9	< 1 (5)
		VEP13	75 ± 15 (7)

MoAb = monoclonal antibody

Coexpression of various antigens on VEP13 positive cells

The newly developed VEP13 antibody which marks cells with LGL morphology
and high NK activity[14] was used to characterize the phenotype of LGL. Lymphocytes obtained by Ficoll-Hypaque centrifugation (depleted of granulocytes) and
marked by VEP13 coexpressed M1 ($84 \pm 6\%$), Leu 2a ($48 \pm 14\%$) and human Lyt-3
($52 \pm 17\%$) antigens. Other antigens (VEP8, VEP9, Leu 1, Leu 3a) were missing
or detectable only on a minor portion of cells (table 4). These experiments are
in accordance with the findings presented in table 3.

TABLE 4

COEXPRESSION OF VARIOUS ANTIGENS ON VEP13$^+$ PBL (3 EXPERIMENTS)

Antigens	% of VEP13$^+$ cells coexpressing other antigens as determined by double marker experiments
Leu 1	< 1
Leu 2a	48 ± 14
Leu 3a	< 1
Human Lyt-3	52 ± 17
M1	84 ± 6
HLA-DR	6 ± 4
VEP8	< 1
VEP9	< 1

DISCUSSION

Characterization of human NK cells has been hampered so far by the fact that these cells are a heterogenous population and represent only a relatively low percentage of peripheral blood mononuclear leucocytes. Enrichment of LGL which are held responsible for all NK activity by means of Percoll gradient centrifugation[3] improved this situation drastically. In our experiments monoclonal antibodies directed against various myelomonocytic or lymphocytic antigens were tested for reactivity with these cells thus providing more information about the surface phenotype and possible origin of LGL. Two monoclonal antibodies reacting exclusively with myelomonocytic antigens (VEP8 and VEP9) were tested. These antibodies recognize mature and a high percentage of immature myeloid cells. Neither of these antibodies was reactive with enriched LGL preparations. When testing monoclonal antibodies against several lymphocytic antigens for activity against LGL no or moderate reactivity was found with anti-Leu 1 and anti-Leu 3a. A high percentage of LGL was found, however, to be reactive with anti-human Lyt-3 and anti-Leu 2a antibodies. These antibodies recognize E receptors (Lyt-3) and the cytotoxic/suppressor T-lymphocyte subset. These findings are in agreement with West et al.[4] and Ortaldo et al.[6] When monoclonal antibodies against common antigens shared by myelomonocytic cells and lymphocytes were used a positive staining was found with OKM1 antibody confirming results of other authors.[9,10,11] Finally, experiments with VEP13 antibody provide evidence that LGL express an antigen which is also shared by granulocytes. When PMNL depleted cell preparations were used the reactivity pattern with VEP13 resembles that observed with HNK-1.[12] The results of the coexpression experiments are in accordance with the data assessing the phenotypes of LGL.

In conclusion our data demonstrate that LGL express antigens commonly found on T cells, myelomonocytic cells or both cell types. There are markers, however, normally reactive with lymphocytes, myelomonocytic cells or both which cannot be found on LGL. It seems as if LGL express phenotypes intermediate between lymphocytes and myelomonocytic cells. Regarding the origin of these cells one could speculate on three possibilities: Firstly, human NK cells might be immature T-cells which do not express the full antigenic profile of mature T cells; secondly, NK cells might represent a separate lymphoid subset reflecting phylogenetically a rest cell population inherited from a time when the full T cell repertoire had not yet developed; thirdly, NK cells might be capable of undergoing differentiation to either lymphocytes or myelomonocytic cells. Experiments inducing terminal differentiation steps will be necessary to clarify this questions.

190

ACKNOWLEDGMENT

This study was supported in part by the Austrian Science Research Fund, Project No. 4568 and Fonds der Österreichischen Nationalbank.

REFERENCES

1. Herberman, R.B., Timonen, T., Ortaldo, J.R., Bonnard, G.D. and Gorelik, E. (1980) in Progr. Immunol. IV, Fougereau, M., Dausset, J. ed., Academic Press London, New York, Toronto, Sydney, San Francisco, p. 691-709.
2. Saksela, E.T., Timonen, T., Ranki, A. and Häyry, P. (1980) Immunol.Rev.44, 71-123.
3. Timonen, T., Ortaldo, J.R. and Herberman, R.B. (1981) J. Exp. Med. 153, 569-582.
4. West, W.H., Cannon, G.B., Kay, H.D., Bonnard, G.D., and Herberman, R.B. (1977) J. Immunol. 118, 355-361.
5. Fast, L.D., Hansen, J.A. and Newman, W. (1981) J. Immunol. 127, 448-452.
6. Ortaldo, J.R., Sharrow, S.O., Timonen, T. and Herberman, R.B. (1981) J. Immunol., 127, 2401-2409.
7. Lohmeyer, J., Rieber, P., Feucht, H., Johnson, J., Hadam, M. and Riethmüller, G. (1981) Eur. J. Immunol. 11, 997-1001.
8. Kraft, D., Rumpold, H., Steiner, R., Radaskiewicz, T., Swetly, P. and Wiedermann G. (1981) in Mechanisms of lymphocyte activiation, Resch, K. and Kirchner, M. ed., Elsevier/North Holland Biomedical Press, Amsterdam, New York, Oxford, p. 279-281.
9. Kay, H.D., and Horwitz, D.A. (1980) J. Clin. Invest. 66, 847-850.
10. Zarling, J.M. and Kung, P.L., (1980) Nature 228, 394-396.
11. Breard, J., Reinherz, E.L., O'Brien, C. and Schlossman, S.F. (1981) Clin. Immunol. Immunopathol. 18, 145-150.
12. Abo, T. and Balch, C.M. (1981) J. Immunol. 127, 1024-1029.
13. Rumpold, H., Obexer, G. and Kraft, D. (1982) in Natural Cell Mediated Immunity, Vol. 2, Herberman, R.B., ed., Academic Press, London and New York, in press.
14. Rumpold, H., Kraft, D., Obexer, G., Böck, G. and Gebhart, W., J. Immunol. in press.
15. Breard, J., Reinherz, E.L., Kung, P.C., Goldstein, G. and Schlossman, S.F. (1980) J. Immunol. 124, 1943-1948.
16. Wang, C.Y., Good, R.A., Ammirati, P., Dymhart, G. and Evans, R.L. (1980) J. Exp. Med. 151, 1539-1544.
17. Evans, R.L., Wall, D.W., Platsoucas, C.D., Siegal, F.P., Testa, S.M. and Good, R.A. (1981) Proc. Natl. Acad. Sci, USA, 78, 544-548.
18. Kamoun, M., Martin, P.S., Hansen, J.A., Brown, M.A., Siadak, A.W. and Nowinsky, R.D. (1981) J. Exp. Med. 153, 207-212.
19. Lampson, L.A. and Levy, R. (1980) J. Immunol., 125, 293-299.
20. Rumpold, H., Kraft, D., Scheiner, O., Meindl, P. and Bodo, G. (1980) Int. Archs. Allergy. appl. Immun. 62, 152-161.
21. Schauenstein, K., Wick, G. and Kink, H. (1976) J. Immunol. Methods, 10, 143-150.

GENETIC AND EXTERNAL REGULATION OF NATURAL KILLER CELL CYTOTOXICITY IN MICE

PHYLLIS B. BLAIR, YVONNE R. FREUND, MARTHA O. STASKAWICZ, YASUKO FUKUDA
AND JUDITH SAM
Department of Microbiology and Immunology, and the Cancer Research Laboratory,
University of California, Berkeley, California 94720, USA

INTRODUCTION

Natural killer (NK) cells, which constitute one of the natural immune
mechanisms postulated to play a role in defense against neoplastic development and metastasis, are regulated by a number of genes controlling not only
NK cell number but also their lytic ability.[1] This basic control can be
significantly altered by environmental influences. Some factors, such as
viral infections[2] (which can increase interferon production), may stimulate
NK activity, whereas others, such as treatment with carcinogens,[3] may cause
a long-lasting depression. In many strains of mice, the normal level of NK
activity diminishes with age. As a consequence, not only the absence of
depressive environmental influences but also the presence of stimulatory
ones may be crucial for this system to function as a useful surveillance
mechanism in the ageing individual.

We present here studies on 11 inbred and recombinant inbred strains of
mice, and some of their hybrids, which demonstrate that the gradual loss of
normal NK activity with ageing is also accompanied by a loss in the ability
to respond to interferon induction with augmented NK activity. Further, we
provide evidence that differences in genotype can produce dramatic differences
in NK activity in mice chronically exposed to a virus in a contaminated mouse
colony. Finally, we present a genetic analysis of the effect of an oncogenic
agent, pristane, on NK activity. Pristane, which induces plasmacytomas in
some strains of mice, such as the BALB/c, suppresses not only T cell and B
cell responses but also NK activity.[4] We now report that there are significant strain differences in the effect of pristane on NK activity, as well as
differences in recovery from that depression. Studies of hybrids reveal that
the genetic mechanisms responsible for the pristane-induced loss of NK
activity in the BALB/c and in the C57BL strains are not the same.

© 1983 Elsevier Science Publishing Co., Inc.
Cancer: Etiology and Prevention, Ray G. Crispen, Editor

MATERIALS AND METHODS

Inbred mice from the colony of the Cancer Research Laboratory (C57BL, BALB/c, I, A, and 7 newly developed recombinant inbred strains, B, AD, AS, ABDS, ABS, ADS, and BPS) were used in these studies. Mice were virgin females in all experiments except the pristane studies, where only males were used.

Natural killer activity of spleen cells was measured in a standard 4-hour ^{51}Cr-release assay using the YAC-1 cell line as targets.[5] Spleen cells from each mouse were tested separately, using effector:target cell ratios of 25:1, 50:1, and 100:1. As expected, the level of cytotoxicity observed correlated with the ratios used; only data for the 100:1 ratio are presented here. Percent cytotoxicity was calculated by subtracting spontaneous isotope release from experimental release and from total release, and then dividing the former by the later calculated figure (x 100).

For augmentation of NK activity by polyinosinic:polycytidylic acid (Poly I:C), mice were injected with 100 mg Poly I:C (Sigma) intraperitoneally 18 hours before spleens were harvested.

In the pristane experiments, 2 month old male mice received one intraperitoneal injection of 0.5 ml pristane (2,6,10,14-tetramethylpentadecane, Aldrich Co.). Control males received an injection of saline.

Exposure to Sendai virus was not experimentally induced. The exposed mice were housed in colony rooms in which the mice were known to be infected with Sendai. Infection was confirmed by complement fixation assays for antibodies to Sendai virus (Microbiological Associates, Bethesda, MD); titers ranged from 10 to 80. Fifty-four mice of the strains included in the data presented here were tested during this time period, and 38 (70%) had positive antibody titers. The incidence of positive responders in mice of the I strain was 83%. Control mice (for comparison with the Sendai-exposed) were housed in different locations in rooms free of Sendai-infected animals, as were all other mice used in our NK studies.

RESULTS AND DISCUSSION

Baseline levels of NK activity and the effect of age

Genetic analyses have demonstrated that NK activity is under polygenic control with a major gene linked to the H-2.[1] Using our recombinant inbred strains, 6 of which carry the H-2^b haplotype derived from the C57BL strain and thus the linked NK activity gene, we have demonstrated that modifier genes can significantly affect the levels of NK activity.[5] In the age study reported here (Table 1), we have included 4 of these H-2^b strains (ABS, AD, ADS, and AS). One of these, ABS, has relatively little natural NK activity, whereas, in contrast, AS is as reactive as the C57BL strain (Table 2). With age, these responses diminish in each strain (Table 1). Nevertheless, at 6 months of age, mice of the AS strain are still more reactive than are mice of the other strains at their peak activity (2 months).

Table 1

EFFECT OF AGE ON NORMAL LEVELS OF NK ACTIVITY*

Strain	Average Percent Cytotoxicity Range in Parentheses)		
	2 months	4 months	6 months
BPS	2.9 (0.5 - 6.0)	1.0 (0 - 2.3)	0.2 (0 - 0.7)
ABS	6.2 (0 - 12.0)	4.6 (2.0 - 8.1)	4.3 (1.4 - 8.2)
AD	11.9 (9.8 - 15.2)	8.9 (4.4 - 14.3)	NT
ADS	15.3 (10.5 - 20.8)	9.5 (7.3 - 11.8)	3.4 (2.0 - 6.0)
AS	23.3 (13.1 - 36.5)	17.6 (15.4 - 20.5)	14.1 (12.8 - 16.3)

*In each group, 4-8 female mice were individually tested. NT = not tested.

Augmentation of NK activity by an interferon inducer and the effect of age

Poly I:C is a potent inducer of interferon production, and, as a consequence, mice treated with Poly I:C rapidly develop a significant increase in NK activity. In studies of our inbred and recombinant inbred strains, we have observed that females of every strain respond dramatically to Poly I:C treatment, even those of such low responder strains as the A, I, or BPS; data for 6 of our strains are presented here (Table 2). With age, this ability to respond to Poly I:C treatment diminishes (Table 3), but the augmentation observed is nevertheless significant, as comparison of the data in Table 3 with the control data in Table 1 will demonstrate.

194

TABLE 2

INDUCTION OF AUGMENTED NK ACTIVITY BY TREATMENT WITH POLY I:C*

Strain	Average Percent Cytotoxicity (Range in Parentheses)	
	Controls	Poly I:C Treated
BALB/c	9.3 (5.2 - 20.1)	39.4 (32.0 - 48.6)
BPS	2.9 (0.5 - 6.0)	33.0 (25.1 - 45.3)
ABDS	7.1 (4.0 - 13.0)	30.6 (24.7 - 37.3)
C57BL	22.1 (11.1 - 27.9)	42.1 (26.6 - 54.8)
I	2.4 (0.8 - 5.1)	25.3 (3.8 - 38.3)
A	0.9 (0 - 2.6)	33.5 (33.3 - 33.6)

*In each group, 4-8 female mice (aged 6-8 weeks) were individually tested, except strain A Poly I:C treated (2 mice), and A controls (3 mice).

TABLE 3

EFFECT OF AGE ON ABILITY TO RESPOND TO POLY I:C TREATMENT*

Strain	Average Percent Cytotoxicity (Range in Parentheses)		
	2 Months	4 Months	6 months
BPS	33.0 (25.1 - 45.3)	20.1 (13.3 - 30.4)	12.8 (9.4 - 15.5)
ABS	32.5 (26.2 - 40.8)	17.7 (12.1 - 20.7)	15.4 (14.4 - 16.5)
AD	40.0 (31.4 - 46.6)	33.8 (32.5 - 34.4)	NT
ADS	32.7 (26.7 - 39.8)	27.0 (17.2 - 31.9)	22.4 (20.7 - 24.7)
AS	54.2 (47.9 - 63.0)	43.5 (36.5 - 50.0)	38.3 (35.0 - 41.0)

*In each group, 4-9 female mice were individually tested. NT = not tested.

Genetic control of NK response to viral exposure

It is common to characterize inbred strains of mice as either high NK responders or low NK responders, but this is clearly a relative matter, since the "normal" NK activity of any strain is determined not just by the genotype of the mouse or the type of target cells used for assay, but is greatly influenced by the environment in which the mice are maintained. We had the undesired opportunity to demonstrate the importance of chronic viral infestations on NK activity when mice in some of our colony rooms became infected with Sendai virus. Presented in Table 4 are comparative data for 6 inbred strains maintained either in rooms in which the mice were known to be infected with Sendai virus or in rooms free of Sendai-infected mice. Three of these strains (BALB/c, BPS, and ABDS) appeared, under the exposed conditions, to be high NK responder strains, with reactivities equivalent to that observed in unexposed C57BL mice. The effect of the exposure on mice of the C57BL strain was not pronounced, and, most importantly, mice of two other strains (the I and the A) remained low NK responders under the exposed conditions. (Mice of the I and A strains can produce high NK activity under other conditions, as was demonstrated by data presented in Table 2.) An important conclusion may be drawn from this "experiment"; exposure to viruses such as Sendai leads to changes in baseline NK activity in some but not all mouse genotypes and thus attempts to compare NK data generated in different laboratories should take into account the conditions under which the animals are maintained in each laboratory.

TABLE 4

EFFECT OF MAINTENANCE IN A SENDAI-INFECTED MOUSE COLONY ON "NORMAL" LEVELS OF NK ACTIVITY*

Strain	Average Percent Cytotoxicity (Range in Parentheses)	
	Controls	Sendai-Exposed
BALB/c	9.3 (5.2 - 20.1)	18.1 (6.5 - 40.4)
BPS	2.9 (0.5 - 6.0)	21.8 (5.9 - 34.0)
ABDS	7.1 (4.0 - 13.0)	21.0 (20.6 - 21.4)
C57BL	22.1 (11.1 - 27.9)	29.2 (23.1 - 35.3)
I	2.4 (0.8 - 5.1)	5.1 (0.6 - 13.4)
A	0.9 (0 - 2.6)	4.1 (1.8 - 4.8)

*In each group, 6-14 female mice (aged 6-8 weeks) were individually tested, except ABDS and C57BL Sendai-exposed (2 mice each), BPS Sendai-exposed (4 mice), and A controls (3 mice). Control data are repeated from Table 2.

Genetic control of NK response to treatment with the oncogen pristane

In our previous studies on the effect of pristane on male BALB/c mice, we have observed that NK activity is significantly reduced within one month after the first pristane injection and remains depressed for at least 3 months. Further, the normal ability to respond with augmented NK activity after in vivo treatment with the interferon inducer Poly I:C is significantly depressed.[4] Lessened production of interferon in the pristant-treated mice is apparently a significant cause of this depression, but we also find that splenic NK cells of the treated mice are deficient in their ability to respond to interferon (unpublished observations). There are considerable strain differences in the effect of pristane treatment (Table 5). Some strains resemble the BALB/c in developing a significant depression of NK activity. However, two of our recombinant inbred strains (AD and AS) show no defect in NK response, and one strain (the I) shows a significant increase in activity.

TABLE 5

STRAIN DIFFERENCES IN EFFECT OF PRISTANE TREATMENT ON NK ACTIVITY*

Strain	Average Percent Cytotoxicity (Range in Parentheses)	
	Saline-Injected	Pristane-Injected
C57BL	18.0 (12.8 - 19.4)	7.6 (6.1 - 9.1)
BALB/c	7.3 (4.0 - 10.4)	1.4 (0 - 3.6)
B	12.2 (2.1 - 17.5)	1.0 (0 - 4.3)
ABS	6.8 (5.2 - 9.1)	0 (0)
AD	6.9 (5.3 - 10.0)	9.2 (6.5 - 11.3)
AS	17.3 (6.7 - 27.8)	21.8 (8.5 - 29.1)
I	0.6 (0 - 1.9)	5.1 (0 - 9.2)

*In each group, 2-12 male mice were individually tested at 3 months of age, 4 weeks after the inoculation of pristane.

Depression of NK activity following pristane treatment does not correlate with susceptibility to plasmacytoma development; both the BALB/c and the C57BL strains show depression, but only the former proceeds to develop tumors. However, hybrid studies reveal that the mechanism by which these two strains develop lack of responsiveness is different (Table 6). Since the hybrid of the C57BL and I strains resembles the C57BL parent in showing NK depression, the C57BL response must be controlled by a dominant gene or genes. However, the hybrid of the BALB/c and I strains does not resemble the BALB/c parent. Depression of NK activity is not seen after pristane treatment, and thus the BALB/c response must be controlled by a different (and recessive) gene or genes than that of the C57BL.

In BALB/c mice, the depression resulting from a single injection of pristane persists for at least 3 months. However, in one of our recombinant inbred strains (the B) recovery from the initial significant depression occurs within less than two months (Table 7). We are currently testing a number of strains to see if the inability to recover NK responsiveness after pristane treatment is correlated with the eventual development of plasmacytomas.

TABLE 6

STRAIN AND HYBRID DIFFERENCES IN EFFECT OF PRISTANE TREATMENT ON NK ACTIVITY*

Strain or Hybrid	Average Percent Cytotoxicity (Range in Parentheses)	
	Saline-Injected	Pristane-Injected
I	0.6 (0 − 1.9)	5.1 (0 − 9.2)
C57BL	18.0 (12.8 − 19.4)	7.6 (6.1 − 9.1)
(C57BL x I) (I x C57BL)	13.5 (5.2 − 33.0)	5.1 (1.2 − 9.6)
BALB/c	7.3 (4.0 − 10.4)	1.4 (0 − 3.6)
(BALB/c x C57BL)	19.4 (11.6 − 22.9)	3.2 (0 − 5.6)
(BALB/c x I)	9.4 (5.7 − 13.4)	8.5 (2.2 − 15.6)

*In each group, 5-12 male mice were individually tested at 3 months of age, 4 weeks after the inoculation of pristane. Data for the parental inbred strains are repeated from Table 5.

)

198

TABLE 7

STRAIN DIFFERENCES IN RECOVERY OF NK CYTOTOXIC ACTIVITY FOLLOWING THE INITIAL
PRISTANE-INDUCED LOSS OF ACTIVITY*

| Strain | Average Percent Cytotoxicity (Range in Parentheses) | | |
| | Saline-Injected | Pristane-Injected | |
		Early Response	Later Response
BALB/c	7.0 (2.0 - 11.5)	1.4 (0 - 3.6)	1.8 (0 - 5.0)
ABS	8.1 (5.2 - 11.7)	0 (0)	1.8 (1.1 - 3.1)
B	12.2 (2.1 - 16.5)	1.0 (0 - 4.3)	9.5 (8.3 - 11.2)

*In each group, 3-15 male mice were individually tested after the inoculation
of pristane. Mice in the early response groups were tested 4 weeks after the
inoculation of pristane, at 3 months of age. BALB/c mice in the later
response group were tested 12 weeks after the inoculation of pristane, and
ABS and B mice in the later response groups were tested 7-8 weeks after the
inoculation of pristane.

ACKNOWLEDGMENTS

These experimental studies were supported by grants from the National
Cancer Institute (CA-05388 and CA 09041), the American Cancer Society
(IM-69), and the Council for Tobacco Research (1490), and by research funds
of the University of California.

REFERENCES

1. Kiessling, R. and Wigzell, H. (1979) Immunological Rev., 44, 165-208.
2. Herberman, R.B., Nunn, M.E., Holden, H.T., Stall, S. and Dieu, J.Y.
   (1977) Int. J. Cancer, 19, 555-564.
3. Gorelik, E. and Herbermann, R.B. (1981) J. Nat. Cancer Inst. 66, 543- 548.
4. Freund, Y.R. and Blair, P.B. (1982) J. Immunol., in press.
5. Blair, P. B. (1980) in Natural Cell-Mediated Immunity Against Tumors,
   Herberman, R.B. ed., Academic Press, New York, pp. 401-410.

MODULATION OF MURINE NK CELL CYTOTOXICITY *IN VITRO*
AND ANTITUMOR ACTIVITY *IN VIVO* BY LOW MOLECULAR
WEIGHT INTERFERON INDUCERS.

EVA LOTZOVA[+], CHERYLYN A. SAVARY AND DALE A. STRINGFELLOW[++]
[+]Department of Clinical Immunology and Biological Therapy, The University of
Texas System Cancer Center, M.D. Anderson Hospital and Tumor Institute, Houston,
Texas; [++]Department of Cancer and Virus Research, The Upjohn Company, Kalamazoo,
Michigan

INTRODUCTION

In recent years it has become increasingly evident that natural killer (NK)
cells may play an important role in surveillance against neoplastic diseases.[1-5]
This implication rests primarily on the observations demonstrating that low NK
cell-responding, NK cell-deficient or NK cell-depleted mice display lower anti-
tumor activity.[6-9] In addition to their involvement in resistance to the establishment of primary malignancies, NK cells were implicated in resistance a-
gainst metastatic tumor growth in mice.[10-11] Most recently, several other functions were ascribed to NK cells. Some of these are natural resistance to micr-
obial, viral and fungal infections[5,12-13] and parasites,[5] natural resistance to
histoincompatible bone marrow transplants[14-16] and the involvement in auto-
immune diseases.[17] NK cells also possess the capability to produce interferon[18-19] and small amounts of T cell growth factor under certain conditions.[20]
Via production of these factors, NK cells may mediate self-regulation as well as
regulation of other components of lympho-hemopoietic systems. In fact, the observation that NK cells inhibited granulopoiesis *in vitro*[21] and enhanced
in vitro T cell colony-forming potential[22] substantiate their regulatory role
in hemopoiesis and lymphopoiesis.

Since NK cells were implicated in multifacet and sometimes diverse biological
functions, modulation of their activity in both positive and negative direction
is of interest. It would be for instance, desirable to augment NK cell activity
in cancer patients and on the contrary, to inhibit it in bone marrow recipients
to prevent rejection of marrow grafts. That such NK cell modulation is possible experimentally, was shown recently by us and others in transplantation
studies. Agents, such as hydrocortisone, glucan, cyclophosphamide, silica,

Cancer: Etiology and Prevention, Ray G. Crispen, Editor

and NK 1.1 antiserum were found to depress NK cell activity and simultaneously to prevent rejection of foreign hemopoietic tissues. [14-16,23-24] Reversely, the agents augmenting NK cell activity, mediated increased resistance to hemopoietic transplants (Lotzová, unpublished observations).

NK cell activity *in vitro* and antitumor resistance *in vivo* was found to be augmented by various natural and synthetic factors. The first category of factors is represented by bacterias, such as *Bacille Calmette-Guerin* and *Corynebacterium parvum* (the latter bacteria however, can also cause NK cell suppression under certain conditions), by various viruses, tumor cells and interferons (IFN). [2,25-27] Agents, such as poly I:C, tilorone, statolon and pyran copolymer are the representatives of the second category of NK cell-augmentors. [2,28-29] Interestingly, most of these NK cell-augmenting agents are also IFN inducers, the observation suggesting that IFN may be of primary importance in regulation of NK cell functions.

In this study, we have investigated the effect of three new IFN-inducing pyrimidinone molecules on murine NK cell activity. The following pyrimidinones were used in our studies: 2-amino-5-bromo-6-phenyl-4-pyrimidinol (ABPP), 2-amino-5-bromo-6-meta fluoro phenyl-4(3H)-pyrimidinol (ABmFPP), and 2-amino-5-iodo-6-phenyl-4-pyrimidinol (AIPP). These molecules do not possess only IFN-inducing properties, but exhibit also antiviral and antineoplastic properties, in animals. [30-31] Moreover, ABPP is being clinically investigated for its cancer therapeutic potential, in Phase I study at our Institute.

MATERIALS AND METHODS

Experimental animals

Inbred females of A/He, C57BL/6 (B6), BALB/c, DBA/2, C3H/Anf, CBA, AKR, [C57BL/6 X DBA/2]F_1 (B6D2F$_1$) and [C57BL/6 X BALB/c]F_1 (B6CF$_1$) strains of mice were used in these experiments. Most of the mice were 10-16 weeks old, except for B6CF$_1$ mice which were both, adult (6-11 weeks old) and infant (13-18 days-old).

Pyrimidinone molecules

Three pyrimidinone molecules were used: ABPP, ABmFPP and AIPP. ABPP and ABmFPP are potent IFN inducers, and AIPP is a weak IFN inducer. [31] Pyrimidinones were suspended in saline and injected in the dose of 250 mg/kg into each mouse, intraperitoneally (i.p.). Because of the poor solubility of pyrimidinones, these agents were ground and vigorously mixed by Vortex to achieve an uniform suspension.

Determination of IFN levels

IFN levels were determined (in Dr. Stringfellow's laboratory) in serum and peritoneal exudate of control and pyrimidinone-treated mice, as described previously.[31] A standard vesicular stomatitis virus plaque reduction assay was performed on murine L929 cells.[31]

Preparation of effector cells

Spleen and bone marrow cell suspensions were prepared as described in detail before.[32] Peritoneal exudate (PE) cells were harvested by massage of peritoneal cavity after injection of 3 ml of saline and aspiration of exudate with a Pasteur pipette. When large numbers of cells were required, the exudates from several animals were pooled.

Target cells

Murine T cell lymphoma, YAC-1, acute myelogenous leukemia, Cl498 and human acute myelogenous leukemia, K-562 were used in these studies. All target cells were grown as continuous cultures in RPMI 1640 medium.[24]

NK cell cytotoxicity assay

NK cell activity was assessed in ^{51}Cr release cytotoxicity assay as reported in detail earlier.[33] Briefly, 10^4 of ^{51}Cr labelled target cells were incubated with effector cells (target-to-effector cell ratio 1:50) at 37°C in a 5% CO_2 humidified atmosphere for 4 hours. Spontaneous release of ^{51}Cr was determined by incubating the target cells with medium alone, and ranged from 5-9%. Maximum release of ^{51}Cr was determined after freezing and thawing tumor cells four times and ranged from 85-95%. The percentage of cytotoxicity was determined according to the following formula:

$$\frac{\% \text{ exp. release} - \% \text{ spont. release}}{\% \text{ max. release} - \% \text{ spont. release}} \times 100$$

Evaluation of tumor-binding cells

Percentage of tumor binding cells was determined according to Roder.[34] Briefly, two million of YAC-1 cells were mixed with 2×10^5 of fluorescein isothiocyanate labeled effector cells in 0.2 ml of RPMI 1640. The mixture of target and effector cells was then centrifuged (200 x G) for 5 min (20°C) and placed on ice for an additional 30 minutes. The percentage of fluorescing effector cells, binding to nonfluorescing target cells was determined after counting 200 cells.

Irradiation

In some experiments, control and pyrimidinone-treated mice were irradiated from a ^{60}cobalt radiation source (at the rate of 40 R/min).

Statistical analysis

The difference between experimental and control groups was evaluated statistically with a Student's t test, and the probability (P) was calculated.

RESULTS

Augmentation of NK cell activity by pyrimidinones

Initially, we have tested the effect of 3 different pyrimidinones, i.e. ABPP, ABmFPP and AIPP on PE NK cell cytotoxicity of B6D2F$_1$ hybrid mice. As illustrated in Figure 1 A, untreated B6D2F$_1$ mice exhibited low levels of PE NK cell cytotoxicity against T cell lymphoma, YAC-1 (mean 6.8% ± 1.0). However, after the injection of either of the pyrimidinones (250 mg/kg, i.p.), a strong and consistent augmentation of NK cell cytotoxicity was demonstrated.

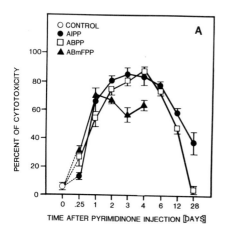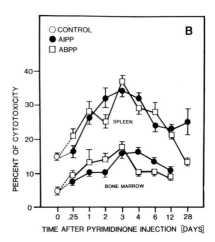

Fig 1. Augmentation of NK cell cytotoxicity in PE (A), spleen and bone marrow (B) of B6D2F$_1$ mice against YAC-1 by pyrimidinones. Symbols represent the mean % of cytotoxicity ± S.E. of 6-12 mice. Augmentation was significant at all points (P values ranged from <0.05-<0.001) except of splenic and bone marrow cytotoxicity at 6 hours after AIPP treatment.

Enhanced NK cell cytotoxicity was evident as early as 6 hrs after a single injection, and progressed with time. The peak of NK cell activity was achieved

2-4 days post treatment, at which time the cytotoxicity reached levels as high as 60-90%. The effect of pyrimidinones was relatively long-lasting, since the augmented PE-NK cell levels were sustained for 12 days after ABPP and 28 days after AIPP administration.

In the next study, we investigated sensitivity of splenic and bone marrow NK cell cytotoxicity of the same mice to modulation by pyrimidinones (Figure 1B). We selected for these experiments older B6D2F$_1$ mice with relatively low splenic NK cell cytotoxicity. Similarly to the PE, both AIPP and ABPP augmented significantly splenic and bone marrow NK cell cytotoxicity to YAC-1 (P value <0.05-<0.001, except of splenic and bone marrow cytotoxicity 6 hours after AIPP injection). Even though the peak and decline of splenic and bone marrow NK cell augmentation was comparable to those of PE, the degree of augmentation in the former organs was lower.

Strain distribution of pyrimidinone-mediated NK cell augmentation

To determine whether pyrimidinone-mediated NK cell augmentation was restricted to B6D2F$_1$ hybrid mice, or represented a more general phenomenon, 7 inbred strains of mice with identical or different H-2 haplotypes were tested. The results of these experiments are illustrated in Figures 2 and 3. As Figure 2 illustrates, NK cell cytotoxic potential in peritoneal cavity of all untreated mouse strains studied, was very low. However, substantial increases in PE NK cell activity were observed in each strain of mice,3 days after i.p. administration of 250 mg/kg of ABPP or AIPP. Interestingly, and perhaps most importantly, PE cytotoxicity was induced not only against allogeneic target cells, but also against syngeneic tumors. Anti-syngeneic reactivity was demonstrated by a 17-fold increase of NK cell cytotoxicity from A strain of mice to YAC-1. NK cell

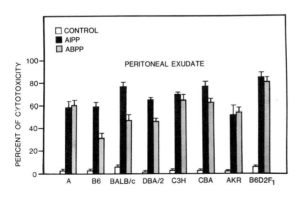

Fig.2. Strain distribution of pyrimidinone-mediated NK cell augmentation. Bars represent mean % of cytotoxicity ± S.E. of 4-12 mice.

cytotoxicity to YAC-1 was also augmented in the spleens of various strains of mice,3 days after injection of both pyrimidinones (Figure 3).

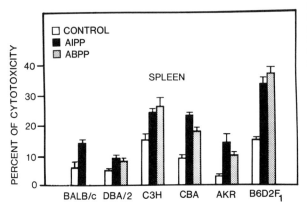

Fig.3. Strain distribu-
tion of pyrimidinone-
mediated NK cell augmen-
tation. Bars represent
mean % of cytotoxicity ±
S.E. of 4-12 mice.

Pyrimidinone-mediated NK cell cytotoxicity was not displayed only to YAC-1, but also to Cl498, another allogeneic target, and to xenogeneic target, K-562 (unpublished data).

Effect of pyrimidinones on NK cell activity of infant mice

Results from our and other laboratories have shown that NK cell activity is not expressed in mice less than 3-4 weeks old. [14,35] Thus, it was of interest to determine whether NK cell activity of young $B6CF_1$ mice could be induced by pyrimidinones. Figure 4A and B indicates that both AIPP and ABPP were effect-ive in inducing NK cell cytotoxicity in the spleen and PE of infant mice (13-18 days old), when injected 1-3 days prior to NK cell test. In the spleen, the pyrimidinone-induced NK cell cytotoxicity (3 days after injection) of in-fant mice resembled that of control adult mice, and in the PE, it was signifi-cantly above that of adult control mice. These experiments indicate that pyri-midinones not only potentiate pre-existing NK cell cytotoxicity, but also in-duce NK cell activity in young, NK cell-lacking mice.

Characterization of effector cells involved in pyrimidinone-mediated augmentation of cytotoxicity

Since pyrimidinones are also macrophage-stimulating agents, [31] it was impor-tant to determine the possible role of macrophages in pyrimidinone-augmented PE and splenic NK cell cytotoxicity. As evaluated by latex-ingesting technique, [36] the AIPP and ABPP-augmented PE and splenic cytotoxicity was not affected by

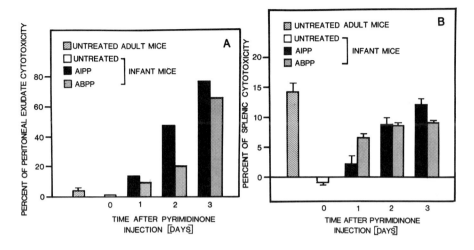

Fig. 4. Induction of PE (A) and splenic (B) NK cell activity of infant B6CF$_1$ mice. Bars represent mean % of cytotoxicity ± S.E. of 2-10 mice. Bars without S.E. represent pool of PE cells from 2 mice.

treatment with carbonyl iron [37] or silica, [38] treatments resulting in <1% of phagocytic cells. Furthermore, the activity was not removed by glass-adherence (Figure 5 and 6). These studies indicate that the pyrimidinone-augmented PE and splenic cytotoxic cells were not of macrophage nature.

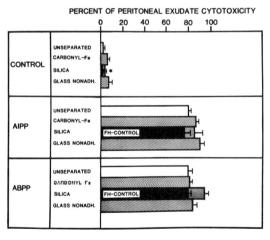

Fig. 5. Effect of macrophage-depleting techniques on pyrimidinone-augmented PE cytotoxicity of B6D2F$_1$ mice (3 days after treatment) against YAC-1. Bars represent the mean % of cytotoxicity ± S.E. of 5 experiments. Silica-ingesting cells were removed from other cell populations on Ficoll-Hypaque gradient, according to Tracey. [38] Asterisk indicates that the control suspensions were also processed on Ficoll-Hypaque gradient.

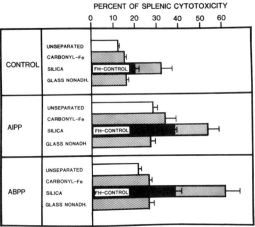

PERCENT OF SPLENIC CYTOTOXICITY

Fig. 6. Effect of macrophage-depleting techniques on pyrimidinone-augmented splenic cytotoxicity of B6D2F$_1$ mice (3 days after treatment) against YAC-1. Bars represent the mean % of cytotoxicity ± S.E. of 5 experiments. Silica treatment was the same as indicated in legend of Figure 5.

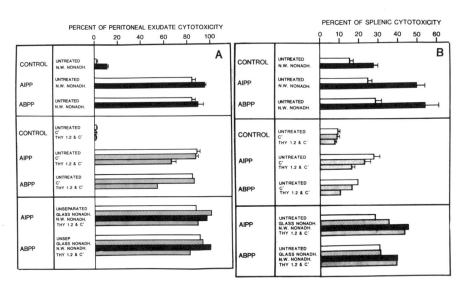

Fig. 7. Effect of B cell and T cell-depleting procedures on pyrimidinone-augmented PE (A) and splenic (B) cytotoxicity of B6D2F$_1$ mice (3 days after treatment). Bars represent mean % of cytotoxicity ± S.E. of 3 experiments. Bars without S.E. indicate a single experiment.

Further characterization studies demonstrated that both splenic and PE cytotoxic potential was not abolished by treatment with Thy-1.2 monoclonal antibodies and complement (Figure 7), despite the fact that such treatment was ef-

fective in removing >95% of thymocytes and 30% of splenocytes. Based on these
experiments, mature cytotoxic T cells did not appear to mediate pyrimidinone-
stimulated cytotoxicity. A slight decrease in cytotoxic potential, observed after Thy-1.2 treatment, was compatible with sensitivity of a subpopulation of NK
cells to Thy-1.2 antisera. [39] Nylon wool fractionation experiments (Figure 7)
revealed that cytotoxic cells were present in the nylon wool-filtered fraction
(composed of <2% of B cells, as determined by direct immunofluorescence technique), thus eliminating B cells as effectors in this system. Moreover, cytotoxicity was fully expressed after exposure of splenocytes and PE cells to combined multiple treatments, composed of glass adherence, nylon wool fractionation, and Thy-1.2 antiserum and complement treatment (Figure 7). These treatments resulted in removal of a majority of macrophages, T cells, and B cells,
and in a substantial enrichment of null cell population(s). Results from all
of these characterization experiments indicated that NK cells are the cytolytic
cells.

Some studies on the mechanism(s) of pyrimidinone-augmented NK cell cytotoxicity

Effect of irradiation and silica. We have shown earlier that pyrimidinone-
augmented cytotoxic cells were radioresistant and were not destroyed by macrophage-depleting agent, silica. In these studies, we tested whether the mechanism of augmentation is sensitive to silica (i.e., is macrophage-dependent)
or to irradiation. Silica was injected into B6D2F$_1$ mice i.p., 1 or 3 days before injection of AIPP; NK cell activity was tested 3 days post AIPP treatment.
Two different doses of silica were used, 3 mg or 10 mg/mouse.

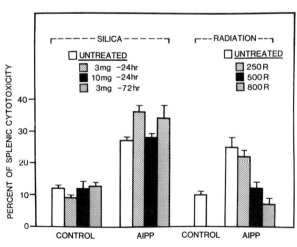

Fig. 8. Effect of silica
and irradiation on py-
rimidinone-mediated
splenic NK cell augment-
ation of B6D2F$_1$ mice.
Bars represent mean % of
cytotoxicity ± S.E. of
2 experiments.

208

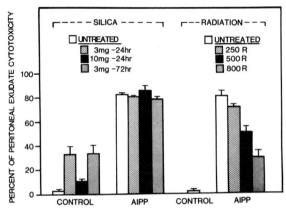

Fig. 9. Effect of silica and irradiation on pyrimid-inone-mediated PE NK cell augmentation of B6D2F$_1$ mice. Bars represent mean % of cytotoxicity ± S.E. of 2 experiments.

As can be seen from Figures 8 and 9, both splenic and PE NK cell augmentation was comparable in silica-pretreated and silica-free mice. These experiments indicate that macrophages are not necessary for AIPP-mediated NK cell augmentation. Similarly, B6D2F$_1$ mice were irradiated with either 250, 500 or 800R of total body irradiation and 1-2 hrs later injected with AIPP. Splenic and PE NK cell cytotoxicity was assayed 3 days post AIPP injection. Pre-irradiation with 250R showed no effect on augmentation of splenic or PE NK cell cytotoxicity; significant reduction in the degree of PE NK cell augmentation was observed after 500 and 800R of irradiation(P<0.05 and <0.01, respectively). In the spleen, no augmentation was observed after irradiation of mice with 500 and 800R, since the NK cell cytotoxicity of pre-irradiated and AIPP treated mice was comparable to control mice (Figures 8 and 9).

Effect of pyrimidinones on NK cell tumor-binding properties. We have also tested the effect of AIPP and ABPP on the capacity of splenic and PE NK cells to bind to YAC-1 tumor. Nylon wool filtered cell populations were used in these studies, to avoid possible non-specific tumor cell binding, which was observed previously in unseparated cells from various tissues.[34]

It can be seen from Table 1 that the efficiency of PE NK cells to bind to YAC-1 tumor was significantly augmented by both pyrimidinones; the augmentation index was 1.5 (P<0.05) and 1.8 (P<0.02) following administration of AIPP and ABPP, respectively. However, the tumor-binding NK cell properties remained unchanged in the spleen.

Involvement of IFN in pyrimidinone-mediated NK cell augmentation. Since IFN has been shown previously to be one of the powerful NK cell stimulators,[18-19,33] and the pyrimidinones are IFN inducers, we considered the possibility that NK cell augmentation by pyrimidinones, may be IFN-mediated. Interestingly, however, ABPP and AIPP were equally effective in NK cell stimulation, despite the fact that the former is a strong and the latter a poor inducer of serum IFN (Figure 10). Additionally, ABmFPP, which also induced significantly higher levels of serum IFN than AIPP, was less efficient as an NK cell augmentor. We reasoned, that this apparent discrepancy cannot be taken to indicate that IFN does not play a role in NK cell induction by pyrimidinones, since locally produced, rather than circulating IFN, may be involved. In fact, our preliminary results illustrated in Figure 10 indicate that AIPP, although not an inducer of circulating IFN, induces significant levels of IFN in peritoneal cavity. The final proof of IFN involvement in pyrimidinone-mediated NK cell augmentation, however, will come from experiments with specific anti-IFN antibodies.

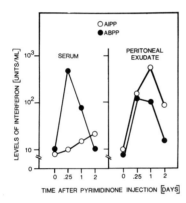

Fig. 10. Interferon levels in serum and peritoneal cavity of control and pyrimidinone-treated $B6D2F_1$ mice. The points represent the mean of serum or PE IFN levels of 7 mice. Standard error of the mean was 20%.

TABLE 1

EFFECT OF PYRIMIDINONES ON NK CELL TUMOR-BINDING AND KILLING PROPERTIES

Tissue	Treatment	Percent of Cytotoxicity[a]	Percent of TBC[a]
Spleen	None	27.7 ± 6.2	20.5 ± 2.1
	AIPP	51.6 ± 4.0	23.2 ± 2.1
	ABPP	55.3 ± 9.6	23.3 ± 4.1
Peritoneal	None	12.3 ± 1.9	19.4 ± 2.7
Exudate	AIPP	92.7 ± 3.7	29.9 ± 0.8
	ABPP	95.5 ± 6.5	35.5 ± 2.7

[a]Cytotoxicity and tumor-binding cell (TBC) potential was tested 3 days after pyrimidinone injection. Values represent mean ± S.E. of 3 experiments. Cytotoxicity was tested in ^{51}Cr release cytotoxicity assay. $B6D2F_1$ mice were used.

Effect of AIPP on the growth of adenocarcinoma 755 *in vivo*

In the next series of experiments, we investigated the effect of AIPP on the growth of ascitic tumors (mammary adenocarcinoma 755) of B6 origin in B6D2F$_1$ hybrid mice. As indicated in Table 2, control mice invariably died within 17 days after tumor injection. In contrast, B6D2F$_1$ mice injected with 2 or 3 injections of AIPP (250 mg/kg, i.p.) survived more than 4 months after tumor inoculation, without any signs of tumor growth. These experiments suggest that AIPP exerts protective effect on tumor growth.

TABLE 2

EFFECT OF AIPP ON THE GROWTH OF ADENOCARCINOMA 755 IN B6D2F$_1$ MICE

No. of Tumor Cells Injected[a]	Treatment (Days)[b]	Survival of Mice (Days)[c]
1.2 X 10^5	None	17
	AIPP −3, + 3	128[d]
	AIPP 0, + 1, + 3	150
5.0 X 10^5	None	14
	AIPP −3, + 3	111
	AIPP 0, + 1, + 3	150

[a]Mammary adenocarcinoma 755 was injected i.p. on day 0.
[b]AIPP was injected i.p. in a dose of 250 mg/kg.
[c]Values represent mean of 16-20 mice.
[d]Mice were sacrificed on indicated days.

In summary, our findings that pyrimidinone molecules are powerful stimulators of NK cells, together with the observation that they exhibit antitumor properties suggest that these agents may be of particular importance in cancer therapy. Indeed, it is plausible to postulate that the antitumor properties of pyrimidinone molecules observed in experimental animals, may, at least in part, be mediated by NK cells.

ACKNOWLEDGEMENT

This work was supported by the Grant CA 31394 from NCI. The technical assistance of A. Khan and G. Spotts and secretarial assistance of J. White is greatly appreciated.

REFERENCES

1. Kiessling, R. and Haller, O. (1978) Contemp. Topics in Immunobiol. 8, 171-201
2. Herberman, R.B. and Holden, H.T. (1978) Adv. Cancer Res. 27, 305-377.
3. Lotzová, E. and McCredie, K.B. (1978) Cancer Immunol. and Immunother. 4, 215-221.

4. Herberman, R.B. (1980) Clinical Immunobiol. 4, 73-88.
5. Herberman, R.B. and Ortaldo, J.R. (1981) Science 214, 24-30.
6. Klein, G.O., Klein, G., Kiessling, R., and Karre, K. (1978) Immunogenetics 6, 561-569.
7. Riccardi, C., Santoni, A., Barlozzari, P., Puccetti, P., and Herberman, R.B. (1980) Int. J. Cancer. 25, 475-486.
8. Karre, K., Klein, G.O., Kiessling, R., Klein, G., and Roder, J.C. (1980) Nature 254, 624-626.
9. Pollack, S.B., and Hallenbeck, L.A. (1982) Int. J. Cancer 29, 203-207.
10. Hanna, N. (1980) Int. J. Cancer. 26, 675-680.
11. Hanna, N. and Fidler, I.J. (1980) J. Natl. Cancer Inst. 65, 801-809.
12. Lopez, C. (1980) in: Genetic Control of Natural Resistance to Infection and Malignancy, Skamene, E. Kingshaun, P.A.L. Landy, M. ed., Academic Press, New York, pp. 253-263.
13. Welsh, R.M. and Kiessling, R.W. (1980) Scand. J. Immunol. 11, 363-367.
14. Lotzová, E. and Savary, C.A. (1977) Biomedicine 27, 341-344.
15. Kiessling, R., Hochman, P.S., Haller, O., Shearer, G.M., Wigzell, H., and Cudkowicz, G. (1977) Eur. J. Immunol. 7, 655-663.
16. Lotzová, E. and Savary, C.A. (1982) Transplantation, in Press.
17. Oshimi, K., Gonda, N., and Sumiya, M. (1980) Clin. Exp. Immunol. 40, 83-88.
18. Trinchieri, G., Santoli, D., Dee, R.R., and Knowles, B.B. (1978) J. Exp Med. 147, 1299-1313.
19. Djeu, J.Y., Timonen, T., and Herberman, R.B. (1981) in: Progression Cancer Research and Therapy, Chirigos, M.A. Mastrangelo, M.J. Mitchel, M. Krim, M. ed., Raven Press, New York, pp. 161-166.
20. Domzig, W., Timonen, T.T., and Stadler, B.M. (1981) Proc. AACR 22, 309.
21. Hanson, M., Beran, M., Andersson, B., and Kiessling, R. (1982) J. Immunol. 129, 126-132.
22. Pistoia, V., Perata, A., Nocera, A., Ghio, R., Leprini, A., and Ferraini, M. Exp. Hematol. 10, 78-89 (Abstract).
23. Lotzová, E. and Gutterman, J.U. (1979) J. Immunol. 123, 607-611.
24. Lotzová, E. and Savary C.A. (1981) Exp. Hematol. 9, 766-774.
25. Wolfe, S.A., Tracey, D.E., and Henney, C.S. (1976) Nature 262, 584-586.
26. Gidlund, M., Orn, A., Wigzell, H., Senik, A., and Gresser, I. (1978) Nature 273, 759-761.
27. Herberman, R.B., Nunn, M.E., Holden, H.T., Staal, S., and Djeu, J.Y. (1977) Int. J. Cancer 19, 555-564.
28. Djeu, J.Y., Heinbaugh, J.A., Holden, H.T., and Herberman, R.B. (1979) J. Immunol. 122, 182-188.
29. Santoni, A., Puccetti, P., Riccardi, C., Herberman, R.B., and Bonmassar, E. (1979) Int. J. Cancer 24, 656-661.
30. Weed, S.D., Kramer, G.D., and Stringfellow, D.A. (1980) in: Current Chemotherapy and Infectious Disease, Nelson, J.D. and Grassi, C. ed., Amn. Soc. Microbiol Wash, D.C., pp. 1408-1409.
31. Stringfellow, D.A., Vanderberg, H.C., and Weed, S.D. (1981) J. Interferon Res. 1, 1-14.
32. Lotzová, E. (1977) J. Immunol. 119, 543-547.
33. Lotzová, E., Savary, C.A., Gutterman, J.U., and Hersh, E.M. (1982) Cancer Res. 42, 2480-2488.
34. Roder, J.C. and Kiessling, R. (1978) Scand. J. Immunol. 8, 135-144.
35. Savary, C.A. and Lotzová, E. (1978) J. Immunol. 120, 239-243.
36. Arala-Chaves, M.P., Key, M., Fett, J.W., Porto, M.T., and Fudenberg, H.H. (1978) Scand. J. Immunol. 8, 81-89.
37. Kiessling, R., Klein, E., Pross, H., and Wigzell, H. (1975) Eur. J. Immunol. 5, 117-121.
38. Tracey, D.E. (1979) J. Immunol. 123, 840-845.
39. Mattes, M.J., Sharrow, S.O., Herberman, R.B., and Holden, H.T. (1979) J. Immunol. 123, 2851-2860.

EFFECT OF BACILLUS CALMETTE GUÉRIN ON NATURAL KILLER CELL ACTIVITY IN
RANDOM BRED RATS

WIM H. DE JONG[+], PIET S. URSEM[++], WIM KRUIZINGA[++], AB D.M.E. OSTERHAUS[++] AND
E. JOOST RUITENBERG[++]
[+]Fellow of the Koningin Wilhelmina Fonds of the National Cancer League;
[++]National Institute of Public Health, Laboratory for Pathology, P.O. Box 1,
3720 BA Bilthoven, The Netherlands.

ABSTRACT

The effect of BCG on natural killer (NK) cell activity was investigated in
male random bred rats. The NK cell activity was determined in a 4 h ^{51}Cr release
assay using a microcytotoxicity system with YAC lymphoma target cells.

Both live and irradiated (600,000 Rad, ^{60}Co) BCG stimulated NK activity in
the spleen at day 4 after i.v. administration. At day 7 after i.v. BCG administration spleen NK cell activity had returned to control levels. Oral and subcutaneous BCG had no effect on spleen NK cell activity. Intraperitoneal administration of live BCG caused apart from a stimulation of peritoneal NK cell activity, an increase in spleen NK cell activity. Plastic adherent peritoneal cells
showed a measurable spontaneous cytotoxicity in the 4 h ^{51}Cr-release assay,
which was enhanced after i.p. BCG.

BCG was found to cause a significant but relatively modest stimulation of NK
cell cytotoxicity. The stimulation was dependent on the route of administration;
i.v. treatment mainly increased spleen NK cell activity, i.p. administration
mainly increased peritoneal NK cell activity.

NK cell stimulation by BCG occurred in the absence of interferon induction,
since in sera of BCG treated rats no interferon could be demonstrated.

INTRODUCTION

For the last decade Bacillus Calmette Guérin (BCG) has been intensively
studied for its immunopotentiating and possible anti-tumor properties. In spite
of the effect of BCG on the immune system and the anti-tumor activity in animal
tumor systems, in clinical studies anti-tumor effects have been described only
occasionally[1-3]. Much effort has been directed to study the influence of BCG on
tumor cytotoxic effector cells since these cells are probably directly related
to a possible anti-tumor effect of BCG. In vitro generation of specific cytotoxic lymphocytes against allogeneic and syngeneic tumors was shown to be potentiated after BCG treatment[4-5]. Not only the phagocytic and killing capacities
of macrophages are enhanced by BCG[6], but also the cytotoxic capacities[7-8].

In mice and rats natural killer (NK) cell activity was found to be stimulated after in vivo treatment with live or heat killed BCG[9-10].

Natural killer (NK) cells are cells capable of tumor cell lysis in vitro without previous sensitization (reviewed in 11). These NK cells are suggested to be part of a surveillance system against malignancies[11-13]. Besides BCG also other substances, experimentally used for immunotherapy of cancer, may cause an increase in NK cell activity such as Corynebacterium parvum, pyran, poly I : C and interferon[14, 15]. Interferon seems to be linked with the augmentation of NK cell activity. Macrophages were found to play an important role in the production of interferon after poly I : C administration[16] and also in the regulation of the enhancement of NK activity after BCG administration[17]. However, each living cell is probably capable to produce interferon dependent on the stimulus used; T-cells[18, 19], non T-cells, probably B-cells[20] and NK cells[21] were reported to be able to produce interferon.

Most of the work in the enhancement of NK cell activity was performed in inbred strains of mice and rats which are known to have a relatively consistent reaction pattern. Since clinical immunotherapy is being applied in a heterogenous population it is relevant to determine whether the stimulation of NK cell activity after BCG administration is also present in individuals from an random bred population.

We studied some functional aspects of NK cell stimulation by BCG in random bred rats. Various dosages of live and irradiated BCG were compared in their ability to stimulate spleen NK cell activity. For live BCG different routes of administration were investigated (intravenous, intraperitoneal, subcutaneous and oral) for effect on spleen NK activity. Peritoneal NK cell activity was studied after intraperitoneal and intravenous BCG treatment.

MATERIALS AND METHODS

Animals. Seven weeks old male random bred rats, Wistar derived and raised in our Institute (Dr.B.C.Kruijt, Department of Breeding of Laboratory animals) under specified pathogen free conditions, were used for all experiments. Prior to and during the experiments the animals were housed in laminar flow cabinets.

BCG preparations. BCG-RIV lots 060A and 065A were produced in our Institute by Dr.R.H.Tiesjema (Laboratory of Vaccine Production) as concentrated preparations, especially intended for experimental immunostimulation[22].

The bacteria were grown in homogeneous culture under continuous stirring in Ungar medium with 0,05% Tween 80[R], harvested by centrifugation, resuspended in a stabilizing medium (containing 83 g/l Haemaccel[R], 50 g/l glucose and 50 mg/l

Tween 80^R), filled in 2 ml portions and lyophilized. Lot 060A contains per vial 36 x 10^6 culturable particles (c.p.) in 0.30 mg dry weight, and lot 065A 200 x 10^6 c.p. in 0.80 mg dry weight. Dead BCG was prepared by irradiating with 600,000 Rad ^{60}Co. BCG was administered by various routes as indicated in the figures.

Effector cells of spleen, mesenteric lymph node and thymus were harvested by pressing organ fragments through nylon gauze (100 μm) with the continuous addition of cold Hank's solution (without Ca^{++} and Mg^{++}). Cell suspensions were pelleted and erythrocytes were lysed by adding 0.3 ml sterile H$_2$O for ten seconds. This process was stopped by adding 5 ml minimal essential medium (MEM). Bone marrow cells were harvested by flushing the marrow of tibia and femur with cold Hank's solution (without Ca^{++} and Mg^{++}) supplemented with DNase (3 mg/100 ml) and heparin (10 IU/ml) to prevent clumping of the cells. Peritoneal exudate cells (PEC) were harvested by washing the peritoneal cavity three times with 5 ml cold Hank's solution (without Ca^{++} and Ng^{++}). Blood lymphocytes (PBL) were isolated with Lymphoprep with a density of 1.077 g/ml (Nyegaard and Co., Oslo, Norway) from heparinized whole blood obtained from the aorta under ether anaesthesia. After washing, the cells were resuspended in RPMI 1640 medium supplemented with penicillin (100 IU/ml), streptomycin (100 μg/ml), fugizone (0.25 μg/ml) and 10% heat inactivated fetal calf serum (Gibco, Grand Island, N.Y. USA). Viable cells were counted by trypan blue (0.5%) exclusion in a hemocytometer. During processing the cell suspensions were kept on melting ice.

^{51}Cr-release assay. The cytolytic activity was determined with a microcytotoxicity system as previously described[23], using xenogeneic murine YAC lymphoma target cells of A/Sn Moloney leukemia origin[24]. In short, ^{51}Cr labeled YAC target cells were incubated with lymphoid cells at various effector to target cell (E : T) ratios for 4 h at 37°C in a humidified atmosphere with 5% CO$_2$. Before and after the incubation period the microtiter trays (Removawell System, Dynateck Companies, Zug, Switzerland) were centrifuged for 3-5 min at 1000 rpm. The percentage ^{51}Cr release was determined by measuring the radioactivity in half of the supernatant and half of the supernatant plus sediment. The radioactivity was determined in a γ counter and expressed as counts per minute (cpm). The percentage release was calculated according to the formula:

$$\% \text{ release} = \frac{2 \times \text{cpm } (\tfrac{1}{2} \text{ supernatant})}{\text{cpm (sediment} + \tfrac{1}{2} \text{ supernatant)} + \text{cmp } (\tfrac{1}{2} \text{ supernatant})} \times 100$$

The cytolytic activity was expressed as specific release i.e. percentage experimental release minus percentage spontaneous release. The spontaneous release was determined by incubating 1 x 10^4 labeled target cells with medium alone (200 µl) and with 1 x 10^6 (ratio 1 : 100) unlabeled target cells. The spontaneous release varied from 3 to 8%. In general, addition of unlabeled target cells caused 1% less spontaneous release when compared with incubation with medium alone.

Interferon induction and assay. For the demonstration of interferon induction in rats by BCG sera were collected before harvesting the lymphoid cell populations. Also six weanling rats were inoculated i.v. with 1.0 ml of each BCG preparation (1 x 10^7 and 1 x 10^8 c.p.). At four hours intervals during 24 hours after BCG administration, serum samples were collected and pooled per six animals and stored at -70°C before testing. For control purposes similar groups of six rats were inoculated with 10^9 plaque forming units (pfu) of sindbis virus obtained from Dr.B.A.M.van Zeist (Institute of Virology, Veterinary Faculty, State University, Utrecht, The Netherlands) or intramuscularly with one human dosis of dog kidney cell rabies vaccine (produced in our Institute). 100 µl volumes of serial twofold dilutions of pooled serum samples were tested in an interferon assay on Ratec cells (kindly supplied by Dr.H.Schellekens, T.N.O., Rijswijk, The Netherlands) by demonstration of the reduction of cytopathic effect (cpe) of 10-30 tissue culture infective doses 50% ($TCID_{50}$) of vesicular stomatitis virus. The assay was carried out in a microtiter system, essentially as described by Billiau and Buckler[25]. Highest serum dilutions showing complete reduction of cpe were determined. Positive samples were retested for cpe reduction on Ratec and baby hamster kidney (BHK) cells after pH_2 treatment and dialysis to demonstrate that the reduction was caused by interferon.

Statistical analysis. Student's-t-test was used to calculate two-sided significance of difference between control and treated groups of animals. For evaluation of the overall results for all experiments in time Fisher's combination test was used[26].

RESULTS

Spontaneous cytotoxicity in random bred rats. In figure 1 the organ distribution is presented of spontaneous cytolytic activity in six weeks old random bred rats. The peritoneal cavity expressed the highest cytolytic activity against YAC target cells. Spleen cells showed less activity and PBL very low activity, whereas cells from bone marrow, mesenteric lymph node and thymus expressed no activity (spec.rel. < 1% at E : T ratio 100).

Dose response studies with BCG. Dose response investigations were performed at day 4 after intravenous (i.v.) administration. At high dose levels both live and irradiated BCG significantly enhanced NK activity in the spleen. As shown in in fig. 2, after live BCG (1×10^7 c.p.) a specific release of $40.5 \pm 6.3\%$ was found versus $17.6 \pm 3.6\%$ in the control group (E : T 100, $p < 0.001$). Irradiated BCG (1×10^7 c.p.) augmented the specific release to $35.1 \pm 3.4\%$ versus $20.6 \pm 6.0\%$ in the control group (E : T 100, $p < 0.01$) after i.v. inoculation (data not shown). An almost equal activation was found after 10^7 or 10^8 live BCG, this was also seen after 10^7 or 10^8 irradiated BCG. A marginal activation was noted after 10^6 live BCG.

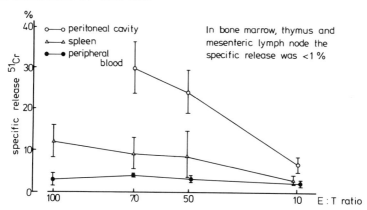

Figure 1.

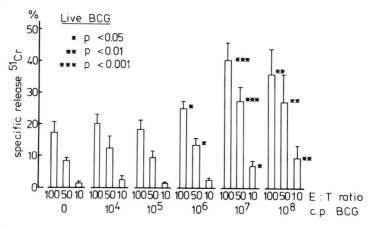

Figure 2.

As rat NK cells have been reported to be non-adherent[27] in both experiments spleen NK cell activity was determined in the total cell population as well as in the adherent and non-adherent fraction. The non-adherent fraction was

isolated from the wells of the microtiter tray by vigorously pipetting. Four
days after i.v. injection of 10^7 or 10^8 live and dead BCG the specific release
in the adherent fraction was increased from < 1% to 5% (data not shown). As
shown in fig. 3, no differences in specific release were found between the total
spleen cell population and the non-adherent fraction of the same spleen cell population. Consequently in the other experiments only the total spleen cell population was investigated for NK cell activity.

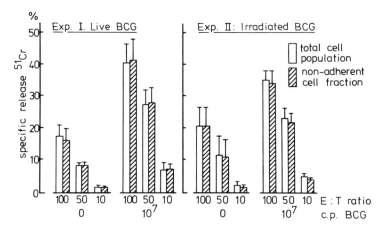

Figure 3.

Effect of route and time interval of BCG administration on spleen NK cell
activity. Live BCG (1 x 10^7 c.p.) was administered by the intravenous (i.v.),
intraperitoneal (i.p.), subcutaneous (s.c.) or oral route. Both i.v. and i.p.
administration of BCG-RIV 060A caused a significant (p < 0.01) increase of
spleen NK cell activity (table 1). With BCG-RIV 065A only i.v. treatment caused
a statistically significant stimulation (p < 0.05) of spleen NK cell activity,
whereas i.p., s.c. and oral administration did not enhance NK cell activity.

Since, in general, a wide range of specific release was found both in the
control group (5.6 - 38.5%) and in the BCG treated animals (13.1 - 49.1%), many
treated animals showed an NK cell activity within the range of the control group.
Fig. 4 shows the distribution of spleen cytolytic activity of control and BCG
treated animals (10^7 c.p. at day -4).

Although in all experiments performed an augmentation of spleen NK cell activity was found at day 4 after i.v. BCG treatment, the results were not always
statistically significant (Student's-t-test). When the results of all experi-

TABLE 1

EFFECT OF BCG (1 x 10^7 C.P. AT DAY -4) ON NK CELL ACTIVITY IN THE SPLEEN OF
7-WEEKS OLD MALE SPF RANDOM BRED RATS (TARGET CELLS: MURINE YAC LYMPHOMA)

	E : T ratio 100		
	control	BCG-RIV 060 IV	BCG-RIV 060 IP
Exp. 1	17.6 + 3.6 (4)[a]	40.5 + 6.3 (4)***	-
2	8.2 + 2.8 (4)	21.5 + 4.3 (4)**	11.5 + 3.4 (4)
3	20.4 + 5.9 (4)	29.6 + 6.3 (4)	21.8 + 3.9 (4)
4	13.9 + 3.3 (4)	23.2 + 6.9 (4)	16.3 + 5.4 (4)
5	18.9 + 4.1 (11)	32.3 + 9.3 (12)**	-
6	20.1 + 3.6 (12)	-	26.6 + 5.7 (12)**
1-6[b]		p < 0.001	p < 0.001
	control	BCG-RIV 065 IV	BCG-RIV 065 IP
Exp. 7	19.9 + 2.9 (7)[a]	28.3 + 11.2 (8)	18.0 + 4.1 (8)
9	17.4 + 4.6 (9)	27.0 + 9.5 (12)	-
10	28.0 + 5.4 (12)	-	31.8 + 5.7 (12)
7-10[b]		p < 0.01	n.s.

[a] specific release, mean + s.d. (n)
[b] Fisher's combination test.
* p < 0.01.
** p < 0.001.

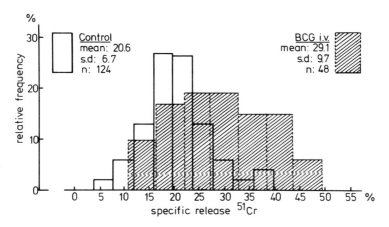

Figure 4.

ments were combined, i.v. treatment of random bred rats with BCG-RIV 060A or
BCG-RIV 065A resulted in highly significant (p < 0.001 and p < 0.01 respectively)
increase of NK cell activity in the spleen (table 1). Also the overall results
of i.p. administration of BCG-RIV 060 showed a significant (p < 0.001) increase
in NK cell activity in the spleen.

At day 7 after i.p. administration, BCG-RIV 065A caused a stimulation
(p < 0.05) of spleen NK activity, whereas i.v. administration had no effect
(data not shown). As the effect of i.v. injection of BCG seemed to be an acute
and short lasting phenomenon, also spleen NK cell activity was determined at
day 2 after injection. However, at that time, no effect on spleen NK cell activity was found (data not shown).

Effect of BCG on PEC NK cell activity. To assess the effect of BCG administration, NK cell activity of the peritoneal cavity was investigated at day 4
after i.v., i.p. and s.c. administration of live BCG. Only i.p. BCG caused significant enhancement (p < 0.01) of NK cell activity in the total cell population. Fig. 5 shows the cytolytic activity of PEC after i.v. and i.p. administration. In an experiment in which also the adherent and non-adherent fractions
were tested, the adherent cell fraction of control animals had not only a measurable activity (ca. 10% spec. rel.) but this activity was significantly
(p < 0.01) enhanced after i.p. treatment with BCG (fig. 5).

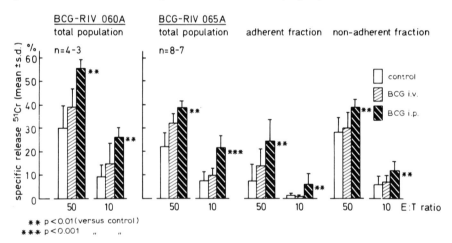

Figure 5.

Interferon induction. In sera of rats used for the determination of NK cell
activity after various routes of BCG administration no interferon activity could

be demonstrated. Also in pooled serum of weanling rats no activity could be shown during a 24 h period after inoculation of 10^7 and 10^8 c.p. BCG. Fig. 6 shows the interferon activity demonstrated in pooled sera of control groups of rats which were inoculated with sindbis virus (10^9 pfu) or rabies vaccine (one human dose). Interferon levels found in rats inoculated with 10^9 pfu sindbis virus showed a course similar to but exceeding those found by other workers using a similar system[25]. This indicates that the sensitivity of the interferon assay was satisfactory.

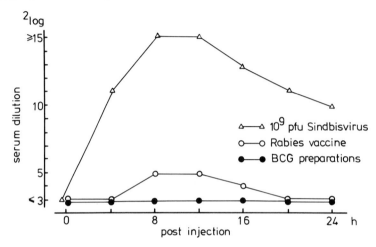

Figure 6.

DISCUSSION

In our experiments the xenogeneic murine YAC lymphoma was used for assaying rat NK cell activity. In mice YAC cells were reported to be a good target for NK lysis[24, 28, 29]. The data presented in this study and the results obtained previously in athymic rats[23] show YAC cells also to be a suitable target for assaying rat NK cell activity with a short term (4 h) ^{51}Cr release assay.

We found consistently the highest spontaneous cytotoxic activity to be present in the peritoneal cavity. This finding is in contrast with results obtained by other workers[10, 30]. Using a Gross virus induced rat lymphoma, Oehler[30] found high cytotoxic activity in blood and spleen. We found low levels of activity in PBL. These differences could be due to strain variation as NK cell activity in rat spleen has been reported to be strain dependent[30, 31]. Also antigenic properties of the target cells could play a role together with the antigen recognition capacities of the NK cells as was reported for human NK cells[32, 33].

At day 4 after intravenous BCG in our random bred rats consistently an increase of NK cell activity in the spleen was found, although the difference with the control group was not always statistically significant. However, considering all experiments together the overall results were highly significant (table 1). Comparing the frequency distribution of the NK cell activity in the spleen of BCG treated animals with the activity of non-treated control animals a shift was found to a higher NK cell activity. However, the activity of both control and BCG-treated animals where found to be overlapping in a large area. Either some animals in this random bred rat colony are non-responders or these animals have normally a (very) low activity and their BCG enhanced NK cell activity lies within the range of control animals. The simultaneous investigation of cell samples from individual animals pre- and post BCG administration could give an answer to this question. Our data indicate BCG to stimulate NK cells both by i.v. and i.p. route, the activation by BCG like Corynebacterium parvum seeming to be mainly a local event[34, 35]. However, BCG seems to be a more consistent NK cell activator since C.parvum also can suppress spleen NK cell activity[34] which was reported to be strictly a dose dependent phenomenon[35]. In contrast with C.parvum, low dosages of BCG had no effect on spleen NK cell activity (fig. 2).

Intraperitoneal application at day-4 also gave a slight increase in NK cell activity of the spleen. This is in agreement with results for BCG in mice[36], and for C.parvum in rats[35]. In contrast, Potter and Moore[10] found no stimulation of spleen NK cell activity in rats after i.p. treatment with BCG. For mice also suppression was described after i.p. treatment with BCG, which was not due to a migration of NK cells from the spleen to the peritoneal cavity, as splenectomy had no influence on the increase of peritoneal NK cell activity[29].

Oral and subcutaneous administration of BCG had no effect on spleen NK cell activity. Although no time sequence study was done after these routes of administration it seems more likely that after these routes of administration in stead of a systemic effect on the spleen, a local effect on the regional lymph nodes might be present.

Intraperitoneal administration of BCG also increased peritoneal NK activity, which was not only restricted to the non-adherent fraction, since also the adherent cell fraction showed enhanced activity. However, the activity of the total cell population was not simply an addition on the adherent and non-adherent fraction. In the athymic rat, the plastic adherent fraction of peritoneal cells was also found to have a considerable cytotoxic activity against YAC cells[23]. This could be due to a technical failure in separating adherent and non-adherent cells. However, the specific ^{51}Cr release might also be due to the activity of spontaneous and BCG stimulated macrophages[37]. For C.parvum also an activation of adherent peritoneal cells was found[35].

Soluble factors, probably interferon, released from macrophages after activation by poly I : C[16] and BCG[17] augment mice NK cell activity. In rats macrophages also mediated the effect of poly I : C enhancement of NK cell activity[38]. This effect of poly I : C suggests a role for interferon in the enhancement of NK cell activity. In sera of rats on day 2, 4 or 7 after BCG treatment no induction of interferon could be detected. Also during the first 24 hours after BCG interferon could not be demonstrated. This absence of demonstrable levels of interferon could not be attributed to an insensitivity of the interferon assay as in control sera from animals treated with sindbis virus levels comparable with those reported by Billiau and Buckler[25] were found. Also interferon could be detected after administration of a weak interferon inducer like rabies vaccine. This lack of interferon induction by BCG could be due to the BCG preparations used. It also could give an explanation for the relatively modest enhancement of NK cell activity after i.v. BCG. However, with regard to immunostimulation and induction of cytolytic activity in PEC of mice, BCG-RIV has similar activity as BCG-Tice and BCG-Pasteur[22, 39].

NK cells are suggested to play a role in the surveillance against neoplasia[11-13], and BCG was found to have an anti-neoplastic effect in experimental tumor systems[1, 2]. However, although activated by BCG, NK cells probably only play a role in the early phase of the anti-tumor effect of BCG, as NK cell activation after BCG is a short-term effect (our data[9, 10, 29, 36]) and limited to the cellular compartment directly stimulated (this study). Furthermore, it has to be considered that progressing tumors already have escaped from NK cell activity in the host.

ACKNOWLEDGEMENTS

We wish to acknowledge the expert technical assistance of Mr.P.de Jong, Mr. H.H.Näring, Mr.C.Moolenbeek and Mr.F.W.van Nimwegen.

REFERENCES

1. Salmon, S.E. (1977) Cancer Res., 37, 1245-1248.
2. Goodnight, J.E., and Morton, D.L. (1978) Ann.Rev.Med., 29, 231-238.
3. Mitchell, M.S., and Murahata, R.I. (1979) Pharmac.Ther., 4, 329-353.
4. Mokyr, M.D., Dennett, J.A., Braun, D.P., Hengst, J.C.D., Mitchell, M.S., and Dray, S. (1980) J.Natl.Cancer Inst., 64, 339-344.
5. Alaba, O., Bernstein, I.D., Wright, P.W. and Hellström, K.E. (1980) Cellular Immunol., 50, 106-114.
6. Ruitenberg, E.J., Steerenberg, P.A., and Noorle Jansen, L.M.van (1978) Dev.biol.Stand., 38, 97-101.

224

7. Florentin, I., Huchet, R., Bruley-Rosset, M., Halle-Panenko, O., and Mathé, G. (1976) Cancer Immunol.Immunother., 1, 31-39.
8. Ruco, L.P., and Meltzer, M.S. (1977) Cellular Immunol., 32, 203-215.
9. Tracey, D.E., Wolfe, S.A., Durdik, J.M., and Henney, C.S. (1977) J.Immunol., 119, 1145-1151.
10. Potter, M.R., and Moore, M. (1980) Immunology, 39, 427-434.
11. Herberman, R.B., and Holden, H.T. (1978) Advan.Cancer Res., 27, 305-377.
12. Kiessling, R., and Wigzell, R. (1979) Immunol.Rev., 44, 165-208.
13. Roder, J.C., and Haliotis, T. (1980) Immunology Today, 1, 96-100.
14. Herberman, R.B., Nunn, M.E., Holden, H.T., Staal, S., and Djeu, J.Y. (1977) Int.J.Cancer, 19, 555-564.
15. Oehler, J.R., Lindsay, L.R., Nunn, M.E., Holden, H.T., and Herberman, R.B. (1978) Int.J.Cancer, 21, 210-220.
16. Djeu, J.Y., Heinbaugh, J.A., Holden, H.T., and Herberman, R.B. (1979) J.Immunol., 122, 182-188.
17. Tracey, D.E. (1979) J.Immunol., 123, 840-845.
18. Wallen, W.C., Dean, J.H., and Lucas, D.O. (1973) Cellular Immunol., 6, 110-122.
19. Stobo, J.I., Green, I., Jackson, L., and Baron, S. (1974) J.Immunol., 112, 1589-1593.
20. Yamaguchi, T., Handa, K., Shimizu, Y., Abo, T., and Kumagai, K. (1977) J.Immunol., 118, 1931-1935.
21. Timonen, T., Saksela, E., Virtanen, I., and Canell, K. (1980) Eur.J.Immunol., 10, 422-427.
22. Ruitenberg, J.E., Jong, W.H.de, Kreeftenberg, J.G., Steerenberg, P.A., Kruizinga, W., and Noorle Jansen, L.M.van (1981) Cancer Immunol.Immunother., 11, 45-51.
23. Jong, W.H.de, Steerenberg, P.A., Ursem, P.S., Osterhaus, A.D.M.E., Vos, J.G., and Ruitenberg, E.J. (1980) Clin.Immunol.Immunol.Immunopathol., 17, 163-172.
24. Kiessling, R., Klein, E., and Wigzell, H. (1975) Eur.J.Immunol., 5, 112-117.
25. Billiau, A., and Buckler, C.E. (1969) Symp.Series Immunobiol.Standard., 14, 37-44.
26. Fisher, R.A. (1948) Statistical method for research workers. Oliver and Boyd, eds., Edinborough, pp. 99-101.
27. Shellam, G.R. (1977) Int.J.Cancer, 19, 225-235.
28. Santoni, A., Pucetti, P., Riccardi, C., Herberman, R.B. and Bonmassar, E. (1979) Int.J.Cancer, 24, 656-661.
29. Ito, M., Ralph, P., and Moore, M.A.S. (1980) Clin.Immunol.Immunopathol., 16, 30-38.
30. Oehler, J.R., Lindsay, L.R., Nunn, M.E., and Herberman, R.B. (1978) Int.J. Cancer, 21, 204-209.
31. Shellam, G.R., and Hogg, N. (1977) Int.J.Cancer, 19, 212-224.
32. Jensen, P., and Koren, H.S. (1979) J.Immunol., 123, 1127-1132.
33. Philips, W.H., Ortaldo, J.R., and Herberman, R.B. (1980) J.Immunol., 125, 2322-2327.
34. Ojo, E., Haller, O., Kimura, A., and Wigzell, H. (1978) Int.J.Cancer, 21, 444-452.
35. Flexman, J.P., and Shellam, G.R. (1980) Br.J.Cancer, 42, 41-51.
36. Pioch, Y., Gerber, M., and Serrou, B. (1979) Cancer Immunol.Immunother., 7, 181-184.
37. Gray, J.D., and Brooks, C.G. (1980) Cellular Immunol., 53, 405-412.
38. Oehler, J.R., and Herberman, R.B. (1978) Int.J.Cancer, 21, 221-229.
39. Kreeftenberg, J.G., Jong, W.H.de, Ettekoven, H., Steerenberg, P.A., Kruizinga, W., Noorle Jansen, L.M.van, Sekhuis, J., and Ruitenberg, E.J. (1981) Cancer Immunol.Immunother., 12, 21-29.

A STIMULUS-SECRETION MODEL FOR NATURAL KILLER CELL MEDIATED CYTOLYSIS.

JOHN C. RODER AND JEROME WERKMEISTER
Department of Microbiology and Immunology, Queen's University, Kingston, Ontario, Canada, K7L 3N6.

INTRODUCTION

Microbes are thought to be killed directly by cell-derived H_2O_2 and possibly O_2^- and certain free radicals. Tumor cells, on the other hand, are destroyed in part by natural killer (NK) cells[1] in a process which does not involve phagocytosis, much like non-phagocytic killing of tumor cells by macrophages. It has previously been shown that murine macrophages utilize H_2O_2 in their cytolytic mechanisms[2], as do human neutrophils[3], but very little is known about the cytolytic mechanism in NK cells. In this paper, we show that the NK-target cell interaction results in an immediate burst of chemiluminescence and O_2^- production and we postulate that these events are necessary but not sufficient for NK mediated cytolysis. In addition, recent data is discussed which supports a "stimulus-secretion" model of NK cytolysis.

MATERIALS AND METHODS

Assays for chemiluminescence[4], cytochrome C reduction[5], and cytolysis[4], as well as methods for the preparation of plasma membrane vesicles[4], and fluorescence activated cell sorting[6] are described in detail in the references cited here and in the table and figure descriptions.

RESULTS

The Generation of Superoxide, O_2^-, in NK enriched populations. Peripheral blood lymphocytes were depleted of monocytes and separated on a discontinuous Percoll density gradient[7]. Lymphocytes from the NK enriched fraction were dark adapted in the presence of luminol, to achieve a stable background, and then stimulated by the addition of tumor cells at a 10:1 tumor cell:lymphocyte ratio. As shown in Fig. 1, the addition of K562

Cancer: Etiology and Prevention, Ray G. Crispen, Editor

cells (a human erythroleukemia) caused a rapid increase in chemiluminescence reaching a peak of 167 x 10^3 CPM within 30 sec. followed by a gradual decline to low levels at 8 min. Parallel experiments using a cytochrome C reduction assay revealed a somewhat slower kinetics with a reaction velocity of 200 pmol cytochrome C reduced/min/10^6 Percoll fractionated cells. No further cytochrome C reduction occurred after 8 min., by which time the chemiluminescence response had returned almost to baseline. Addition of P815-2 cells (a murine mastocytoma) to Percoll fraction 2 cells caused a low chemiluminescence response (35 x 10^3 CPM) and little cytochrome C reduction (< 200 pmol) (Fig. 1). The area under the anti-P815-2 chemiluminescence curve was 36% of the area under the anti-K562 curve. Addition of 100 ug (280 Units) of superoxide dismutase (SOD) caused an 80-90% inhibition of both chemiluminescence and cytochrome C reduction.

The chemiluminescence response was directly proportional to the concentration of effector cells or targets as shown in Fig. 2. In the presence of a fixed number of 10^7 target cells, 10^6 NK-enriched lymphocytes generated a peak chemiluminescent response of 2 x 10^6 counts over the 10-minute assay period (Fig. 2, left panel). The reason for the decline in the chemiluminescence response when the effectors were increased to 2 x 10^6 is not known but could conceivably arise due to the release of SOD or scavengers from cells killed at this higher E:T ratio. When the effector cells were held constant at 0.5 x 10^6, a near maximum chemiluminescence response was observed upon addition of 10^7 intact K562 cells (Fig. 2, right panel).

Plasma membrane vesicles of K562 were less able to induce chemiluminescence at high concentrations compared to intact K562 cells whereas low numbers of vesicles (0.01 x 10^6 cell equivalents, 0.028 ug protein) generated markedly more chemiluminescence than intact K562 cells. Since each K562 cell yields many plasma membrane vesicles, one would expect intact cells to be more limiting than vesicles, as we observed. These results imply that a given number of hits is necessary to trigger the NK cells regardless of particle size. Vesicles prepared from an NK-insensitive target, P815, failed to induce any detectable chemiluminescence response.

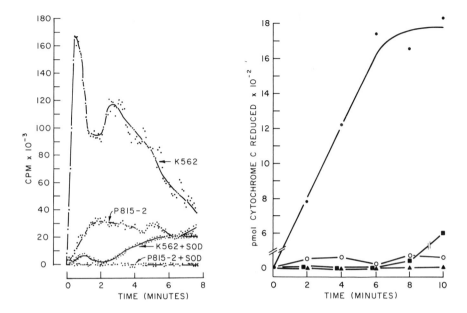

Figure 1.   Chemiluminescence and Cytochrome C reduction in large granular lymphocytes (LGL) induced by NK sensitive tumor cells.   Peripheral blood was treated for 30 min.   at 37° with carbonyl-iron and a magnet to remove monocytes.   Mononuclear cells were isolated by centrifugation on Ficoll-Hypaque (1.077 g/cm^3) and further depleted of monocytes by adherence on autologous-serum coated plastic dishes for 1 hr at 37°.   The non-adherent lymphocytes were layered on a 5 step, discontinuous, Percoll density gradient and centrifuged for 30 min.   at 20° as described by Timonen and Saksela[7].   Fraction 2 cells were enriched 5 fold in cytolytic activity against K562.   60% of fraction 2 cells were LGL as detected morphologically in Giemsa smears, whereas < 0.1% phagocytosed antibody coated erythrocytes.

   LEFT PANEL: 10^6 Percoll fraction 2 cells were dark adapted for 30 min.   in 1.0 ml of 10% luminol-saturated, fetal calf serum in plastic scintillation vials. 10^7 tumor cells, medium alone, or tumor cells + 100 ug superoxide dismutase (280 units, Sigma type I, EC 1.15.1.1) was added in 0.1 ml volumes and mixed.   Chemiluminescence was measured at ambient temperature (20°) in an LKB liquid scintillation counter in the out-of-coincidence mode. Values represent CPM above background, measured in successive 5 sec intervals.   Luminol alone gave 35 x 10^3 CPM and Percoll fr.   2 cells + luminol gave a stable background ot 50 x 10^3 CPM throughout the 8 min.   of the assay.   This experiment was repeated 10 times with similar results and in replicate samples within each experiment the area under the curves varied < 3%.

228

RIGHT PANEL: 10^6 Percoll fraction 2 cells were combined with 10^7 K562 cells (●), 10^7 P815-2 cells (○), 10^7 K562 cells + 100 ug/ml SOD (280 units) (■), 10^7 P815-2 cells + 100 ug/ml SOD (280 units) (▲) in 1 ml of balanced salt solution (BSS) containing 0.2% BSA, 10μM KCN, 200 units catalase (Sigma 11,500 units/mg, thymol-free) and 0.01 mM Cytochrome C (Sigma, type III). After varying periods of incubation at 20°C the reaction was stopped at 0°. Supernatants were measured spectrophotometrically at A_{550}. Maximum, reducible cytochrome C was determined with an excess of sodium dithionite. OD readings were converted to pmol Cyt. C reduced after substracting a small background response (< 500 pmol) by tumor cells alone. Percoll fr. 2 cells gave 0 background over the 10 min period of assay. This experiment was repeated 5 times with similar results and values for replicate samples at each point varied < 10%.

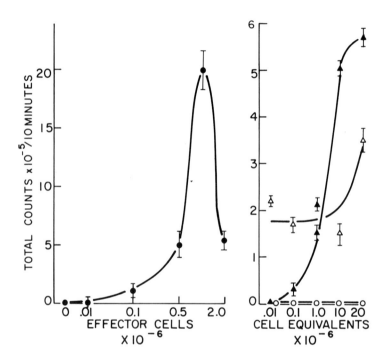

Figure 2: Effector-Target Titrations in the Chemiluminescence Assay. Monocyte-depleted peripheral blood lymphocytes were separated on Percoll density gradients and the fraction highest in NK-mediated cytotoxicity was selected for further study. **LEFT PANEL:** Varying numbers of these lymphocytes were mixed with 10^7 K562 cells at a time 0, in the presence of

luminol and CPM were recorded every 5 seconds on an LKB liquid scintillation counter in the out-of-coincidence mode ($\bullet$———$\bullet$). RIGHT PANEL: Varying numbers of intact K562 cells were mixed with 5 x 10^5 , NK-enriched Percoll fraction lymphocytes ($\blacktriangle$———$\blacktriangle$). Cell-free plasma membrane vesicles were prepared from K562 ($\triangle$———$\triangle$) and P815 ($\bigcirc$———$\bigcirc$) cells and mixed with 5 x 10^5 NK-enriched Percoll fraction lymphocytes. 10^7 cell quivalents of plasma membrane vesicles contained 28 ug of protein. Target cells or vesicles alone did not generate chemiluminescence. Values represent mean total CPM above background ± s.e. over a 10-minute period in triplicate samples. This experiment was repeated 3 times with similar results.

DISCUSSION

NK cells produce oxygen intermediates. Within seconds of mixing HNK-1[+], large granular lymphocytes with K562 tumor cells a burst of O_2^- and chemiluminescence is observed (Fig. 1)[5]. The fact that oxygen radicals were induced by glutaraldehyde-fixed target cells[4] and cell-free, plasma membrane vesicles made from NK-sensitive but not NK-insensitive targets (Fig. 2) shows that it is the effector cells rather than the targets that are responsible for the generation of these oxygen radicals. Extensive target panel studies have shown a direct correlation (r > 0.93) between target-effector conjugate formation, induction of oxygen radical production in NK cells and susceptibility to NK-mediated cytolysis[4]. Highly sensitive NK target cells (human fetal fibroblasts, K562) induce a large amount of oxygen radicals whereas insensitive NK targets (P815, L5178Y) induce very little. In addition, glutaraldehyde-fixed K562 cells that differ in the degree of preservation of the NK target structure, as determined by ability to compete with unfixed K562 cells in a cold target inhibition assay, show a strong correlation (r > 0.98) between the ability to compete for the NK receptor and the ability to trigger oxygen radical production. Finally, several differentiated K562 clones which were selectively resistant to NK-mediated cytolysis [8] also induced less oxygen radicals[5]. These data suggest that it is the target structure binding to the NK receptor itself that may be the trigger for oxygen radical production.

Oxygen intermediates are a necessary step in the NK cytolytic pathway. We then asked whether oxygen intermediates were merely an epiphenomena or if they were involved directly in the NK cytolytic pathway. Specific enzymes and scavengers were used to selectively remove these highly reactive molecules from the system.

Superoxide dismutase (SOD) is an enzyme whose apparent sole function is to scavenge free superoxide radical, O_2^-, by the dismutation reaction $O_2^- + O_2^- + 2H^+ \longrightarrow O_2 + H_2O_2$ [9,10] whereas mannitol[11], benzoate[11,12] or DMSO[13] are $OH^\bullet$ scavengers. All of these agents cause a marked decrease in the chemiluminescence resulting from the NK-target cell interaction. Catalase[14], an enzyme which specifically degrades H_2O_2 to $H_2O + O_2$, has a lesser effect on the chemiluminescence. These results indicate that all three molecular species (O_2^-, H_2O_2, $OH^\bullet$) are generated during NK activation.

The addition of SOD, mannitol, benzoate or DMSO to the NK cytolytic assay markedly inhibited cytolysis (80%) in a dose-dependent reversible reaction. Catalase, on the other hand, had no effect on NK-mediated cytolysis. Further analysis has shown that none of these agents, with the possible exception of DMSO, interfered with the ability of the NK cell to recognize and bind to its target cell. This data suggests that the highly reactive molecular species (O_2^- and $OH^\bullet$) are necessary for cytolysis to proceed. It is also interesting to note that this is the converse of what is known to occur in monocyte mediated cytolysis where H_2O_2 has been shown to be important[2]. In our hands, catalase but not SOD, mannitol, benzoate nor DMSO inhibited cytolysis of tumor cells by human monocytes.

Production of oxygen intermediates is dependent on the state of NK activation. Since oxygen intermediates are essential in NK cytolysis, it was not surprising to find that the state of NK activation and the generation of oxygen intermediates are closely related. Interferon pre-treatment of NK cells caused a concomitant increase in oxygen intermediate production and cytolysis[5]. In addition, the degree of augmentation in both oxygen intermediate production and cytolysis by interferon-boosted effectors versus non-boosted effectors correlated directly.

An examination of low-NK responsiveness in humans has shown that individuals with this stable, selective defect have normal frequencies of HNK-1[+] NK cells which bind normally to the tumor targets and are boosted normally by interferon, but fail to become activated as judged by a 60% decrease in the burst of oxygen intermediates that are normally generated following target-effector interaction[5]. Preliminary data suggest that these low NK responders are also more sensitive to SOD-induced inhibition of their NK-mediated cytolysis than normals.

Possible mechanisms for generation of oxygen intermediates. Since NK recognition and binding to target determinants induces the NK cell to generate oxygen intermediates, we also investigated the possible mechanisms of the triggering event. Agents that effect the NK cell's ability to generate oxygen intermediates and kill tumor cells include azide and chloroquine. Sodium azide inhibits oxidative metabolism completely and consequenly blocks the generation of oxygen intermediates[15] and NK-mediated cytolysis[16]. Chloroquine, on the other hand, is a selective inhibitor of lysosomes and also leads to a parallel decrease in oxygen intermediate production[15] and NK-mediated cytolysis[16]. Neither of these agents inhibits target-effector binding. Therefore, both oxidative metabolism and normal lysosome function are necessary for stage 2 and 3 in the cytolytic pathway as postulated previously[16].

In leukocytes, the oxidase enzyme which generates these oxygen intermediates appears to be associated with the plasma membrane[17,18]. In these cells, an appropriate perturbation of their plasma membrane leads to activation of the oxygen-intermediate producing system. The depolarization of the membrane and resultant Ca^{++} influx caused by the perturbation are felt to be responsible for this activation[19,20,21]. Therefore, we studied the effect of inducing a calcium ion influx on the NK cell. It was found that when a calcium ionophore, A 23178, was added to the NK cells in the presence of Ca^{++}, there was a production of oxygen intermediates[15]. This presumed triggering of the oxidase enzyme system in the NK cell is accomplished without the need for the NK receptor-target structure interaction and suggests that with the NK cell, as with other leukocytes, the appropriate perturbation of their plasma membrane, (as would occur following NK-target cell binding or interferon-interferon receptor binding) leads to (i) depolarization of the membrane; (ii) calcium ion flux; (iii) activation of the oxidase enzyme system; and (iv) the subsequent generation of oxygen intermediates.

The data suggest that the generation of oxygen intermediates is an early event in the triggering and activation of the lytic mechanism. A further piece of evidence to support this hypothesis comes from studies of patients with Chediak-Higashi disease who have normal frequencies of HNK-1[+] cells[6] which do not function[22]. The block in NK cytolysis appears to be in a later stage since binding to the target (stage 1) is normal and is followed by normal triggering and production of oxygen intermediates thereby indicating that the oxygen intermediates normally appear prior to the late step in the cytolytic pathway which is blocked in the Chediak-Higashi syndrome.

Oxygen intermediates are known to be intimately involved in the biosynthesis of several important compounds by triggering and participating in both the lipooxygenase and cyclooxygenase pathway of arachidonic acid oxidation[23,24]. These two independent pathways which generate such potent biological compounds as 5HETE, leukotrienes, hydroxy fatty acids, prostaglandins, prostacyclins and thromboxanes have already been implicated in the NK cytolytic pathway. Steroids[25] and phospholipase inhibitors[26] inhibit NK acitivity and also block the production of arachidonic acid by the phospholipases. ASA (aspirin) and NSAID's block the cyclooxygenase step and are known to inhibit NK[27]. cAMP, theophylline, and PGE also inhibit NK function[28] and are known to inhibit phospholipase A[29] and may inhibit prostaglandin synthesis later in the pathway[30].

The role of Calmodulin in the NK cytolytic pathway. Calmodulin is a ubiquitous, multifunctional regulatory protein, 148 amino acids long, which can bind intracellular Ca^{2+} and activate a number of physiological responses[31]. When calmodulin binds to Ca^{2+}, a highly lipophilic region of the molecule is exposed which is essential for interaction with its receptor proteins. This same lipophilic region also binds a variety of phenothiazines, thus blocking calmodulin-receptor interactions[32]. As shown in Table 1 a marked (76%) inhibition of NK activity was observed after a 1 hr pre-treatment of nylon wool non-adherent, splenic effector cells with 2.5×10^{-5}M trifluoperazine or fluphanozine, a non toxic dosage[33]. The biologically inactive sulphoxide derivative, was not inhibitory and the efficacy of inhibition of other compounds was directly correlated (r=0.96, p < 0.02) with their reported affinities for calmodulin. Fluphenazine (FP) may act on the earliest stages of the target-effector interaction since conjugate formation between CBA effectors and YAC targets decreased from 20% to 6% (p < 0.02) upon pre-treatment with this drug. However, FP was not selective for NK cells since cytotoxic T lymphocytes, derived from both mixed lymphocyte culture and by concanavalin A stimulation, also revealed depressed cytolytic activity against P815 tumor targets after FP treatment. Tumoricidal activity by activated macrophages, and effectors of antibody-dependent cell-mediated cytotoxicity were also blocked. Similar concentration of FP caused striking changes in cell morphology as well as in microtubule and calmodulin distribution in 3T6 fibroblasts as detected by indirect immunofluorescence using anti-tubulin or anti-calmodulin antibody. Addition of 1.25 - 5 ug/ml A23187, a calcium ionophore, to FP-treated effectors, restored NK binding and cytolytic functions to normal levels.

These data are compatible with the suggestion that FP inhibits NK function by inactivating the calcium-calmodulin complex, thereby altering the organization of the cytoskeleton so that early binding events in target-effector interaction are impaired.

TABLE 1

COMPARISON OF NK INHIBITION AND CALMODULIN-BINDING EFFICIENCIES OF VARIOUS COMPOUNDS.

Compound	%NK Inhibition[a]	IC_{50} (uM)[b]	Relative CaM binding Capacity
Control	0	0	0
Trifluoperazine	76.3	1.5	100.0
trans-Flupenthixol	65.6	2.5	60.0
cis-Flupenthixol	59.2	4.0	37.0
(+)-Butaclamol	40.7	75.0	2.0
(-)-Butaclamol	1.0	350.0	0.4

[a] Nylon non-adherent spleen cells from CBA mice were pre-treated for 1 hr at 37°C with various compounds and then reacted with ^{51}Cr-labelled YAC-1 cells in a 6-hr ^{51}Cr release assay. Values are expressed as percent inhibition of control lysis with no drug added, at effector:target ratios of 100:1. Actual control lysis was 40% ± 4%.
[b] IC_{50} is the concentration of drug required to displace 50% of ^{3}H-trifluoperazine from CaM, (taken from Weiss et al.[7]) indicating CaM-binding efficiency. This experiment was repeated 2 additional times with similar results. (r = 0.96, p< 0.02). This table is adapted from Laing et al.[33].

Evidence for acceptor sites on tumor cells for the NK derived toxin. Recent results lead to the inference of an acceptor site on the target cell which binds the putative NK-lymphotoxin released during the lethal hit[34]. Clones of NK-resistant (NK[R]) mutants (YAC-6, YAC-6.28) derived from YAC, expressed normal NK-target structures and were bound by NK cells but not lysed as shown in Table 2. The NK[R] clones however were equally susceptible to lysis mediated by alloimmune cytotoxic T lymphocytes or antibody and complement thereby suggesting that they were selectively resistant to NK cytolysis only. It is reasonable to assume therefore that this mutation has occurred in an acceptor site for the NK-lymphotoxin-like substance. It is interesting to note that these NK[R] lines also resist lysis by a soluble NK-derived toxin first described by Wright and Bonavida[35] and that YAC lines selected for toxin resistance also resist NK mediated cytolysis[36]. Further work will be aimed at isolating the toxin acceptors on tumor cells.

TABLE 2

SELECTIVE NK RESISTANCE IN A CLONE OF MUTAGENIZED YAC CELLS.

	YAC parent	YAC-19	YAC-6	YAC-6.28
Lysis $(LU/10^7)^a$ by				
(a) NK	85	100	10	5
(b) CTL	3000	2800	2500	2700
(c) Lectin-CTL	1100	800	1000	900
Competition vs YAC parent[b]	0.6	0.5	0.8	0.6
% TBC[c]	20	22	23	24

Effectors were derived from nylon passed fresh spleen (NK), mixed lymphocyte cultures (CTL) or spleen cells cultured in the presence of Con A (lectin-CTL).
[a] Data is expressed as the number of lytic units/10^7. 1 LU was defined as the number of effector cells required to yield 25% cytolysis.

[b] Data is expressed as the unlabelled competitor/labelled target cell ratio required for 50% inhibition of ^{51}Cr release from YAC parent cells in an NK assay.
[c] The frequency of nylon-passed CBA spleen cells binding to the various targets.
These data are summarized from Roder et al.[34].

Evidence for a Stimulus-Secretion Model of NK cytolysis. The "stimulus-secretion" model for NK cytolysis was first proposed in 1978[37] and later elaborated upon[16]. Under this model specific target cell contact[38,39] results in a change in the cyclic nucleotide balance[28], or some other second messenger $(O_2^-$?)[5], which triggers secretion of the lethal toxin.

The evidence that secretion may be important in the cytolytic pathway of human NK cells can be summarized as follows: (i) pre-treatment of LGL with Sr^{2+} led to degranulation and following washing, there was a concomitant loss of cytolytic activity[40]; (ii) cytotoxicity was inhibited by monensin, a carboxylic ionophore, which blocked cellular secretion in LGL[41]; (iii) a calcium flux across the membrane was necessary for cytolysis as shown by use of verapamil[42], a Ca^{2+} channel blocker, and a calcium ionophore (A23187)[33]; (iv) agents which inhibit cytolysis (cAMP,PGE1, theophylline, histamine)[28] also block lysosome secretion in other cells[28,43], at the same concentrations, and conversely, agents which increase lysosomal discharge (cGMP, carbamylcholine) augment NK cytolysis[28,44]; (v) chloroquine, a selective inhibitor of lysosomes, simultaneously decreased NK cytolysis and N-acetyl-B-glucosaminidase levels in mouse spleen and human peripheral blood lymphocytes (PBL)[16]; (vi) secretion is energy dependent, and DNP and CCCP, uncouplers of oxidative phosphorylation, block both NK cytolysis[37] and secretion; and (vii) CH patients and biege mice carry a gene mutation which selectively impairs both the lethal-hit stage of NK-mediated cytolysis[22,46] and the secretion of lysosomal enzymes in the kidney and into the phagolysosome of leukocytes[47]. In addition the secretion of plasminogen activator, a neutral serine protease, from CH LGL was impaired[48]. Since HNK-1+ LGL from CH patients have a single giant granule rather than many small granules[6], it is likely that lack of secretion may also explain this genetic NK insufficiency. Neither monocytes nor T cells from these patients exhibited giant granules, and both effector-cell types had normal cytolytic functions [22,49]. It seems likely, therefore, that the giant granules in NK may be linked to the functional defect in CH patients.

Two hypotheses have been put forward for the nature of the lethal-hit phase of NK-mediated cytolysis. First, it was suggested that a lysosomal protease was the lethal substance since secretion of lysosomal or granule contents may be involved (above) and since inhibitors of serine esterases (PMSF, DIFP), blocked killing but not binding to the target[37]. Subsequent work using a larger panel of more specific inhibitors has revealed that chymotrypsin-like activity, as opposed to a trypsin activity, may be involved in early activation events rather than the lethal hit itself[50]. The second hypothesis suggests that soluble toxic molecules are released by the NK cell and bind to specific acceptor sites on the target-cell membrane[1,34]. Human PBL stimulated by lectins release soluble factors which are toxic to NK-sensitive, but not NK-resistant, targets[35]. The existence of toxin acceptor sites on the target-cell membrane has been inferred from data discussed above. It is conceivable that the toxin contains a hexose phosphate residue which binds to the acceptor sites since mannose-6-phosphate, and stereochemically similar fructose-1-phosphate, inhibit NK-mediated cytolysis at the target-cell level, and gelonin conjugated to mannose-6-phosphate was highly toxic to NK-sensitive, but not NK-resistant targets[45]. In a similar manner various carbohydrates competed with toxins derived from PBL in another system[35]. The inability of NK cells to kill NK-insensitive targets (innocent bystanders) after triggering with NK-sensitive targets does not exclude the existence of soluble toxins. The insensitive target may lack acceptor sites for the toxin as there may be a specilized mode of delivery that prevents leakage.

Late Events. A later event in the cytolytic pathway, measurable directly at 1 hr postbinding, involves the methylation of phospholipids within the NK cell[26]. Inhibitors of transmethylation (3-dezaadenosine) blocked cytolysis, and it is conceivable that transmethylation may enhance signal transduction across the plasma membrane of NK cells as occurs in many other systems[51]. A concurrent increase in phospholipase A_2 activity was also measured directly and could be blocked by several specific inhibitors of this enzyme including DL-(2.3-disteroyloxy propyldimethyl-2-hydroxyl) ethylammonium acetate. These results have been confirmed in the mouse[50] but it remains to be shown if phospholipase A_2 or its detergent-like product, lysophosphatidylcholine, is the lethal substance.

SUMMARY

The mechanism of NK cytolysis is summarized in Fig. 3, in the form of a stimulus-secretion model.

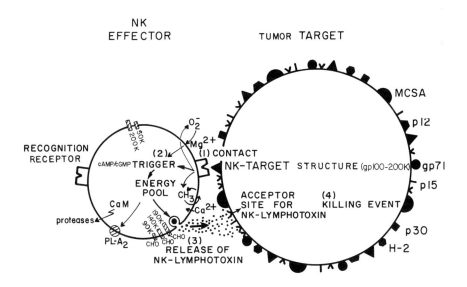

Figure 3.   Stimulus–secretion model of NK cytolysis.   The target structure glycoprotein has been isolated and described[38,39] and the NK receptor is known to be a de novo synthesized protein[37].   STEP 1 involves a Mg^{2+} dependent, calmodulin controlled contact between the target and effector. STEP 2 Following this interaction four necessary events are triggered including the generation of O_2^-,[5] an influx of Ca^{2+},[42] the transmethylation of membrane phospholipids and the activation of phospholipase A_2 ($PL-A_2$)[26].[37] STEP 3 Secretion of NK–lymphotoxin begins by an energy dependent process[37]. STEP 4   The lytic molecules bind to acceptor sites on the target membrane[1,34] and thereby deliver the lethal hit.   Target cell death is thought to result from colloid osmotic lysis.   Neutral serine proteases are also released[48] and seem to be necessary for NK cytolysis[16,48] but there is no evidence yet to show that this event is stimulus-coupled.   Antibodies against 190, 140 and 90K effector cell glycoproteins block the lethal hit stage[52] and it is presumed therefore that these molecules lie in close proximity to the secretory vesicles.   Monoclonal antibodies against a 200k and 50k effector cell proteins also block cytolysis[53,54].

238

REFERENCES

1. Roder, J.C., Karre, K. and Kiessling, R. (1981) Prog. Allergy 28, 66-159.
2. Nathan, C.F., Silverstein, S.C., Brukner, L.H. and Cohn, Z.A. (1979) J. Exp. Med. 149, 100.
3. Clark, R.A. and Klebanoff, S.J. (1975) J. Exp. Med. 141, 1442.
4. Helfand, S.L., Werkmeister, J. and Roder, J.C. (1982) J. Exp. Med. 156, 492-505.
5. Roder, J.C., Helfand, S.L., Werkmeister, J., McGarry, R, Beaumont, T.J. and Duwe, A. (1982) Nature 298, 569-572.
6. Abo, T., Roder, J.C., Abo, W., Cooper, M.D. and Balch, C.M. (1982) J. Clin. Invest. 70, 193-197.
7. Timonen, T. and Saksela, E. (1980) J. Immunol. Methods 36, 285-291.
8. Werkmeister, J.A., Helfand, S.L., Haliotis, T., Pross, H.F. and Roder, J.C. (1982) J. Immunol. 129, 413-418.
9. McCord, J.M. and Fridovich, I. (1969) J. Biol. Chem. 244, 6049.
10. McCord, J.M., Keele, B.B. Jr., and Fridovich, I. (1971) PNAS USA 68, 1024.
11. Kellogg, E.W. and Fridovich, I. (1975) J. Biol. Chem. 250, 8812.
12. Neta, P. and Dorfuran, L.M. (1968) Adv. Chem. Ser. 81, 1, 222.
13. Anabor, M. and Neta, P. (1967) Int. J. Appl. Radiat. Isot. 18, 493.
14. Beers, R.F. and Sizer, I.W. (1952) J. Biol. Chem. 195, 133.
15. Helfand, S.L., Werkmeister, J. and Roder, J.C. (1982) In "Natural Cell Mediated Immunity Against Tumors" Herberman, R.B., ed., Academic Press, N.Y. vol. 2 1011-1020.
16. Roder, J.C., Argov, S., Klein, M., Petersson, C., Kiessling, R., Andersson, K. and Hanssen, M. (1980) Immunology, 40, 107.
17. Dewald, B., Baggiolini, M., Curnutte, J.T., Babior, B.M. (1979) J. Clin. Invest. 63, 21-29.
18. Cohen, H.J., Chovaniec, M.E. and Davies, W.E. (1980) Blood 55, 355-363.
19. Lew, P.D., and Stossel, T.P. (1981) J. Clin. Invest. 67, 1, 9.
20. Whitin, J.C., Chapman, C.E., Simons, E.R., Chovaniec, M.E., and Cohen, H.J. (1980) J. Biol. Chem. 255, 1874-1878.
21. Seligman, B.E., and Grallin, J.I. (1980) J. Clin. Invest. 66, 493-503.
22. Roder, J.C., Haliotis, T., Klein, M. Korec, S., Jett, J., Ortaldo, J., Herberman, R., Katz, P. and Fauci, A.S. (1980) Nature 284, 553.
23. Lewis, R.A. and Austen, K.F. (1981) Nature 293, 103-108.
24. Kuehl, F.A., Jr., and Egan, R.W. (1980) Science 210, 978-984.
25. Hochman, P. and Cudkowicz, G. (1977) J. Immunol. 119, 2013.
26. Hoffman, T., Hirata, F., Bougnoux, P., Fraser, B.A., Goldfarb, R.H., Herberman, R.B. and Axelrod, J. (1981) PNAS USA 78, 3839-3843.
27. Grohman, P.H., Prozsolt, F., Quirt, I., Miller, R.G. and Phillips, R.A. (1981) Clin. Exp. Immunol. 44, 611.
28. Roder, J.C. and Klein, M. (1979) J. Immun. 123, 2785.
29. Gerrard, J.M., Peller, J.D., Krick, T.P. and White, J.G. (1977) Prostaglandin 14, 39-50.
30. Lepetina, E.G., Schmitges, C.J., Chandrabose, K. and Cuatrecasus, P. (1977) Biochem. Biophys. Res. Commun. 76, 3, 828-835.
31. Cheung, W.Y. (1980) Science 207, 19.

32. Weiss, B., Prozialeck, W. and Cimino, M. (1980) Adv. Cyclic Nucleotide Res. 12, 213.
33. Laing, L.P., Boegman, R.J. and Roder, J.C. (1982) submitted for publication.
34. Roder, J.C., Beaumont, T.J., Kerbel, R.S., Haliotis, T. and Kozbor, D. (1981) PNAS USA 78, 6396-6400.
35. Wright, S.C. and Bonavida, B. (1981) J. Immunol. 126, 1516-1521.
36. Bonavida, B. and Wright, S. (1982) First International Workshop on NK Cells. (abstract).
37. Roder, J.C., Kiessling, R., Biberfeld, P. and Andersson, B. (1978) J. Immunol. 121, 2509-2517.
38. Roder, J.C., Rosen, A. Fenyo, E.M. and Troy, F.A. (1979) PNAS USA 76, 1405.
39. Roder, J.C., Ahrlund-Richter, L. and Jondal, M. (1979) J. Exp. Med. 150, 471.
40. Neighbour, A.P., and Huberman, H.S., Sr. (1982) J. Immunol. 128, 1236-1240.
41. Carpen, O., Virtanen, I., and Saksela, E. (1981) Cell Immunol. 58, 97-106.
42. Hiserodt, J.C., Britvan, L.J. and Targan, S.R. (1982) First International NK Workshop (abstract).
43. Weissman, G., Goldstein, F., Hoffstein, S., and Tsung, P.K. (1975) Ann N.Y. Acad. Sci. 253, 750-762.
44. Katz, P., Zaytoun, A.M. and Fauci, A.S. (1982) J. Immunol. 129, 287-296.
45. Forbes, J.T., Bretthauer, R.K. and Oeltmann, T.N. (1981) PNAS USA 78, 5797-5801.
46. Roder, J.C. and Duwe, A.K. (1979) Nature 278, 451.
47. Brandt, E.J., Swank, R.T. and Novack, E.K. (1980) In "Immunologic Defects in Laboratory Animals I". Gershwin, M.E. and Merchant, B., eds., New York Plenum Press pp 99-117.
48. Goldfarb, R.H., Timonen, T., and Herberman, R.B. (1982) First International NK Workshop (abstract).
49. Roder, J.C., Haliotis, T., Laing, L., Kozbor, D., Rubin, P., Pross, H.F., Boxer, L.A., White, J.G., Fauci, A.S., Mostowski, H. and Matheson, D.S. (1982) Immunol. 46, 555-560.
50. Quan, P.C., Ishizaka, T. and Bloom, B.R. (1982) J. Immunol. 128, 1786-1791.
51. Hirata, F., and Axelrod, J. (1980) Science 209, 1082-1090.
52. Bonavida, B., Kahle, R. and Hiserodt, J.C. (1982) First International Workship on NK Cells (abstract).
53. Newman, W. (1982) PNAS USA 79, 3858.
54. Newman, W., Martin, P. Hansen, J.A. and Fast, L.D. (1982) First International NK Workshop (abstract).

INHIBITORS OF SKIN TUMOR PROMOTION

AJIT K. VERMA+

+Department of Human Oncology, Division of Clinical Oncology, University of
Wisconsin, Center for Health Sciences, 600 Highland Avenue, Madison, WI 53792,
USA

INTRODUCTION

Inhibitors of the process of tumor formation are useful agents to obtain
clues about the mechanism of carcinogenesis. The two-stage model of the
induction of murine skin cancer is an excellent quantitative model for the
investigation of the biochemical mechanism of carcinogenesis as well as for the
study of the nature of the mechanism of action of agents which modify
carcinogenesis. This introduction section will deal with the features of the
two-step model of mouse skin carcinogenesis.

The process of tumor formation in mouse skin can be divided into at least
two defined stages, initiation and promotion (1-6). Initiation can be
accomplished by a single application of a carcinogen (e.g., 7,12-dimethyl-
benz[a]anthracine (DMBA)), at a sufficiently small dose so that it will not
lead to the induction of visible tumors during the life span of the animal.
However, many tumors develop following repeated and prolonged applications to
the initiated skin of another chemical known as a tumor promoter. Applications
of tumor promoter alone rarely elicit tumors; it is only their applications
following initiation that elicit tumors. Treatment with the initiator and the
promoter in reverse order should cause no more tumors than either agent
alone. Initiation is essentially an irreversible process; a long time can be
elapsed between initiation and promotion steps without diminution of the tumor
yield. In contrast, promotion is relatively reversible; if the period between
applications of a promoter is extended too long, the ultimate tumor yield is
decreased. Thus, initiation and promotion are qualitatively different
components of the process of tumor formation and also have been shown to be
operative in organs other than the skin (7-11). Initiation of tumor formation,
which requires a single exposure to a low level of a carcinogen and is
irreversible, appears to be inevitable. On the other hand, the promotion stage
of tumor formation, which requires repeated and prolonged exposures to a
promoter for autonomous tumor growth and is essentially reversible, offers a
great potential for the control of cancer. In human beings, this promotion

phase of tumor development may be many years. Currently, there is a great interest for the investigation of antipromoters which may antagonize the promotion of tumor formation (12, 13). 12-0-Tetradecanoylphorbol-13-acetate (TPA), a component of croton oil is a very potent skin tumor promoter (14-16). TPA, in nanomole quantity, can promote mouse skin tumor formation and is a useful compound to study the phenomenon of tumor promotion.

The type of neoplastic lesions that develop first in mouse skin with initiation with DMBA and promotion with TPA are the epithelial papillomas. The papillomas are benign lesions; some of them regress, others persist, and a few develop into invasive carcinomas (17-19). A variety of chemicals (a few of them are listed in Table 1) inhibit the formation of skin cancer when applied to the initiated mouse skin in conjunction with promotion treatments with TPA. In this chapter, I would primarily discuss our results of the effects of polyamine synthesis inhibitor α-difluoromethylornithine (DFMO) and retinoids on tumor promotion by TPA (20-28).

TABLE 1

INHIBITORS OF MOUSE SKIN TUMOR PROMOTION

Inhibitors	References
1. Anti-inflammatory steroids	12, 51
2. Retinoids	13, 21-28
3. Protease inhibitors	53, 54
4. Prostaglandin synthesis inhibitors	58
5. Polyamine synthesis inhibitor DFMO	20, 57
6. Cyclic nucleotide phosphodiesterase inhibitors	59
7. Poly I:C	60

EXPERIMENTS AND RESULTS

The Experiments and the Results section is divided into six subsections. The first deals with the biochemical and biological processes linked to tumor promotion by TPA. The second and third summarizes the effects of DFMO (an irreversible inhibitor of ornithine decarboxylase (ODC)) and retinoids on TPA-induced polyamine biosynthesis and tumor promotion by TPA, respectively . The fourth reviews the mechanism of inhibition by retinoic acid of ODC induction. The fifth presents evidence indicating that the effect of retinoic acid on skin carcinogenesis is not universal and the mechanism by which retinoic acid inhibits carcnogenesis involves its ability to inhibit the induction of ODC.

Finally, the results, that the mode of inhibition of tumor promotion by steroids and protease inhibitors is different than that of retinoids, are presented.

1. Biochemical and biological processes linked
   to tumor promotion by TPA

There are two obvious objectives to identify the early biochemical pertur-bations linked to the promotion of tumor formation. First, it will provide means to devise a rapid test to identify tumor promoters in the environment. Second, knowledge of the early marker(s) of tumor promotion is essential for the rational approach for the design of drugs for the intervention of the promotion of tumor formation. Thus, a great interest has been aroused to investigate the biochemical mechanism(s) of tumor promotion by TPA, and this has been a subject of many reviews (29-33). Briefly, a single topical applica-tion of TPA to mouse skin leads to enhanced incorporation of ^{32}P into phospho-lipids, increased accumulation of prostaglandins, and to sequential activation of RNA, protein and DNA synthesis. Other biochemical changes observed following TPA treatment include enhanced phosphorylation of nuclear histones, decreased histidase activity, altered cyclic nucleotide metabolism, induction of ODC and S-adenosylmethionine (SAMD) decarboxylase activities, and the accu-mulation of putrescine and spermidine in mouse epidermis (Figure 1). Among the numerous biological effects of TPA in mouse epidermis are hyperplasia, altered terminal differentiation, and the induction of dark keratinocytes (34, 35). TPA also induces similar cellular and biochemical changes when added into cultured cells in vitro (30-32). TPA binds specifically to membrane fractions but, it is still not clear whether the TPA responses are triggered by its initial specific binding to the plasma membrane receptors (36-40).

Now, the question that needs immediate attention is how to identify a specific TPA response(s) which is related to tumor promotion. Various approaches are employed to obtain clues about the relevance of TPA response to the mechanism of tumor promotion. Examples include structure-activity and, dose-response relationship, and the effects of the agents which block certain of the TPA-induced changes and also block tumor promotion. Thus, it has been shown that the induction of ODC activity and the resultant accumulation of putrescine is one of the important components of the mechanism of tumor promo-tion by TPA (23, 33). Among the morphological changes induced by TPA, the induction of dark cells by TPA may be specifically related to tumor promotion (35).

244

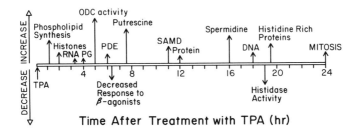

Time After Treatment with TPA (hr)

Figure 1. A simplified presentation of temporal biochemical changes elicited following topical application of TPA to mouse skin. Double line indicates the time in hours, and the direction of an arrow indicates whether a particular phenotypic change is increased or decreased as compared to the controls not treated with TPA. PG, prostaglandin; PDE, phosphodiesterase; SAMD, S-adenosyl-methionine decarboxylase.

2. Inhibition of TPA-promoted mouse skin

   tumor formation by DFMO

Decarboxylation of ornithine to putrescine, as catalyzed by ODC, is the first and the rate-limiting step in the pathway of polyamine biosynthesis (41, 42). SAMD, a second enzyme in the polyamine biosynthetic pathway, decarboxy-lates S-adenosylmethionine; the propylamine moiety derived from S-adenosyl-methionine condenses with putrescine to form spermidine (41). The activities of polyamine biosynthetic enzymes, especially ODC, and the levels of their biosynthetic products (putrescine, spermidine and spermine) are elevated in various tissues and cultured cells which are stimulated to proliferate (41, 42) and to differentiate (43, 44), as well as in transformed cells (41, 42, 45). Polyamines play important roles in the regulation of the synthesis of nucleic acid and protein (25, 41).

Topical application of TPA to mouse skin leads to a dramatic induction of epidermal ODC activity between 4 and 6 hr and the enhanced accumulation of putrescine at about 7 hr after treatment (33). Available data indicate that

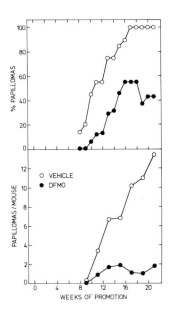

Figure 2. The effect of oral administration of DFMO in the drinking water on promotion of mouse skin papillomas by TPA. All mice were initiated with 0.2 µmol of DMBA. Two weeks after initiation, all mice were promoted twice a week with 10 nmol of TPA for the duration of the experiment. Administration of 1% DFMO (w/v) in the drinking water was started 2 days before the first TPA treatment (●). The same source of tap water was given to control mice (O). Both drinking waters were constantly available for the duration of the experiment. There were 20 mice in each group housed with 5 mice per cage. Average intake of drinking water was as follows: TPA only, 9.1 ± 0.3 ml/mouse/day; TPA + DFMO, 9.0 ± 0.2 ml/mouse/day. Average body weight at 20 weeks as follows: TPA only 32.6 ± 2.7 g; TPA + DFMO, 34.5 ± 0.9.

TABLE 2

EFFECT OF DFMO ON TPA-CAUSED ACCUMULATION OF POLYAMINES IN MOUSE EPIDERMIS

A. DFMO applied to the skin. Groups of mice were treated with 0.3 mg of DFMO
    or vehicle 1 hr after application of 10 nmol of TPA or acetone.
B. DFMO administered in drinking water. DFMO was dissolved in water at a
    concentration of 1% (w/v) and administered 72 hr before application of 10
    nmol of TPA. The same source of tap water was given to control mice. Both
    drinking waters were constantly available for the duration of the
    experiment.
    In both cases, the mice were killed at the indicated times after the TPA or
    acetone treatment. Each value represents the mean ± S.E. of determinations
    carried out on 3 groups of mice with 2 mice per group.

Treatment	Polyamines (nmol/mg DNA)		
	Putrescine (at 8 hr)	Spermidine (at 24 hr)	Spermine (at 24 hr)
A. DFMO applied to the skin			
Acetone + acetone:ethanol:H_2O	24 ± 7	146 ± 14	68 ± 4
Acetone + DFMO	6 ± 2	118 ± 18	56 ± 6
TPA + acetone:ethanol:H_2O	50 ± 1	264 ± 12	61 ± 2
TPA + DFMO	13 ± 3	201 ± 13	61 ± 8
B. DFMO administered in drinking water			
Acetone	21 ± 3	120 ± 11	50 ± 4
Acetone + DFMO	12 ± 4	95 ± 14	69 ± 7
TPA	51 ± 5	223 ± 15	53 ± 6
TPA + DFMO	6 ± 1	91 ± 13	61 ± 3

ODC induction and the accumulation of putrescine by TPA, although not sufficient (46, 47), are important components of the mechanism of skin tumor promotion by TPA (13, 20, 23, 25). The availability of DFMO, an enzyme activated
irreversible inhibitor of ODC (48), has enabled us to establish an essential
role for TPA-stimulated polyamine biosynthesis in skin tumor promotion (20).

    DFMO, either applied to mouse skin or administered in the drinking water in
conjunction with applications of TPA to DMBA-initiated mouse skin inhibited the
formation of mouse skin papillomas. Thus, application of 0.3 mg of DFMO in
0.2 ml vehicle (acetone:ethanol:H_2O, 2:1:1, v/v) 1 hr after each twice weekly
application of 10 nmol of TPA to DMBA (0.2 μmol) initiated mouse (female CD-1)
skin inhibited the formation of skin papillomas by 50%. The number of
papillomas per mouse in the vehicle and DFMO treatment groups was 6.90 and
3.50, respectively, and the percentages of mice with papillomas were 97 and
61%, respectively. The survival rate was greater than 90% in all groups.

DFMO, when given in the drinking water (1% w/v), was a very effective inhibitor of mouse skin tumor promotion (Figure 2). Drinking water containing DFMO was started 2 days before the first of the twice weekly applications of 10 nmol of TPA and was given throughout the promotion period. DFMO treatment inhibited by 90% the number of papillomas per mouse and by 56% the number of mice bearing papillomas (Figure 2).

DFMO treatment completely inhibited TPA-induced ODC activity and the accumulation of putrescine. Application of DFMO to skin did not inhibit epidermal spermidine levels, but did inhibit when given in the drinking water (Table 2).

3. Inhibition by retinoids of TPA-stimulated polyamine
   biosynthesis and tumor promotion by TPA

The mechanism of inhibition by retinoic acid of tumor promotion by TPA involves its ability to inhibit the induction of ODC activity and the resultant accumulation of putrescine (13, 25). As shown in Figure 3, application of

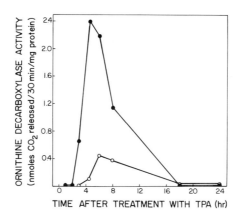

Figure 3. The effect of pretreatment with retinoic acid on the induction of epidermal ODC activity by TPA. Groups of mice were treated with 1.7 nmols of retinoic acid (O) or acetone (●) 1 hr before treatment with 17 nmoles of TPA. Mice were killed for enzyme assay at the indicated times after application of TPA. Each point on the graph represents the average of triplicate determinations of enzyme activity from soluble epidermal extracts prepared from 4 mice.

1.7 nmol of retinoic acid 1 hr before application of 17 nmol of TPA to the shaved backs of mouse skin, inhibited the induction of ODC activity. Furthermore, it should be noted that the degree of induction of ODC by TPA increased with increasing numbers of applications of TPA; retinoic acid treatment 1 hr before each TPA treatment to DMBA-initiated skin inhibited the induction of ODC activity by 80% (Figure 4).

Topical applications of retinoic acid in acetone 1 hr before each twice weekly applications of TPA to DMBA-initiated mouse skin inhibited skin tumor formation but, application of retinoic acid in conjunction with an initiating dose of DMBA failed to inhibit tumor formation elicited by repeated applications of TPA (Figure 5). The results indicate that retinoic acid treatment inhibits tumor formation by interference with the promotion stage and not with the initiation stage of skin carcinogenesis.

It has been shown that 5,6-epoxyretinoic acid may be an active metabolite of retinoic acid (24). 5,6-Epoxyretinoic acid inhibited the induction of ODC

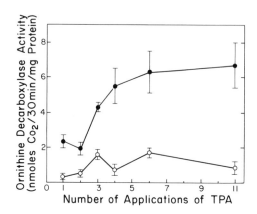

Figure 4. The effect of repeated applictions of TPA on induction of epidermal ODC activity and its inhibition by retinoic acid pretreatments. Mice were initiated with 0.2 µmol of DMBA in 0.2 ml of acetone; 14 days later, mice were treated with either 0.2 ml of acetone (●) or 1.7 nmol of retinoic acid (○) in 0.2 ml of acetone 1 hr before treatment with 17 nmol of TPA on days 1 and 4 of each week. Mice were killed 4.5 hr after TPA treatment, and ODC activity in soluble epidermal homogenates was determined. Each point is the mean ± S.E. (bars) of the determinations carried out in 3 groups of 3 mice each. ODC activity was not determined beyond the 11th application of TPA because the mice started bearing papillomas.

activity as effectively as retinoic acid (24). Furthermore, both 5,6-epoxy-retinoic acid and retinoic acid, when applied 1 hr after each application of TPA to the initiated mouse skin, inhibited the formation of both skin papillomas and carcinomas to the same extent (Figure 6).

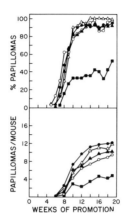

Figure 5. The effect of retinoic acid on mouse skin tumor formation. Groups of mice were treated as follows: 68 nmol of retinoic acid were applied 1 hr before initiation with 0.2 μmol of DMBA (▲); 68 nmol of retinoic acid were applied 1 hr after treatment with DMBA as well as every day for 7 days following initiation (O); 68 nmol of retinoic acid were applied every day for 5 days starting 7 days after initiation with DMBA (△). Treatment of mice concurrently with 68 nmol of retinoic acid and DMBA did not inhibit the incidence of formation of papillomas (not shown). Two weeks following initiation, all mice were promoted twice a week with 17 nmol of TPA. Mice were treated with either acetone (●) or 68 nmol of retinoic acid (■) 1 hr before each promotion with TPA.

Application of certain retinoids in conjunction with TPA inhibited the induction of ODC activity as well as skin tumor formation (Table 3). Retinoids, which inhibited skin tumor promotion, inhibited the accumulation of putrescine, but inhibited neither the induction of SAMD activity nor spermidine by TPA (23). Thus, there appears to be a correlation between the ability of retinoids to inhibit the induction of ODC activity and their ability to inhibit the formation of skin papillomas (23).

4. How does retinoic acid inhibit the induction
   of ODC activity by TPA?

The inhibitory effect of retinoic acid on ODC induction was neither the result of nonspecific cytotoxicity nor due to the production of soluble

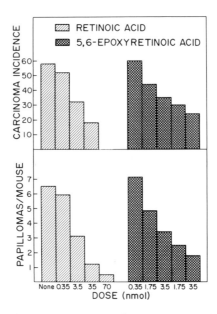

Figure 6. The effect of retinoid dose on skin tumor promotion by TPA. The sencar mice were initiated with 10 nmol of DMBA and promoted twice weekly with 1.6 nmol of TPA plus the retinoid for the duration of the experiment. Bottom, papillomas/mouse at 16 weeks after promotion; top, carcinoma incidence (percentage of mice with carcinomas) at 45 weeks after promotion.

inhibitor of ODC enzyme. Inhibition of ODC induction was not the result of an inhibitory effect of retinoic acid on general protein synthesis. TPA-caused increase in ODC activity is inhibited by inhibitors of protein (cycloheximide) and RNA (5-azacytidine) synthesis (33). This suggests that ODC induction involves new protein and RNA synthesis. To prove that retinoic acid inhibits the net amount of ODC protein increased by TPA, one has to demonstrate a decrease in immunoprecipitable protein after treatment with antibodies monospecific to ODC. Since the efforts to purify TPA-induced ODC and to raise antibodies to ODC are still being made, the availability of radiolabeled DFMO, enzyme-activated irreversible inhibitor of ODC, has provided means to quantitate ODC from a partially purified ODC sample. The results are summarized in Table 4. Application of 17 nmol of retinoic acid 1 hr before application of 10 nmol of TPA to mouse skin inhibited ODC induction which was paralleled by decreased binding of [^{3}H]DFMO.

TABLE 3

THE EFFECT OF VARIOUS RETINOIDS ON THE INDUCTION OF EPIDERMAL ODC AND SAMD
ACTIVITIES, AND TUMOR PROMOTION BY TPA

All mice were initiated by topical application to skin of 0.2 μmol of DMBA in
0.2 ml of acetone; 2 weeks after initiation, mice were treated twice a week
with either 0.2 ml of acetone or a retinoid in 0.2 ml of acetone 1 hr before
each treatment with 8 nmol of TPA. The analyses were made after the seventh
TPA treatment and the tumor data were recorded at the twentieth week of
promotion. For determination of ODC and SAMD activities, mice were killed 4.5
and 24 hr after TPA treatment, respectively. Each value represents the mean ±
S.E. of determinations of enzyme activity from 3 groups of mice, and each group
contained the combined supernatant prepared from 3 or 4 mice.

Treatment	Dose (nmol)	ODC activity	SAMD activity	A 20 weeks of promotion	
		(nmol CO_2/30 min/mg protein)		Pa[a]/mouse	% with Pa
None		0.02	0.04 ± 0.01	None	None
Acetone		3.5 ± 0.4	0.14 ± 0.01	9.9	90
β-Retinoic acid	34	0.04	0.12 ± 0.00	1.7	54
13-cis-Retinoic acid	34	0.5 ± 0.1	0.14 ± 0.01	3.7	48
TMMP[b] analog of ethyl retinoate	140	0.5 ± 0.1	0.14 ± 0.01	1.5	42
TMHP[c] analog of ethyl retinoate	140	3.3 ± 0.7	0.14 ± 0.01	12.9	92
13-Trifluoromethyl-TMMP analog of ethyl retinoate	140	3.8 ± 0.7	0.13 ± 0.01	9.6	100

[a]Papillomas
[b]Trimethylmethoxyphenyl
[c]Trimethylhydroxyphenyl

5. Retinoic acid fails to inhibit ODC induction and
   skin tumor formation by the complete carcinogen DMBA

The experiments summarized below provide evidence that indicate the failure
of retinoic acid to inhibit ODC induction as well as tumor formation by DMBA
(26-28).

As shown in Figure 7, 17 nmol of retinoic acid, when applied 1 hr before
treatment with 5 nmol of TPA, inhibited by about 90% the induction of ODC
activity. In contrast, the application of retinoic acid 1 hr before 3.6 μmol
of DMBA failed to inhibit at any point but, rather, paradoxically potentiated
the induction of ODC activity at 24 hr (P<0.01) after treatment.

252

TABLE 4

SUPPRESSION BY RETINOIC ACID OF TPA-CAUSED INCREASED ODC PROTEIN QUANTIFIED BY
ITS BINDING TO $\alpha-[5-^3H]$DFMO

Acetone or 17 nmol of retinoic acid in acetone was applied 1 hr before
application of acetone or 10 nmol of TPA in acetone to mouse skin. Mice were
killed 4.5 hr after the second treatment. Epidermis from 20-30 mice was
homogenized and centrifuged at 100,000 g for 60 min; soluble epidermal ODC was
partially purified by ammonium sulphate (35-55%) precipitation and dialysis.
This partially purified ODC fraction was used for $[^3H]$DFMO binding assay (49).
Each value is the mean of determinations carried out from duplicate assays.

Treatment	ODC activity (nmol CO_2/60 min/mg protein)	$[^3H]$DFMO bound (dpm/mg protein)
Acetone	0.3	2,411
Acetone-TPA	62.8	14,531
Retinoic acid-TPA	4.5	4,300

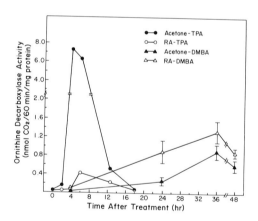

Figure 7. Effect of retinoic acid pretreatment on the induction of ODC
activity by TPA as well as by DMBA. Groups of mice were treated with 17 nmol
of retinoic acid (RA) or acetone 1 hr before the application of 3.6 μmol of
DMBA or 5 nmol of TPA. Epidermal ODC activity was determined at the indicated
times following DMBA or TPA treatment. Each point represents the mean or the
mean ± S.E. of determinations carried out from 3 groups of 3 mice each.

ODC induction by a single application of 3.6 μmol of DMBA, measured at 36 hr after treatment, was not inhibited by topical application of retinoic acid 1 hr before and 24 hr after treatment. Even more extensive treatments with 0.017, 0.17 or 1.7 nmol of retinoic acid were ineffective; 4 applications of either dose at 3 hr intervals immediately preceding and 4 applications at 2 hr intervals immediately following 3.6 μmol of DMBA did not inhibit ODC induction. Furthermore, orally administered retinoic acid did not inhibit ODC induction by DMBA (26).

Induction of skin tumors elicited by a single large dose (3.6 μmol) of DMBA could not be inhibited by application of a dose as large as 68 nmol of retinoic acid. However, application of 367 nmol of 7,8-benzoflavone inhibited both DMBA-induced ODC activity and tumor formation (Table 5).

TABLE 5

EFFECTS OF THE TOPICAL APPLICATION OF RETINOIC ACID AND 7,8-BENZOFLAVONE ON THE INDUCTION OF ODC ACTIVITY AND THE FORMATION OF SKIN TUMORS CAUSED BY A SINGLE LARGE DOSE OF DMBA

Groups of mice were treated only once with 68 nmol of retinoic acid or 367 nmol of 7,8-benzoflavone in 0.2 ml acetone 30 min before a single application of 3.6 μmol of DMBA in 0.2 ml acetone. ODC activity in the soluble epidermal extracts was determined at 36 hr, and the formation of skin papillomas was determined at 20 weeks after DMBA treatment. Each value of ODC activity is the mean ± S.E. of determinations carried out on 4 groups of 2 mice each. In the tumor experiment, there were 30 mice in each group. % Papillomas refers to the % of mice with papillomas in each treatment group.

Pretreatment	ODC activity (nmol CO_2/ 60 min/ mg protein)	Papillomas/ Mouse	% Papillomas
Acetone	1.35 ± 0.11	0.17	14
Retinoic acid	1.30 ± 0.14	0.41	33
7,8-Benzoflavone	0.29 ± 0.15	0.00	0

Topical application of retinoic acid did not inhibit tumor formation by weekly repeated doses of 0.2 μmol of DMBA. In the same experiment, the same solution of retinoic acid inhibited tumor formation by TPA applied to DMBA-initiated skin (Figure 8). In an experiment, where retinoic acid was applied both 1 hr before and 24 hr after each 0.2 μmol of DMBA treatment, paradoxical augmentation of DMBA carcinogenesis was observed. Application of 34 nmol of retinoic acid 30 min before each twice weekly application of 1, 10, 50 nmol of DMBA did not inhibit tumor formation. Intraperitoneal administration of retinoic acid in corn oil 30 min before each weekly application of 0.2 μmol of

254

DMBA failed to inhibit, but rather potentiated DMBA carcinogenesis. Retinoic
acid not only failed to inhibit tumor formation by the carcinogen DMBA, but it
also failed to inhibit tumor formation by twice weekly applications of 0.1 μmol
of either 3-methylcholanthrene or benzo[a]pyrene (27).

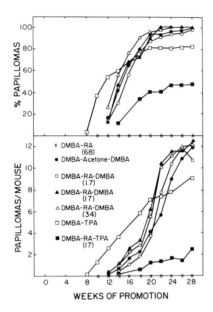

Figure 8. Effect of retinoic acid (RA) on skin tumor formation by either DMBA
or TPA. 0.2 μmol of DMBA in 0.2 ml acetone was applied to the shaved backs of
CD-1 mice. Beginning 2 weeks after initiation, mice were treated twice weekly
with 68 nmol of RA only, acetone or the indicated dose of RA 1 hr before once
weekly application of 0.2 μmol of DMBA or twice weekly applications of 5 nmol
of TPA.

It is interesting to note that retinoic acid inhibited skin tumor promotion
as well as ODC induction by 7-bromomethylbenz[a]anthracene (BrMBA), a congner
of DMBA (Figure 9 and Table 6). BrMBA is a weak complete carcinogen and a skin
tumor initiating agent but is a good tumor promoter when applied to DMBA-
initiated skin (50).

These results indicate that the nature and the mechanism of the biochemical
events elicited by the presumed promoting component of carcinogenesis by a
complete carcinogen are different from that of the tumor promoter TPA.

Retinoic acid inhibited both ODC induction and tumor promotion by TPA as
well as by BrMBA. This suggests that there may be a common pathway for TPA and

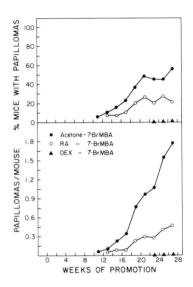

Figure 9. Inhibition of skin tumor promotion by retinoic acid and dexametha-sone. Skin tumors were initiated by a single application of 0.2 μmol of DMBA in 0.2 ml acetone to the shaved backs. Beginning 14 days after initiation, acetone, 17 nmol of retinoic acid, or 76 nmol of dexamethasone in 0.2 ml acetone was applied 30 min before each twice weekly application of 100 nmol of BrMBA.

TABLE 6

EFFECT OF RETINOIC ACID AND DEXAMETHASONE ON THE INDUCTION OF ODC ACTIVITY BY BrMBA

Acetone, retinoic acid or dexamethasone in acetone was applied 1 hr before a single application of 200 nmol of BrMBA. Soluble epidermal ODC activity was determined at 5 hr after BrMBA treatment. Each value is the mean ± S.E. of determinations carried out on preparations made from 3 groups of 3 mice each.

Pretreatment	Dose (nmol)	ODC Activity (nmol CO_2/60 min/mg protein)
Experiment 1		
Acetone	--	0.45 ± 0.09
Retinoic acid	1.7	0.07 ± 0.03
Retinoic acid	17.0	0.04 ± 0.02
Experiment 2		
None	--	0.64 ± 0.19
Retinoic acid	17.0	0.13 ± 0.04
Dexamethasone	76.0	0.05 ± 0.00

BrMBA for ODC induction and tumor promotion. However, the inability of BrMBA to compete for the specific binding of [³H]TPA to epidermal cell membranes as well as the observation that BrMBA did not inhibit ODC induction by TPA may argue against a completely common pathway for the promotion of tumor formation.

The results presented herein strengthen the concept that the mechanism by which retinoic acid inhibits tumor promotion is by its ability to inhibit ODC induction. Thus, retinoic acid inhibits ODC induction by TPA and BrMBA and also inhibits tumor promotion; retinoic acid does not inhibit ODC induction by DMBA and does not inhibit tumor formation (27).

6. Inhibition of skin tumor promotion
by steroids and protease inhibitors

Steroidal anti-inflammatory agents dexamethasone and fluocinolone acetonide are potent inhibitors of skin tumor promotion by TPA (12, 51). The mechanism by which anti-inflammatory steroids inhibits skin tumor promotions is related to their ability to inhibit DNA synthesis, inflammation and hyperplasia induced by TPA. It is also important to note that applications of dexamethasone or fluocinolone acetonide in conjunction with TPA during tumor promotion lead to a considerable loss in the body weight of animals (12, 51). Application of dexamethasone did not inhibit the induction of ODC activity by TPA; accumulation of putrescine and spermine remained unaltered but, dexamethasone inhibited the enhanced levels of spermidine by TPA (12, 52).

A number of protease inhibitors (e.g., tosyl lysine chloromethylketone, tosylphenylalanine chloromethylketone, tosyl alanine methyl ester, antipain, leupeptin) has been shown to inhibit skin tumor promotion (53, 54). The mechanism by which protease inhibitors inhibit tumor promotion is not clear. We have shown that protease inhibitors inhibit neither ODC induction nor enhance DNA synthesis by TPA (52). Recently, it has been shown that the promotion stage of mouse skin tumor formation can be further subdivided into two different components (55); protease inhibitors and the anti-inflammatory steroid fluocinolone acetonide inhibit the first stage of tumor promotion while retinoic acid and DFMO inhibit the second stage of mouse skin tumor promotion (56, 57).

SUMMARY

1. DFMO, a suicide inhibitor of ODC, applied to mouse skin or administered in drinking water in conjunction with applications with TPA to DMBA-initiated mouse skin inhibited the formation of mouse skin papillomas;

TPA-induced ODC activity and the accumulation of putrescine are completely inhibited.

2. Antipromoting activity of retinoic acid is related to its ability to inhibit the induction of ODC and the resultant accumulation of putrescine by TPA.

3. Application of retinoic acid in conjunction with a single 3.6 μmol dose or weekly repeated doses (1, 10, 50 or 200 μmol) of DMBA inhibited neither the induction of epidermal ODC activity nor tumor formation.

4. Application of retinoic acid 1 hr prior to application of 100 nmol of BrMBA to DMBA-initiated skin inhibited skin tumor formation. Retinoic acid treatment inhibited ODC induction by BrMBA.

5. Antipromoting steroids and protease inhibitors did not inhibit ODC induction by TPA.

CONCLUSIONS

1. The mechanism of inhibition by retinoic acid of tumor promotion is due to its ability to inhibit the induction of ODC activity and the resultant accumulation of putrescine. Retinoic acid inhibits TPA-caused synthesis of ODC protein.

2. The mechanism of inhibition of tumor promotion by steroids and protease inhibitors are different from that of retinoids.

3. There may not be a common biochemical pathway that leads to tumor formation by TPA, BrMBA and DMBA. Thus, one should not expect a general inhibitory effect of a modifier of carcinogenesis on tumor formation by diverse carcinogenic agents.

4. The use of combination of drugs may be a better approach in the chemoprevention of cancer. Combinations of inhibitors may show enhanced inhibition at levels below the threshold for undesirable side effects of each when used singly.

258

ACKNOWLEDGEMENTS

The author thanks C. T. Garcia, R. C. Simsiman, H. M. Rice, B. G. Shapas and E. A. Conrad for technical assistance. These investigations were supported by U.S. Public Health Service Grants CA-22484 and CA-07175 from the National Cancer Institute, NIH. The encouragement of Dr. R. K. Boutwell throughout the course of this work is gratefully acknowledged.

REFERENCES

1. Berenblum, I. (1954) Cancer Res, 14, 471-477.
2. Berenblum, I. and Shubik, P. (1947) Br. J. Cancer, 1, 379-382.
3. Mottram, J.C. (1944) J. Pathol. Bacteriol., 56, 181-187.
4. Boutwell, R.K. (1964) Progr. Expt. Tumor Res., 4, 207-250.
5. Boutwell, R.K. (1974) CRC Critical Rev. Toxicol. 2, 419-443.
6. Scribner and Süss (1978) Int. Rev. Expt. Pathol. 18, 137-187.
7. Peraino, C., Fry, R.J.M., Staffeldt, E. and Kisieleski, W.E. (1973) Cancer Res., 33, 2701-2705.
8. Pitot, H.C. and Sirica, A.E. (1980) Biochim. Biophys. Acta, 605, 191-215.
9. Fukushima, S., Friedell, G.H., Jacobs, J.B. and Cohen, S.M. (1981) Cancer Res., 41, 3100-3103.
10. Hicks, R.M. and Chowaniec, J. (1977) Cancer Res., 37, 2943-2949.
11. Reddy B.S., Weisburger, J.H. and Wynder, E.L. (1978) in Carcinogenesis--A Comprehensive Survey, Vol. 2, T.J. Slaga, A. Sivak and R.K. Boutwell (eds.), Raven Press, New York, pp. 453-464.
12. Slaga, T.J., Fischer, S.M., Weeks, C.E., Nelson, K., Mamrack, M. and Klein-Szanto, A.J.P. (1982) in Carcinogenesis--A Comprehensive Survey, Vol. 7, E. Hecker, N.E. Fusenig, W. Kunz, F. Marks and H.W. Thielmann, (eds.), Raven Press, New York, pp. 19-34.
13. Verma, A.K. (1981) in Retinoids, C.E. Orfanos, O. Braun-Falco, E.M. Farber, C. Grupper, M.K. Polano and R. Schuppli (eds.), Springer-Verlag, New York, pp. 117-131.
14. Hecker, E. and Schmidt, R. (1974) in Progress in the Chemistry of Organic Natural Products, Vol. 31, W. Heiz, H. Griseback and G.W. Kirby (eds.), Springer-Verlag, New York, pp. 377-467.
15. Van Duuren, B.L. (1969) Progr. Expt. Tumor Res., 11, 31-68.
16. Van Duuren, B.L. and Orris, L. (1965) Cancer Res., 25, 1871-1875.
17. Burns, F.J., Vanderlaan, M., Sivak, A. and Albert, R.E. (1976) Cancer Res., 36, 1422-1427.
18. Burns, F.J., Vanderlaan, M., Snyder, E. and Albert, R.E. (1978) in Mechanisms of Tumor Promotion and Co-carcinogenesis, Vol., 2, T.J. Slaga, A. Sivak and R.K. Boutwell (eds.), Raven Press, New York, pp. 91-96.
19. Verma, A.K. and Boutwell, R.K. (1980) Carcinogenesis, 1, 271-276.
20. Takigawa, M., Verma, A.K., Simsiman, R.C. and Boutwell, R.K. (1982) Biochem. Biophys. Res., Commun., 105, 969-976.
21. Verma, A.K. and Boutwell, R.K. (1977) Cancer Res., 37, 2196-2201.
22. Verma, A.K., Rice, H.M., Shapas, B.G. and Boutwell, R.K. (1978) Cancer Res., 38, 793-801.
23. Verma, A.K., Shapas, B.G., Rice, H.M. and Boutwell, R.K. (1979) Cancer Res., 39, 419-425.
24. Verma, A.K., Slaga, T.J., Wertz, P.W., Mueller, G.C., Boutwell, R.K. (1980) Cancer Res., 40, 2367-2371.
25. Verma, A.K. and Boutwell, R.K. (1980) in Polyamines in Biomedical Research, J.M. Gaugus (ed.), John Wiley and Sons, Ltd., England, pp. 185-201.

26. Verma, A.K., Conrad, E.A. and Boutwell, R.K. (1980) Carcinogenesis, 1, 607-611.
27. Verma, A.K., Conrad, E.A. and Boutwell, R.K. (1982) Cancer Res., 42, 3519-3525.
28. Verma, A.K. (1982) in Carcinogenesis--A Comprehensive Survey, Vol. 7, E. Hecker, N.E. Fusenig, W. Kunz, F. Marks and H.W. Thielmann (eds.), Raven Press, New York, pp. 35-39.
29. Boutwell, R.K., Verma, A.K., Ashendel, C.L., Astrup, E. (1982) In Carcinogenesis--A Comprehensive Survey, Vol. 7. E. Hecher, N.E. Fusenig, W. Kunz, F. Marks and H. W. Thielmann (eds.), Raven Press, New York, pp. 1-12.
30. Diamond, L., O'Brien, T.G. and Rovera, G. (1978) Life Sci., 23, 1979-1988.
31. Weinstein, I.B., Wigler, M. and Pietropaolo, C. (1978) in Origins of Human Cancer, Book B, H.H. Hiatt, J.D. Watson and J.A. Winstein (eds.), Cold Spring Harbor Laboratory, Cold Spring Harbor, New York, pp. 751-772.
32. Blumberg, P.M. (1980) CRC Crit. Rev. Toxicol., 8, 153-197.
33. O'Brien, T.G. (1976) Cancer Res., 36, 2644-2653.
34. Raick, A.N. (1974) Cancer Res., 34, 2915-2925.
35. Klein-Szanto, A.J.P., Major, S.M. and Slaga, T.J. (1980) Carcinogenesis, 1, 399-406.
36. Delclos, K.B., Nagle, D.S. and Blumberg, P.M. (1980) Cell, 19, 1025-1032.
37. Ashendel, C.L. and Boutwell, R.K. (1981) Biochem. Biophys. Res. Commun., 99, 543-549.
38. Solanki, V., Slaga, T.J. (1982) Carcinogenesis, 3, 993-998.
39. Wheldrake, J.F., Marshall, J., Ramli, J. and Murray, A.W. (1982) Carcinogenesis, 3, 805-807.
40. Froscio, M., Tapley, P.M., Guy, G.R., Pappalardo, S., Jones, M.J. and Murray, A.W. (1982) Carcinogenesis, 7, 837-839.
41. Jänne, J., Pösö, H. and Raina, A. (1978) Biochim. Biophys. Acta, 473, 241-293.
42. Russell, D.H. (1973) Polyamines in Normal and Neoplastic Growth, Raven Press, New York, pp. 1-13.
43. Takigawa, M., Ishida, H., Takano, T. and Suzuki, F. (1980) Proc. Natl. Acad. Sci. USA, 77, 1481-1485.
44. Gazitt, Y. and Friend, C. (1980) Cancer Res., 40, 1727-1732.
45. Bachrach, U. (1976) Ital. J. Biochem., 25, 77-93.
46. Mufson, R.A., Fisher, S.M., Verma, A.K., Gleason, G.L., Slaga, T.J. and Boutwell, R.K. (1979) Cancer Res., 39, 4791-4795.
47. Marks, F., Fürstenberger, G. and Kownatzki, E. (1981) Cancer Res., 41, 696-702.
48. Metcalf, B.W., Bey, P., Danzin, C., Jung, M.J., Casara, P. and Vevert, J.P. (1978) J. Am. Chem. Soc., 100, 2551-2553.
49. Pritchard, M.L., Seeley, J.E., Pösö, H., Jefferson, L.S. and Pegg, A.E. (1981) Biochem. Biophys. Res. Commun., 100, 1597-1603.
50. Scribner, N.K. and Scribner, J.D. (1980) Carcinogenesis, 1, 97-100.
51. Scribner, J.D. and Slaga, T.J. (1973) Cancer Res., 33, 542-546.
52. Verma, A.K., Conrad, E.A. and Boutwell, R.K. (1980) Proc. Am. Assoc. Cancer Res., 21, 91.
53. Troll, W., Klassen, A. and Janoff, A. (1970) Science, 169, 1211-1213.
54. Hozumi, M., Ogawa, M., Sugimura, T., Takeuchi, T. and Umezawa, H. (1972) Cancer Res., 32, 1725-1728.
55. Slaga, T.J., Fisher, S.M., Nelson, K. and Gleason, G.L. (1980) Proc. Natl. Acad. Sci. USA, 77, 3659-3663.
56. Slaga, T.J., Klein-Szanto, A.J.P., Fisher, S.M., Weeks, C.E., Nelson, K. and Major, S. (1980) Proc. Natl. Acad. Sci. USA, 77, 2251-2254.
57. Weeks, C.E., Herrmann, A.L., Nelson, F.R. and Slaga, T.J. (1982) Proc. Natl. Acad. Sci. USA, 79, 6028-6032.

260

58. Verma, A.K., Ashendel, C.L. and Boutwell, R.K. (1980) Cancer Res., 40, 308-315.
59. Perchellet, J.P. and Boutwell, R.K. (1982) Carcinogenesis, 3, 53-60.
60. Gelvoin, H.V. and Levy, H.B. (1970) Science, 167, 205-207.

BIOLOGICAL RATIONAL OF USING α-TOCOPHEROL

(VITAMIN E) IN THE TREATMENT OF CANCER

KEDAR N. PRASAD AND BHOLA N. RAMA
Department of Radiology, College of Medicine,
University of Colorado Health Sciences Center,
Denver, Colorado 80262

INTRODUCTION

The transformation from normal cells to cancer cells due to the effect of ionizing radiation, chemical carcinogens, viruses or any combination of these probably frequently occur in the body; however, these transformed cells do not always establish themselves in the host as a clinical cancer. This suggests that the host exerts considerable selection pressure against the first or first few transformed cells. This selection pressure is exerted by the host's immune system and by certain endogenous substances. The transformed cells probably escape the selection pressure of the host by undergoing additional mutations. Since the transformed cells escape the selection pressure exerted by certain endogenous substances at physiological concentrations, these substances at pharmacological concentrations should exhibit antitumor activity either by inducing normal phenotype and/or by causing cell death. Indeed, recent studies suggest that vitamin A, vitamin C and α-tocopherol (vitamin E) may represent some of the endogenous substances which exert the selection pressure against the transformed cells. We would discuss here only the possible roles of vitamin E in the prevention and treatment of cancer.

© 1983 Elsevier Science Publishing Co., Inc.
Cancer: Etiology and Prevention, Ray G. Crispen, Editor

VITAMIN E IN THE PREVENTION OF CANCER

Some animal experiments and human epidemiological studies suggest [1-7] that the high intake of vitamin E reduces the risk of cancer. However, this suggestion can not be considered conclusive in humans until the intervential trial of vitamin E among high risk population confirms the above observation. The role of vitamin E in the treatment of cancer has just begun.

VITAMIN E IN THE TREATMENT OF CANCER

Induction of normal phenotype and growtn inhibition. Several in vitro studies suggest that vitamin E induces morphological changes and/or growth inhibition (due to cell death and inhibition of cell division) in tumor cells in culture [8-12]. The extent and the type of effect depend upon the type of tumor cells and the type of vitamin E. For example, D- or DL-α-tocopherol acid succinate is more effective in causing morphological changes and/or growth inhibition than DL-α-tocopherol free alcohol, DL-α-tocopherol acetate and DL-α-tocopherol nicotinate [10].

Vitamin E succinate at similar concentrations ($\leq$ 5 µg/ml) does not effect the growth rate or morphology of mouse fibroblasts [10] and 8-day old chick embryo retinal cells (Gremo et al, unpublished observation) in culture.

D-α-tocopherol (vitamin E) acid succinate induces irreversible morphological changes and growth inhibition in mouse melanoma cells (B-16) in culture [10]. The morphological changes include enlargement of soma, enlongation of bipolar cytoplasmic processes, and tendency of cells to arrange themselves in parallel to

each other. The treated melanoma cells look like normal melan-
ocytes. D- and DL- form (Figure 1C) of vitamin E succinate
were equally effective. The untreated melanoma cells form
clumps during growth and exhibit mostly round cell morphology
(Fig. 1A). A concentration of 10 μg/ml of D- or DL- form of
vitamin E succinate was lethal. Sodium succinate at similar
concentrations with or without an equivalent volume of ethanol
was ineffective (Fig. 1B). Other forms of vitamin E such as
aquasol DL-α-tocopherol acetate (up to 10 μg/ml), DL-α-tocopherol
nicotinate (up to 200 μg/ml), DL-α-tocopherol free alcohol (up
to 10 μg/ml) were also ineffective. Higher concentrations of
vitamin E acetate and vitamine E free alcohol could not be used
because of the toxicity of specialized solvents at these
concentrations.

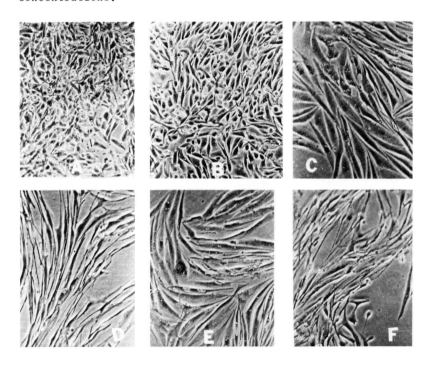

264

Fig. 1. Photomicrographs of melanoma cells were taken 4 days

after treatment. Control cutlure contains fibroblastic cells

as well as round cells in clumps (A). Cultures treated with

ethanol (1%) and sodium acid succinate (6 µg/ml) also exhibited

fibroblastic morphology with fewer round cells (B). DL-α-toco-

pherol acid succinate (6 µg/ml, C)-; butylated hydroxyanisole

(6 µg/ml, D)-; butylated hydroxyanisole (10 µg/ml, E)- and

torolox C (10 µg/ml, F)- treated cultures showed a dramatic change

in morphology.

Our results [10] show that vitamin E succinate was more potent

than vitamin E acetate, vitamin E free alcohol and vitamin E

nicotinate (Fig. 2).

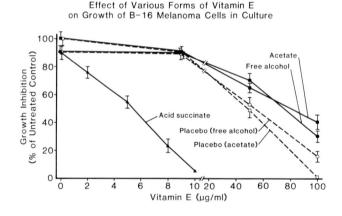

Fig. 2. Effect of various forms of vitamin E on the growth of

mouse melanoma (B-16) cells in culture (Prasad et al, 1982).

A recent study [13] has also shown that vitamin E acid succinate

is more effective than vitamin E acetate in protecting adriamycin

-reduced skin lesion in rats. Recently, we have found that DL- and D-isomer of vitamin E succinate were equally effective in melanoma cells (Table 1).

TABLE 1

EFFECT OF D- AND DL- FORM OF VITAMIN E SUCCINATE AND OTHER LIPID SOLUBLE ANTIOXIDANTS ON THE GROWTH INHIBITION OF MOUSE MELANOMA (B-16) CELLS IN CULTURE

Treatments	Growth Inhibition (% of untreated controls)	
	Cell No.	Colony
Sodium succinate (5 µg/ml) + ethanol (0.5%)	109±7[a]	96±6[a]
DL- vitamin E succinate (5 µg/ml)	59±6	42±4
D- vitamin E succinate (5 µg/ml)	55±5	36±5
Butylated hydroxytoluene (5 µg/ml)	85±5	66±5
Butylated hydroxyanisole (5 µg/ml)	73±4	76±5
Torolox C (5 µg/ml)	83±6	66±6

a=mean ± S.D

Melanoma cells (50,000 cells for counting cell number; 100 cells for colony formation) were plated in Lux culture dishes (60 mm). The growth inhibition was determined on the basis of number of cells per dish and number of colonies per dish. The values of untreated control cultures (62 ± 6 x 10^4; plating efficiency 55%) were considered to be 100%. The growth inhibition was determined as percentage of untreated controls. Each value represents an average of 9 samples.

The effect of vitamin E on melanoma cells in culture is primarily irreversible [10]. This is shown by the observation that when vitamin E acid succinate is removed after 4 days of treatment, the growth does not begin for a period of 24 hours. However, a slight increase in growth is observed at 2 days after removal of vitamin E [10]. This may be due to the existence of vitamin E acid succinate-resistant melanoma cells as well as only partially affected cells which eventually grow to confluency. The reasons for the resistance of melanoma cells to vitamin E succinate are unknown.

Effect of vitamin E in serum free medium. Our results show that vitamin E acid succinate-induced morphological changes and growth inhibition in hormone-supplemented serum free medium were similar to those observed in serum-supplemented medium [10]; however, the concentration needed to produce the effect was about 5 times less. This suggests that the effect of vitamin E is indeed mediated by vitamin E and not by some complex formed in the serum.

Effect of vitamin E on other tumors. To study the generality of the effect of vitamin E acid succinate on mammalian cells in culture, we investigated the effect of vitamin E acid succinate on mouse fibroblast (L-cells), 8-day old chick embryo retinal cells, rat glioma (C-6) and mouse neuroblastoma (NBP$_2$) cells in culture. Results show that vitamin E acid succinate at a concentration of 5 µg/ml did not affect the morphology or growth of mouse fibroblasts [10] and embryonic retinal cells in culture (Gremo et al, unpublished observation), however, it inhibited the growth and increased the size (not shown) of mouse NB cells in culture. In addition, it inhibited the growth of rat glioma (C-6) cells in culture (Fig. 3). D- and DL- form of vitamin E succinate was equally effective on NB cells, but D- form was more effective than DL- form on glioma cells in culture.

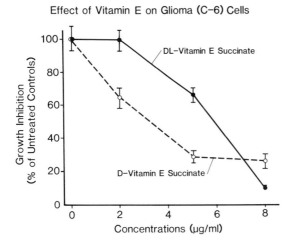

Fig. 3. Relative effect of D- and DL-α-tocopherol succinate on the growth of glioma (C-6) cells in culture.

A recent study [11] has shown that DL-α-tocopherol induces morphological differentiation in mouse myeloid leukemia cells in culture without affecting the growth rate. These studies show that vitamin E could induce differentiation as well as growth inhibition in tumor cells.

MECHANISMS OF THE EFFECTS

Tocopherol has been recognized as a biological lipid anti-oxidant in vitro and in vivo [14-17]. In addition, vitamin E has been suggested to have the following additional functions: vitamin E stabilizes membrane by physiochemical interactions between its phytyl side chain and the fatty acyl chains of polyunsaturated phospholipids [18-22] it stimulates host's immune system [23], it inhibits the synthesis of prostaglandins [24]

it prevents platelet agregation [25-26] and release [27], and it
reduces adriamycin-induced cardiac and skin toxicity [13,28-31]
and bleomycin-induced lung fibrosis [32].

Effect of lipid soluble antioxidants. To study whether the
effects of vitamin E succinate on tumor cells in culture are
mediated by antioxidantion, three lipid soluble antioxidants,
butylated hydroxytolouene (BHT), butylated hydroxyanisole (BHA),
and torolox (contains only tocopherol ring) were used. We
have found that BHT, BHA and torolox at a concentration of
6 µg/ml also inhibit the growth and caused morphological
changes similar to those produced by a concentration of 6 µg/ml
of vitamin E succinate (Fig. 1C); but the extent of the effect
was much less (Fig. 1D). At a concentration of 10 µg/ml,
vitamin E succinate produces lethal effect on melanoma cells
in culture [10]; whereas BHA, BHT and torolox only inhibited
growth and caused more extensive changes in morphology. The
effects of BHA at a concentration 10 µg/ml (Fig. 1E) resemble
that (Fig. 1C) seen at 6 µg/ml of vitamin E succinate. Antioxidants BHA, BHT and torolox also inhibited the growth of
neuroblastoma and glioma cells in cultures. These data show
that the effects of vitamin E succinate on melanoma, neuroblastoma and glioma cells at least in part are mediated by
antioxidation mechanism.

EFFECT OF VITAMIN E IN VIVO

Our preliminary data show (unpublished observation) that
vitamin E acid succinate reduces the growth of transplanted

mouse neuroblastoma (NBP_2) and mouse melanoma (B-16). Vitamin

E free alcohol also reduces the growth of human neuroblastoma

cells in nude mice [12]. It has been reported that vitamin E

produces a beneficial effect in patients with chronic cystic

mastitis, the most common benign lesion of the female breast [33-34]

however, it was not apparent from this study whether vitamin E

caused any regression of tumor. Dr. L. Helson of Sloan Kattering

Research Institute has initiated phase 1 clinical trial of

vitamin E in the treatment of neuroblastomas.

MODIFICATION OF THE EFFECT OF TUMOR THERAPEUTIC AGENTS BY VITAMIN
E IN VITRO AND IN VIVO

In vitro studies. Vitamin E acid succinate enhances the

growth inhibitory effect of vincristine in a synergistic fashion;

but it does not modify the effect of DTIC on melanoma cells in

culture (our unpublished data). Aquasol vitamin E acetate mod-

ifies the effect of several pharmacological agents and ionizing

radiation on mouse neuroblastoma and rat glioma cells in

culture [9]. For example, vitamin E acetate enhances growth

inhibitory effect of 5-FU, adriamycin, 4-(3-butoxy-4-methoxy-

benzyl)-2-imidazolidinone (RO 20-1724), vincristine, sodium

butyrate, chlorozotocin, and prostaglandin E_1 in a synergistic

manner on neuroblastoma cells in culture, whereas it enhances

the growth inhibitory effect of only RO 20-1724, vincristine,

and CCNU on glioma in a similar manner [9]. Vitamin E acetate

in combination with bleomycin, CCNU, ·DTIC, mutamycin and cis-

platinum produces an additive effect on neuroblastoma cells

in culture, whereas it in combination with bleomycin, mutamycin and cisplatinum produced a similar effect on glioma cells. Vitamin E acetate failed to enhance the effect of sodium butyrate, prostaglandin E_1 and chlorozotocin on glioma cells in culture [9]. These results show that the extent of modification of the effect of pharmacological agents on tumor cells by vitamin E depends upon the type of tumor cell and the type of pharmacological agent.

In vivo studies. The modification of the effect of tumor therapeutic agents by vitamin E has not been tested on any tumors growing in vivo.

MODIFICATION OF THE EFFECT OF TUMOR THERAPEUTIC AGENTS BY VITAMIN C IN VITRO AND IN VIVO

In vitro studies. We have also investigated the modification of the effect of tumor therapeutic agents by a water soluble antioxidants, vitamin C [35-36]. Sodium ascorbate modifies the effect of tumor therapeutic agents on tumor cells in a manner which is, in part, different from that produced by vitamin E. Sodium ascorbate (vitamin C) at a nontoxic concentration in combination with certain pharmacological agents and ionizing radiation produced a synergistic or an additive effect on the growth inhibition of mouse neuroblastoma (NBP_2) cells in culture; it did not produce such an effect on rat glioma (C-6) cells in culture [35]. For example, sodium ascorbate at a nontoxic concentration potentiated the growth inhibitory effect of 5-FU, bleomycin sulfate, RO 20-1724 (an inhibitor of cyclic nucleotide phosphodiesterase), and sodium butyrate on neuroblastoma cells in culture, but it does not produce such an effect on glioma cells in culture. Sodium ascorbate did not enhance the growth inhibitory effect of vincristine, 6-thioguanine or CCNU; however, at higher drug concentrations, it potentiated the effect of these drugs in a synergistic fashion [36]. The potentiating effect of sodium ascorbate in combination with certain tumor therapeutic agents was not prevented by the addition of catalase in the growth medium. This suggests [35] that the effect of the combined treatment is not mediated by H_2O_2. Sodium ascorbate enhanced the growth inhibitory effect of electron affinic compounds on Chinese hamster ovary cells in culture [37].

Sodium ascorbate also reduces the cytotoxic effect of certain pharmacological agents [35]. For example, it reduces the cytotoxic effect of methotrexate and DTIC on neuroblastoma cells in culture. The mechanism of this effect is unknown.

The modification of the effect of ionizing radiation by vitamin E is dependent upon the type of tumor cell. For example, sodium ascorbate increased the effect of ionizing radiation on neuroblastoma cells in culture [35], whereas, it protected Chinese hamster ovary cells against radiation damage [38], but it did not modify the effect of irradiation on survival of glioma cells [35].

In vivo studies. A recent study shows that sodium ascorbate when combined with CCNU, enhanced the survival of mice with CNS leukemia by 2-fold in comparison to that observed in CCNU treated mice [39]. Vitamin C, when combined with ionizing radiation, also increased the survival of mice with ascites tumor cells in comparison to those treated with x-irradiation alone [40]. Ascorbate significantly reduced the adriamycin-induced cardio-myopathy [41]. These studies confirmed the concept developed in vitro systems [36-37] that ascorbate may modify the effect of pharmacological agents in a variety of ways. The effect of ascorbate in combination with other tumor therapeutic agents on tumor cells have not been tested as yet.

CONCLUSION

Experimental studies suggest that vitamin E may help in the management of tumors in following manner: (a) It may cause cell death, inhibition of cell division and cell differentiation. (b) It may potentiate the effects of certain tumor therapeutic agents. (c) It may reduce the toxic-effects of certain agents. (d) It may stimulate the host's immune system. Some of these effects of vitamin E are mediated by antioxidation mechanism. Sodium ascorbate (vitamin C) also modifies the effect of tumor therapeutic agents on tumor cells. The extent of the effects of tumor therapeutic agents by vitamins depends upon the type of vitamin, the type of tumor therapeutic agents and the type of tumor cells.

ACKNOWLEDGEMENT

This work was supported by a grant from HOffmann La Roche, Nutley, N.J. We thank Dr. Hemmy Bhagwan of Hoffman La Roche for providing vitamin E and torolox C. We also thank EM Labor-atories, Elmford, N.Y. for providing DL- vitamin E succinate.

REFERENCES

1. Dion, P.W., Bright-See, E., Smith, C.C. and Bruce, W.R. (1982) Mutation Res. in press.
2. Newmark, H.L. and Mergens, W.J. (1981) in Inhibition of Tumor Induction and Development, Zedeck, M.S. and Lipkins, M. ed., Plenum, New York, pp. 127-168.
3. Bright-See, E. and Newmark, H.L. (1982) in First International Conference on Modulation and Mediation of Cancer by Vitamins, Meyskens Jr., F.L. and Prasad, K.N. ed., Karger, New York, in press.
4. Cook, M.G. and McNamara, P. (1980) Cancer Res. 40, 1329-1331.
5. Jaffe, W. (1946) Exp. Med. Surg. 4, 278-282.
6. Haber, S.L. and Wissler, R.W. (1962) Proc. Soc. Exp. Biol. Med. 111, 774-775.
7. Shamberger, R.J., Baughman, F.F., Kalchert, S.L., Willis, C.E. and Hoffman, G.C. (1973) Proc. Natl. Acad. Sci. USA 70, 1461-1463.
8. Prasad, K.N., Ramanujam, S. and Gaudreau, D. (1979) Proc. Soc. Exp. Biol. Med. 16, 570-573.
9. Prasad, K.N., Edwards-Prasad, J., Ramanujam, S. and Sakamoto, A. (1980) Proc. Soc. Exp. Biol. Med. 164, 158-163.
10. Prasad, K.N. and Edwards-Prasad, J. (1982) Cancer Res. 42, 550-555.
11. Sakagami, H., Asaka, K., Abe, E., Miyaura, C., Suda, T. and Konno, K. (1981) J. Nutr. Sci. Vitaminol. 27, 291-300.
12. Helson, L., Verma, M. and Helson, C. (1982) Neuroblastoma, in First International Conference on the Modulation and Mediation of Cancer by Vitamins. Meyskens, F.L. and Prasad, K.N. eds; Karger Press, New York, in press.
13. Svingen, B.A., Powis, G., Appel, P.L. and Scott, M. (1981) Cancer Res. 41; 3395-3399.
14. Dam, H. and Granados, H. (1945) Peroxidation of Body Fat in Vitamin E Efficiency. Acta Physiol. Scand. 10, 162-171.
15. McCay, P.B. and King, M.M. (1980) in Vitamin E. Machlin L.J., ed., Marcel Dekker, Inc, pp. 289-317.
16. Tappel, A.L. (1972) New York Acad. Sci. 203, 12-27.
17. Alcott, H.S. and Matill, H.A. (1941) Chem. Res. 29, 257-268.
18. Lucy, J.A. (1978) in Tocopherol, Oxygen, and Bionutrients. C. deDuve, C., and Hayaishi, O., eds., Elsevier/North-Hollang Biomedical Press, New York, pp. 109-120.
19. Diplock, A.T. and Lucy, J.A. (1973) FEBS Letters 29, 205-210.
20. Molenaar, I., Vos, J., Hommes, F.A. (1972) Vitamin. Horm. 30, 45-82.
21. Huang, C. (1977) Chem Physic. Lipids 191, 150-158.
22. Marusich, W.L. (1980) in Vitamin E. Machlin, L.J., ed., Marcel and Dekker, New York, pp. 445-466.
23. Tengerdy, R.P. (1980) in Vitamin E. Machlin L.J. ed., Marcel Dekker, Inc, New York, pp. 429-444.
24. Machlin, L. (1978) in Tocopherol, Oxygen, and Biomembranes, deDuve C. and Hayaishi O., eds., Elsevier/North-Holland, Biomedical Press, New York, pp. 179-189.

25. Steiner, M. (1978).in Tocopherol, Oxygen, and Biomembranes. deDuve C. and Hayaishi, O., ed., Elsevier/North-Holland Biomedical Press, New York, pp. 143-163.
26. Fong, J.S.C. (1976) Experimentia 32, 639-641.
27. Machlin, L.J., Filipski, R., Willis, A.L., Kuhn, D.C., and Brin, M. (1975). Proc Soc. Exp. Biol. Med. 149, 275-277.
28. Myers, C.E., McGuire, W., and Young, R. (1976) Cancer Treat. Rep. 60, 961-962.
29. Sonnevald, P. (1978) Cancer Treat Rep. 62, 1033-1036.
30. Van Vleet, J.F., Greenwood, L., Ferrans, V.J., and Rebar, A.H. (1978) Am. J. Vitamin Res. 39, 997-1010.
31. Wang, Y.M., Madanat, F.F., Kimball, J.C., Gieiser, C.A., Ali, M.K., Kaufman, M.W., and Van Eys, J. (1980) Cancer Res. 40, 1022-1027.
32. Yamanaka, N., Fukushima, M., Koizumi, K., Nishida, K., Kato, T., and Ota, K. (1978) in Tocopherol, Exygen, and Biomembranes, de Duve C. and Hayaishi, O. eds., Elsevier/North-Holland Biomedical Press, New York, pp. 59-69.
33. Abrams, A.A. (1965) N. Eng. J. Med. 272, 1080-1088.
34. London, R.S., Sundaram, G.S., Manimekalai, S., Strummer, D., Schaltz, M., Nair, P.P., and Goldstein, P.J., (1982) Nutrition Res. 2, 243-247.
35. Prasad, K.N., Sinha, P.K., Ramanujam, M. and Sakamoto, A. (1979) Proc. Natl. Acad. Sci. USA 76, 829-832.
36. Prasad, K.N. (1980) Life Sciences 27, 275-280.
37. Josephy, P.D., Paleic, B., and Skarsgard, L.D. (1978) Nature 271, 370-372.
38. O'Connor, M.K., Malone, J.F., Moriarty, M. and Mulgrew, S. (1977) Brit. J. Radiol. 50, 587-591.
39. Moore, C., Chu, M., Tibbits, and Chalabresi (1979) The Pharmacologist 21, 233.
40. Tewfik, F.A., Riley, E.F. and Mital, C.R. (1977) Presented at the Annual Meeting of the Radiation Research Society, May 8-12.
41. Fujita, A., Shinpo, K., Sato, T., Niime, H., Shamoto, M., Nagatsu, T., Takeuchi, T., and Umezawa, H. (1982) Cancer Res. 42, 309-316.

SUPPRESSION OF MAMMARY CANCER BY RETINOIDS

RICHARD C. MOON, RAJENDRA G. MEHTA AND DAVID L. McCORMICK
Laboratory of Pathophysiology, Life Sciences Division, IIT Research Institute,
10 West 35th Street, Chicago, Illinois, 60616, USA

INTRODUCTION

The role of vitamin A (retinol and its esters) in regulating epithelial cell differentiation and maintenance was first demonstrated over fifty years ago by Mori[1] and by Wolbach and Howe[2]. The classical observations of these workers showed that feeding a diet deficient in retinoids [vitamin A (retinol) and its natural and synthetic analogs] to experimental animals resulted in hyperkeratinization, squamous metaplasia, and the appearance of gross tumors in a variety of epithelial tissues. The development of such retinoid deficient squamous metaplasia is a process closely akin to that induced by certain chemical carcinogens[3]. However, all epithelia do not respond similarly. The epidermis becomes hyperkeratotic whereas the intestinal mucosa exhibits a decrease in the number of goblet cells but no keratinization. Although these epithelia respond differently to the deficient state, the systemic administration of retinoids reverses the process and restores the epithelium to a normal functional capacity. More recently, other investigators have shown that animals fed a diet deficient in retinoids and subsequently exposed to chemical carcinogens, develop a greater than normal incidence of cancers and putative precursors to these malignancies[4-6]. Since retinoids have been shown to inhibit metaplasia of several epithelial tissues and since carcinogen-induced metaplasia appears similar to that resulting from retinoid deficiency, several investigators have extended these studies to show that exogenous retinoids can inhibit tumor induction in epithelia at several organ sites when administered during the preneoplastic period[7-9].

Most primary human cancers arise in epithelial tissues that depend upon retinoids for normal cellular differentiation[10,11] and several epidemiological investigations have noted an inverse relationship between vitamin A intake and risk for developing cancer[12,13]. Over the past few years, considerable effort has been directed towards the modulation of tumorigenesis of these epithelia by retinoids and although reports have appeared relative to inhibition of carcinogenesis of many epithelial tissues[14], the majority of such studies have dealt with chemoprevention of cancer of the skin, mammary gland and urinary bladder.

Cancer: Etiology and Prevention, Ray G. Crispen, Editor

Since our interests have focused on the chemoprevention of mammary and urinary bladder cancer and since the general aspects of the chemoprevention of cancer of these structures has been reviewed recently[15], we shall limit this report to a brief discussion of experiments conducted in our laboratory concerning the interrelationship of retinoids and hormones on chemical carcinogenesis of the breast of experimental animals.

STRUCTURE, ACTIVITY AND ORGAN SPECIFICITY

The basic structure of the retinoid molecule consist of a hydrocarbon ring, side chain and polar end group (Figure 1). Each portion of the molecule can be modified to yield biologically active analogs.

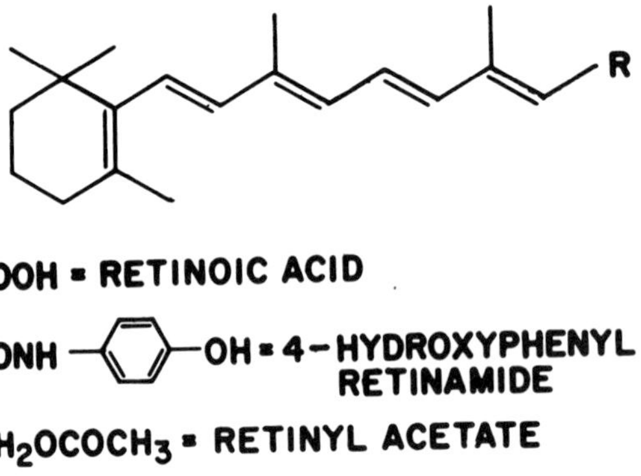

R = COOH = RETINOIC ACID

R = CONH —⟨ ⟩—OH = 4–HYDROXYPHENYL RETINAMIDE

R = CH₂OCOCH₃ = RETINYL ACETATE

Fig. 1. Structure of retinoids.

Several hundred synthetic analogs have been assayed *in vitro*[16] whereas only a few dozen compounds have been evaluated for cancer chemopreventive activity *in vivo*. However, such studies have indicated that modification of the hydrocarbon ring, side chain, or polar terminal group of the molecule can have a dramatic effect on the organ distribution[17] and specificity, and hence, the cancer inhibitory activity of the retinoid.

Figure 2 illustrates the relative efficacy of non-toxic doses of several retinoids in the inhibition of mammary carcinogenesis induced in the rat by MNU. Retinyl acetate and N-(4-hydroxyphenyl)retinamide (4-HPR) are highly effective in reducing mammary cancer incidence and increasing the latency of induced mammary cancers[8,17-19]. Furthermore, the number of mammary carcinomas can be significantly reduced by the administration of retinyl acetate or 4-HPR.

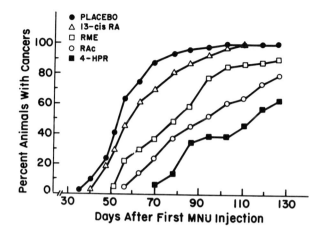

Fig. 2. Effect of retinoids on the incidence of MNU-induced mammary carcino-genesis. ● - no retinoid; Δ - 13-*cis*-retinoic acid; □ - retinyl methyl ether; o - retinyl acetate; ■ - 4-hydroxyphenyl retinamide. (Reproduced with permission of Plenum Press[23]).

However, 13-*cis*-retinoic acid has little effect on the appearance of MNU-induced mammary carcinomas; retinyl methyl ether is of intermediate efficacy, although the latter compound is extremely effective against 7,12-dimethylbenz-(a)anthracene-induced mammary carcinogenesis[20]. Thus, it is readily apparent that minor alterations in the basic retinoid structure can significantly alter the activity of the molecule with respect to the inhibition of chemical carcinogenesis of the mammary gland.

Although the synthetic retinoid 13-*cis*-retinoic acid is ineffective in the chemoprevention of mammary cancer, the retinoid is highly effective in inhibit-ing phorbol ester-induced tumor promotion in mouse skin[11] and in the prevention of urinary bladder cancer induced in rats and mice by the carcinogens N-methyl-N-nitrosourea (MNU)[9] or N-butyl-N-(4-hydroxybutyl)nitrosamine (OH-BBN)[21]. The trimethylmethoxyphenyl analog of ethyl retinoate is highly effective against mouse skin carcinogenesis[11], but this compound has little effect against either bladder carcinogenesis in mice or mammary cancer in rats. On the other hand, retinyl acetate is extremely active in the rat mammary tumor system[8] but exhibits little chemopreventive protection against two-stage skin tumorigenesis in mice[22]. Thus, it is apparent that the retinoids not only exhibit a high degree of organ specificity but that they also appear to be somewhat species specific.

The polar terminal group also has a significant effect on tissue distribution and toxicity of the retinoid. While retinyl acetate and 4-HPR are both effective inhibitors of chemical carcinogenesis of the rat mammary gland, the patterns of metabolism and organ distribution of the two compounds are quite different[23]. Chronic dietary administration of high doses of retinyl acetate results in the accumulation of retinyl esters in the liver, a process frequently accompanied by significant hepatotoxicity[24]. By contrast, dietary administration of 4-HPR results in a much higher level of retinoid in the mammary gland, with relatively little liver accumulation[17]. It thus appears that, on the basis of its organ distribution, 4-HPR is preferable to retinyl acetate for use in the prevention of experimental breast cancer.

CHEMOPREVENTION OF MAMMARY CANCER

As indicated in Figure 2, several retinoids possess mammary anticarcinogenic activity when administered chronically in the diet to experimental animals. Since in all cases retinoid treatment was initiated after carcinogen exposure, it is likely that the retinoid is inhibiting the promotion or progression of carcinogenesis. However, evidence exists which suggest that retinoids may also be effective inhibitors during the initiation phase of carcinogenesis[25].

A significant interaction between retinoids and other modifiers of mammary carcinogenesis has also been noted, with combined treatment being significantly more effective in cancer inhibition than treatment with either agent alone. Chief among these is the interaction between hormonal manipulation and retinoids. As shown in Figure 3, both retinyl acetate and ovariectomy inhibit mammary cancer induction by MNU; however, the combination of ovariectomy plus retinyl acetate is significantly more effective in cancer inhibition than is either treatment regimen alone. Similar results have been obtained with 4-HPR and ovariectomy. As is evident from Table 1, not only is the latency of tumor appearance greatly lengthened but cancer incidence and tumor multiplicity are dramatically reduced in animals treated with 4-HPR. Moreover, combined retinoid administration and ovariectomy are effective in inhibiting the development of subsequent mammary tumors when treatment is begun at the time of surgical removal of the host's first mammary tumor[26]. In our prolactin studies, we[27] have also found a synergistic inhibition of MNU-induced mammary carcinogenesis by the concomitant administration of retinyl acetate and 2-bromo-α-ergocryptine (CB-154), an inhibitor of pituitary prolactin secretion (Figure 4). Combination chemoprevention of mammary cancer has also been demonstrated with retinyl acetate and the antiestrogen, tamoxifen[28].

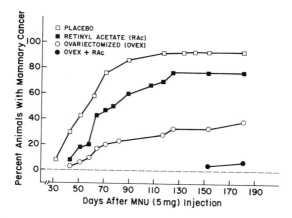

Fig. 3. Effect of retinyl acetate and ovariectomy on latency of appearance of MNU-induced mammary cancer. □ - intact-placebo; ■ - intact-retinyl acetate (328 mg/kg diet); o - ovariectomized-placebo; ● - ovariectomized-retinyl acetate diet. (Reproduced with permission of Plenum Press[23]).

TABLE 1

INFLUENCE OF N-(4-HYDROXYPHENYL)RETINAMIDE (4-HPR) AND/OR OVARIECTOMY ON MAMMARY CANCER INDUCTION BY MNU[a]

Group	No. of Animals	Cancer Incidence (%)	Cumulative Cancers per Rat	T_{50} (days)
Intact - Placebo	25	100	4.50	55
Intact - 4-HPR	25	92[c]	3.29[c]	85
Ovex[b] - Placebo	50	18[c]	0.24[c]	_[e]
Ovex - 4-HPR	50	2[c,d]	0.02[c,d]	_[e]

[a] Animals sacrificed at 225 days post-carcinogen.
[b] Ovex = ovariectomy.
[c] Significantly different from intact-placebo group, $p < 0.05$ or better.
[d] Significantly different from ovex-placebo group, $p < 0.01$ or better.
[e] Group never reached 50% cancer incidence.

These data would tend to suggest the existence of populations of neoplastic cells displaying differential sensitivity to the retinoids and hormones, with the retinoids preferentially affecting the hormone independent tumors or those which do not regress following ovariectomy.

280

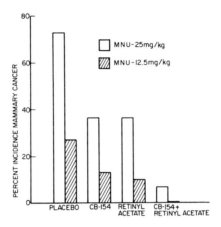

Fig. 4. Effect of retinyl acetate and/or a prolactin inhibitor (CB-154) on the incidence of mammary cancer. (Reproduced with permission of Cancer Res.[27]).

MECHANISM OF INHIBITION

The mechanism(s) by which retinoids inhibit carcinogenesis is presently unclear, although some insight into the process has been gained from the variety of influences of the retinoids on the mammary gland *per se*. Retinyl acetate and 4-HPR both exert an antiproliferative effect and significantly inhibit ductal branching and end bud proliferation in the mammary glands of rats[17]. Retinyl acetate has been also shown to inhibit chemical carcinogen-induced increases in mammary gland DNA synthesis[29] and the induction by carcinogens of terminal ductal hyperplasias, a putative precancerous lesion[18]. The addition of 4-HPR or retinoic acid to organ culture of mouse mammary glands inhibits prolactin-induced increases in DNA synthesis in such glands[30] which is reflected in a decreased structural differentiation. Furthermore, our recent *in vivo* studies[15] in C_3H mice also suggest an antiproliferative effect for 4-HPR in that hyperplastic alveolar nodulogenesis is reduced by approximately 50 percent in animals maintained on a diet supplemented with the retinoid. These effects on the mammary gland are probably not mediated via an influence on host hormonal levels, since retinoid administration has little effect upon either circulating prolactin levels[27] or normal ovarian function[19]. Moreover, the additive or synergistic effect of the retinoid plus hormonal manipulation in the combination studies cited above would also appear to substantiate this view.

Bashor *et al.*[31] were the first to demonstrate the presence of a specific retinol (vitamin A) binding protein sedimenting as a 2S component on sucrose density gradients in tissues highly sensitive to vitamin A deficiency. This finding led these investigators to suggest that the action of retinoids on the cell may be mediated in a manner similar to that of the steroid hormones, in which there is association with a specific cytosolic receptor protein, translocation of steroid-receptor complex to the nucleus, interaction with chromatin, and alteration of the cellular response[32,33].

Since the report of Bashor *et al.*, investigators have found both retinol and retinoic acid binding proteins in many normal and neoplastic tissues[34-36]. Consistant with these studies, we have reported the presence of both retinol and retinoic acid binding proteins in mammary tissue during several physiological states[37,38] as well as in both animal and human breast cancers. As shown in the left panel of Figure 5, the cytosolic retinoic acid binding protein complex of carcinogen-induced mammary cancer sediments as a 2S component. Unlabeled all-*trans*-retinoic acid at a 25 fold excess concentration competes effectively for the binding sites. Certain retinoids which are effective against mammary carcinogenesis (4-HPR, retinyl acetate) failed to compete for retinoic acid binding sites[23,37,38]. This finding is supported by evidence showing that radioactive 4-HPR does not bind with any protein of the tumor cytosol (Figure 5, right panel). These results suggest that 4-HPR requires metabolism to an active component within the mammary cell which then allows it to effectively bind to cytoplasmic retinoic acid binding protein (CRABP). Although a number of metabolites of 4-HPR have been found in mammary gland extracts of the animals consuming 4-HPR supplemented diets when analyzed by high pressure liquid chromatography[17], the active metabolite is, however, presently unknown.

As mentioned above, some of our studies indicated that ovarian hormone independent tumors may be more responsive to retinoid treatment than ovarian hormone dependent tumors[39]. Thus, tumors appearing in intact animals (both ovarian hormone dependent and independent tumors) as well as those arising in ovariectomized rats (ovarian hormone independent tumors) were analysed for their ability to bind retinoic acid specifically. As shown in Table 2, mammary cancers arising in animals which were ovariectomized (hormone-independent) one week after MNU administration contained significantly greater concentrations of CRABP than did cancers appearing in intact animals.

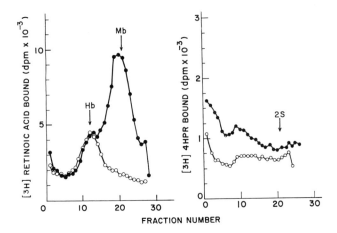

Fig. 5. Retinoid specificity for retinoic acid binding sites. Left Panel – Tumor cytosol was incubated with 1 mM [3H] retinoic acid either alone (●) or in the presence of a 25 fold excess of unlabeled retinoic acid (o). Right Panel - Tumor cytosol incubated with 1 mM [3H] N-(4-hydroxyphenyl)retinamide (4-HPR) either alone (●) or in the presence of a 25 fold excess of unlabeled 4-HPR (o).

TABLE 2

LEVELS OF CRABP IN MNU-INDUCED MAMMARY ADENOCARCINOMAS EXCISED FROM INTACT AND OVARIECTOMIZED HOSTS.

Host	No. of Tumors	CRABP (pmol/mg protein) mean ± SEM
Intact	18	3.24 ± 0.51
Ovariectomized	15	4.62 ± 0.42[a]

Source: Mehta *et al.*[40]
[a] $p < 0.05$ vs. intact group.

Similar results were also obtained when animals bearing palpable tumors were ovariectomized; the tumors which regressed in size (dependent tumors) contained significantly lower levels of CRABP than the ovarian hormone independent tumors which continued to grow (Table 3). Thus, an apparent correlation exists between the ability of retinoids to suppress mammary carcinogenesis and the level of CRABP in the cytoplasm of mammary cancers[40].

TABLE 3

TUMOR RESPONSE TO OVARIECTOMY AND LEVELS OF CRABP IN MNU-INDUCED MAMMARY
CARCINOMAS

Status of cancer after ovariectomy	No. of Tumors	CRABP (pmol/mg protein) mean ± SEM
Regressing	5	0.65 ± 0.16^a
Static	4	1.91 ± 0.35^b
Growing	6	4.02 ± 0.37^c

Source: Mehta *et al.*[40]
[a] vs. [b] $p < 0.025$. [a] vs. [c] $p < 0.01$. [b] vs. [c] $p < 0.01$.

A few investigators have studied the role of the retinoid binding proteins
on the interaction of the retinoid with the nucleus of target cells. Studies
on the role of retinol binding proteins in the interaction of retinoids with
the nucleus, as well as the presence of retinoic acid binding proteins in the
nuclei of retinoblastoma cells, Lewis lung tumors and embyonal carcinoma cells
have been reported[41-44]. Recent studies from our laboratory have indicated
that formation of a retinoic acid-receptor complex in the mammary tumor
cytoplasm is essential for the interaction of retinoic acid with the nucleus.
Retinoic acid *per se* does not bind to nuclei or to nuclear components. The
RABP which is isolated from purified nuclei of mammary cancers, following
incubation of nuclei with cytoplasmic retinoic acid-receptor complex sediments
as a 2S component when subjected to sucrose density gradient analysis[45].
Furthermore, incubation of a constant amount of nuclei (constant DNA concentration, ∿ 100 µg) with an increasing concentration of cytoplasmic retinoic
acid-receptor complex results in saturable nuclear binding (Figure 6B).
The data, when analyzed by a Scatchard plot, indicates that the nuclei bind
retinoic acid with a high affinity ($Kd = 1.7 \times 10^{-9}M$) and that the number of
nuclear binding sites approximates 4-5 pmoles per 100 µg DNA (Figure 6C).
Although our results do not explain whether the retinoic acid-receptor complex
enters the nucleus or simply delivers retinoic acid to the nucleus, they do
provide evidence that the formation of cytoplasmic retinoic acid-receptor
complex is essential for the interaction of retinoic acid with the nucleus
of mammary cancer cells.

284

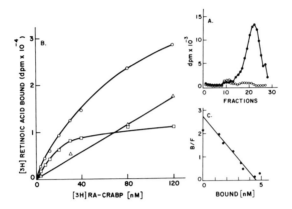

Fig. 6. Titration of [³H]retinoic acid binding sites in the nuclear fraction.
A) Sucrose density gradient profile of carcinogen-induced mammary tumor;
cytosol was incubated with [³H]retinoic acid either alone (●) or in presence of
25 fold excess unlabeled RA (o). Note: No 5S component was present.
B) Increasing concentrations of [³H]RA-CRABP were incubated with constant
amounts of nuclei either alone or in presence of 10 fold excess unlabeled RA-
CRABP. Radioactivity in ethanol extract of nuclei was measured. Total (o),
nonspecific (Δ) and specific (□) binding of [³H]RA to the nuclear fraction is
presented. C) The data on specific nuclear [³H]RA-CRABP complex were evaluated
by Scatchard analysis. The experiment was repeated 3 times. (Reproduced with
permission of Biochem. J.[45]).

At present, it is speculative to suggest that the interaction of retinoic

acid with the nucleus results in altered genomic expression. However, there

are numerous reports which indirectly support such a view. For example,

retinoids inhibit tumor promoter-induced ornithine decarboxylase activity[11],

carcinogen-induced DNA synthesis[29] and growth factor-induced transformation[46].

Our recent studies of RNA polymerase activity of mammary tumor nuclei are also

suggestive of such an effect: nuclei isolated from mammary cancers preincubated

with retinoic acid exhibited reduced RNA polymerase activity compared to

tissues incubated under similar conditions without the retinoid. Furthermore,

the nuclei which were preincubated with mammary cytosol containing retinoic

acid-receptor complex also showed reduced RNA polymerase activity, as compared

with that of nuclei incubated with either buffer or with free retinoic acid

(Table 4). Activity of both RNA polymerase I and II were reduced as a result

of retinoid treatment[47]. These results indicate that retinoids may be active at

the chromatin level, and that retinoic acid-retinoic acid receptor complexing

may be an important step in the mediation of retinoid action.

TABLE 4

INFLUENCE OF RA-CRABP ON NUCLEAR RNA POLYMERASE ACTIVITY

Condition	Percent Enzyme Activity	
	Mn Dependent	Mg Dependent
Control	100	100
RA-CRABP	79	42

Based on the data presented above, a proposed interaction of retinoids at the cellular level is summarized in Figure 7.

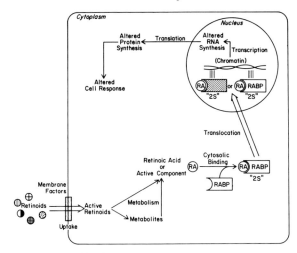

Fig. 7. Proposed steps in the interaction of retinoids in the target cell.

The active retinoid may enter the target cell as an authentic retinoid or as a metabolite; some membrane factors[48,49] may influence the entry of these compounds into the cell. Once in the cell, the retinoid may require further metabolism to an active component which may bind to a 2S cytoplasmic binding protein which specifically binds retinoic acid. The retinoic acid-receptor complex then translocates to the nucleus; unlike steroid receptors, this step does not require temperature activation[45]. The retinoic acid or the retinoic acid-receptor complex in the nucleus may interact with the chromatin and alter the synthesis of specific messenger RNA which, in turn, may influence trans-lation of an enzyme or a protein responsible for the chemoprotective effect of

the retinoid. The entire sequence of events, however, is poorly understood
and is highly speculative at this stage.

ACKNOWLEDGEMENTS

This work was supported in part by Grant CA-26030 and Contracts NO1-CP-23292,
NO1-CB-74207, NO1-CP-75939, NO1-CP-05718 and NO1-CP-15742 from the National
Cancer Institute. We wish to thank our staff for expert technical assistance
and Mrs. Josephine Cavanaugh for the preparation of this manuscript. Radio-
active retinoids were supplied by the Chemoprevention Program, Chemical and
Physical Carcinogenesis Branch, National Cancer Institute, Bethesda, Maryland.
Unlabeled retinoids were generously supplied by Dr. Michael Sporn, National
Cancer Institute, Hoffmann-LaRoche, Inc., Nutley, NJ, BASF Aktiengesellschaft,
Ludwigshafen, Germany and Johnson and Johnson, New Brunswick, NJ.

REFERENCES
1. Mori, S. (1922) Johns Hopkins Hosp. Bull. 33, 357-359.
2. Wolbach, S.D. and Howe, P.R. (1925) J. Exp. Med. 42, 753-777.
3. Harris, C.C., Sporn, M.B., Kaufman, D.G., Smith, J.M., Jackson, F.E. and
   Saffiotti, U. (1972) J. Natl. Cancer Inst. 48, 743-761.
4. Cohen, S.M., Wittenberg, J.F. and Bryan, G.T. (1976) Cancer Res. 36,
   2334-2339.
5. Rogers, A.E., Herndon, B.J. and Newberne, P.M. (1973) Cancer Res. 33,
   1003-1009.
6. Sporn, M.B., Dunlop, N.M., Newton, D.L. and Smith, J.M. (1976) Fed. Proc.
   35, 1332-1338.
7. Bollag, W. (1972) Europ. J. Cancer 8, 689-693.
8. Moon, R.C., Grubbs, C.J., Sporn, M.B. and Goodman, D.G. (1977) Nature 267,
   620-621.
9. Sporn, M.B., Squire, R.A., Brown, C.C., Smith, J.M., Wenk, M.L. and
   Springer, S. (1977) Science 195, 487-489.
10. Moore, T. (1957) Vitamin A. Amsterdam, Elsevier.
11. Verma, A.K., Shapas, B.G., Rice, H.M. and Boutwell, R.K. (1979) Cancer Res.
    39, 419-425.
12. Bjelke, E. (1975) Int. J. Cancer 15, 561-565.
13. Mettlin, C., Graham, S. and Swanson, M. (1979) J. Natl. Cancer Inst. 62,
    1435-1438.
14. Sporn, M.B. and Newton, D.L. (1981) in Inhibition of Tumor Induction and
    Development, M.S. Zedeck and M. Lipkin ed., Plenum Press, New York,
    pp. 71-100.
15. Moon, R.C., McCormick, D.L. and Mehta, R.G. (1983) Cancer Res. (in press).
16. Newton, D.L., Henderson, W.R. and Sporn, M.B. (1980) Cancer Res. 40,
    3413-3425.
17. Moon, R.C., Thompson, H.J., Becci, P.J., Grubbs, C.J., Gander, R.J.,
    Newton, D.L., Smith, J.M., Phillips, S.R., Henderson, W.R., Mullen, L.T.,
    Brown, C.C. and Sporn, M.B. (1979) Cancer Res. 39, 1339-1346.
18. McCormick, D.L., Burns, F.J. and Albert, R.E. (1981) J. Natl. Cancer Inst.
    66, 559-564.
19. Moon, R.C., Grubbs, C.J. and Sporn, M.B. (1976) Cancer Res. 36, 2626-2630.

20. Grubbs, C.J., Moon, R.C., Sporn, M.B. and Newton, D.L. (1977) Cancer Res. 37, 599-502.
21. Grubbs, C.J., Moon, R.C., Squire, R.A., Farrow, G.M., Stinson, S.F., Goodman, D.G., Brown, C.B. and Sporn, M.B. (1977) Science 198, 743-744.
22. Verma, A.K. and Boutwell, R.K. (1977) Cancer Res. 37, 2196-2201.
23. Moon, R.C. and Mehta, R.G. (1982) in Hormones and Cancer, Leavitt ed., Plenum Press, New York, pp. 231-249.
24. Smith, F.R. and Goodman, D.S. (1976) New Engl. J. Med. 294, 805-808.
25. McCormick, D.L., Burns, F.J., and Albert, R.E. (1980) Cancer Res. 40, 1140.
26. Moon, R.C., McCormick, D.L., Sowell, Z.L. and Fugmann, R.A. (1981) Proc. Amer. Assoc. Cancer Res. 22, 124.
27. Welsch, C.W., Brown, C.K., Goodrich-Smith, M., Chuisano, J. and Moon, R.C. (1980) Cancer Res. 40, 3095-3098.
28. McCormick, D.L. and Moon, R.C. (1982) Proc. 13th International Cancer Congress, 682.
29. Mehta, R.G. and Moon, R.C. (1980) Cancer Res. 40, 1109-1111.
30. Mehta, R.G., Cerny, W.L., Ronan, S.S. and Moon, R.C. (1981) Proc. Amer. Assoc. Cancer Res. 22, 112.
31. Bashor, M.M., Toft, D.O. and Chytil, F. (1973) Proc. Natl. Acad. Sci. 70, 3482-3487.
32. Jensen, E.V. and DeSombre, E.R. (1973) Science 182, 126-133.
33. Chan, L. and O'Malley, B.W. (1976) New Eng. J. Med. 294, 1322-1327.
34. Sani, B.P. and Corbett, T.H. (1977) Cancer Res. 37, 209-213.
35. Ong, D.E. and Chytil, F. (1975) J. Biol. Chem. 250, 6113-6117.
36. Chytil, F. and Ong, D.E. (1978) in Receptors and Hormone Action, B.W. O'Malley and L. Birnbaumer, ed., Academic Press, New York, pp. 573.
37. Mehta, R.G., Cerny, W.L. and Moon, R.C. (1980) Cancer Res. 40, 47-49.
38. Mehta, R.G. and Moon, R.C. (1981) Biochem. J. 200, 591-595.
39. McCormick, D.L., Mehta, R.G., Thompson, C.A., Dinger, N., Caldwell, J.A. and Moon, R.C. (1982) Cancer Res. 42, 509-512.
40. Mehta, R.G., McCormick, D.L., Cerny, W.L. and Moon, R.C. (1982) Carcinogenesis 3, 89-91.
41. Takase, S., Ong, D.E. and Chytil, F. (1979) Proc. Natl. Acad. Sci. (USA) 76, 2204-2208.
42. Wiggert, B., Russell, P., Lewis, M. and Chader, G. (1977) Biochem. Biophys. Res. Com. 39, 218-225.
43. Sani, B.P. and Donovan, M.K. (1979) Cancer Res. 39, 2492-2496.
44. Jetten, A.N. and Jetten, M.E.R. (1979) Nature 278, 180-182.
45. Mehta, R.G., Cerny, W.L. and Moon, R.C. (1982) Biochem. J. (in press).
46. Todaro, G.J., DeLarco, J.E. and Sporn, M.B. (1978) Nature 276, 272.
47. Mehta, R.G., Cerny, W.L. and Moon, R.C. (1982) Proc. Am. Assoc. Cancer Res. 23, 21.
48. Smith, J.E. and Goodman, D.S. (1979) Fed. Proc. 38, 2504-2509.
49. DeLuca, L.M. (1977) Vitamins and Hormones, 35, 1-57.

HEPATITIS B VIRUS. PATHOGENESIS AND PREVENTION
OF PRIMARY CANCER OF THE LIVER

BARUCH BLUMBERG AND W. THOMAS LONDON
Institute for Cancer Research
Fox Chase Cancer Center
Philadelphia, Pennsylvania 19111

INTRODUCTION

A goal of cancer research is the prevention of cancers, particularly those
that are common in the world, by the discovery of factors that are necessary
for their development and reducing or eliminating these factors in a manner
which is not, overall, harmful (primary prevention). A second goal is to
arrest the progress of the disease if it has already started by removing very
small tumors that have not spread (secondary prevention). A third approach,
which may be more easily and gently accomplished than secondary prevention, is
to slow the advance of a potential clinical cancer to a pace that avoids
disease perceptible to the individual until very late in his or her possible
life span, by which time the host would have died for another reason. This we
have called "prevention by delay." Developments over the past decade make it
very likely that primary prevention for one of the most common cancers in the
world, primary cancer of the liver, may be feasible, and current work is
directed to an understanding of the other two forms of prevention.

In sub-Saharan Africa, Taiwan, and the populous coastal and southern provinces of mainland China, the incidence of primary hepatocellular carcinoma
(PHC) is 25 to 150 cases per 100,000 population. An annual mortality of
100,000 for all of China (population base 850 million) has recently been
reported. The incidence of PHC is 3 to 9 times higher in males than females.
Hence, the estimated incidence of deaths from PHC in males would be about 17 to
20 per 100,000. Extrapolating these figures to other regions of the world
where PHC is a common cancer, we can estimate a worldwide annual incidence of
about 1/4 to 1 million cases in men and 50 to 200,000 cases in women. Since
PHC is almost always lethal, the incidence and mortality rates per year are
about the same.[1]

In 1975,[2] we pointed out that advances in our knowledge of the pathology,
epidemiology and clinical characteristics of PHC on the one hand, and of the
hepatitis B virus on the other made it possible to test the hypothesis that

Published 1983 by Elsevier Science Publishing Co., Inc.
Cancer: Etiology and Prevention, Ray G. Crispen, Editor

persistent infection with the hepatitis B virus was necessary for the development of (most cases) of PHC. Since that time, a substantial body of evidence which strongly supports this hypothesis has been collected. The quantity and quality of this data are such that it is reasonable to assume that the hypothesis is more likely to be right than wrong and to proceed with the next step; that is, the design of strategies to prevent infection with hepatitis B virus in order to prevent PHC as well as other consequences of HBV infection. Blumberg and Millman, in 1969, introduced a vaccine to protect against hepatitis B infection,[3] and this has now been produced in large quantities in the United States and other countries. Based to a large extent on the study of Szmuness and his colleagues in New York, it has been shown within the limits of the studies that the vaccine is safe and effective. It is likely that the vaccine will constitute a major part of public health programs to prevent hepatitis B infection which will be introduced in the near future. The use of such a vaccine which could ultimately prevent PHC could be economically and medical justified because of its effect on other diseases associated with HBV, and its predicted role as a "cancer vaccine" would be added to this.

In addition to the potential practical importance of this body of scientific information bearing on the HBV-PHC relation, it will be useful in basic studies on how viruses "cause" cancer. Since (if the accumulated evidence is accepted as convincing) HBV is required for the development of PHC, an understanding of how it does so will provide an explanation of the role of a virus in human carcinogenesis independent of its similarity or difference to existing models derived from other species or experimental observations. This explanation could then form the basis for discovering similar virus relations in other species (which has already happened (see below)) and in humans.

Evidence to support the hypothesis that persistent infection with HBV is required for the development of PHC

In this section, the method of "independent evidence" is used. Although any single item cited may have an alternative explanation, the total body of data taken together is best explained by the stated hypothesis. We have published more detailed discussions of these data, and additional bibliographic references are given in them.[1,4]

1) First of all, PHC occurs commonly in regions where chronic carriers of HBV are prevalent and much less frequently in areas where they are not.

2) Secondly, case-control studies have shown that 90 percent or more of patients with PHC who live in areas where HBV is endemic have HBsAg or high

titers of antibody against the core antigen in the blood (anti-HBc). These markers can be considered evidence of current or previous persistent HBV infection. In the same areas, controls have markedly lower frequencies of HBsAg and anti-HBc. Even in the United States, where PHC is uncommon, patients with the disease have higher prevalences of HBsAg and anti-HBc than do controls. In other words, in areas of both high and low PHC incidence, serologic evidence of persistent infection with HBV is more common in patients with PHC than in controls (Table 1).

Prince[5] has estimated that the relative risk of developing PHC for chronic carriers in the United States and western Europe is about the same as the relative risk for carriers in Asia and Africa. If this is correct, then factors (such as aflatoxins and nitrosamines) which are thought to be related to the development of PHC but which presumably are not as common in the western countries as in the high incidence countries, may not be essential for the development of PHC. They may play a role in increasing the frequency of hepatitis carriers, but there is little direct information about this.

3) Most cases of PHC (approximately 80 percent) arise in a liver already affected with cirrhosis or chronic active hepatitis or both. If chronic hepatitis and cirrhosis are steps toward the development of liver cancer, then case-control studies of these two diseases should also show higher prevalence of chronic infection with HBV in the cases. Studies in Africa and Korea have confirmed this prediction (Table 2).

4) HBV proteins can usually be demonstrated with histochemical stains or immunologic techniques in the hepatic tissues of patients with PHC. HBsAg and hepatitis B core antigen (HBcAg) are undetectable or present only in small quantities in the tumor cells themselves, but are found in the nonmalignant cells adjacent to the expanding tumor and elsewhere in the liver. These antigens are not found in the livers of uninfected persons nor in persons with antibody to HBsAg in their serum. A particularly pertinent study by Nayak et al. (6) in India, which is a low incidence area for PHC, showed that if multiple sections of the liver are examined, HBsAg can be found in some hepatocytes in over 90% of the cases of PHC. Thus, HBV proteins are present in the livers of most patients with PHC from areas endemic for HBV and PHC, and they are also found in the livers of many patients from low incidence areas.[6,7]

5) If persistent HBV infection causes PHC, such infection should precede the occurrence of PHC. To test this hypothesis, it is necessary to identify asymptomatic chronic carriers of HBV and controls who are not carriers and to follow them for several years to see whether PHC develops. A major study of

this type is being conducted by Beasley and Lin in male civil servants between the ages of 40 and 60 years in Taiwan.[8] Aproximately 3500 carriers were identified. The controls are an equal number of HBsAg-negative men matched by age and place of origin. Approximately 18,500 additional non-carriers were also identified. The subjects have been followed for two to four years. Fifty cases of PHC have occurred during the follow-up period, and all but one have been in chronic carriers. The one exception arose in a man who had both anti-HBc and anti-HBs, indicating that he had probably been infected in the recent past. Thus far, the relative risk of PHC is more than 250 times greater in carriers than in non-carriers, and 98 percent (the attributable risk) of the cases have occurred in carriers. This is probably the highest risk known for any of the common cancers.

6) Because PHC usually develops in a liver that is affected by cirrhosis or chronic hepatitis or both, some investigators have argued that any hepato-toxic agent that causes cirrhosis is associated with an increased risk of PHC, and that hepatitis B virus is one such agent. A rigorous test of the hypo-thesis that chronic infection with hepatitis B virus increases the risk of PHC in addition to producing cirrhosis is to compare the incidence of PHC in patients with cirrhosis who are or are not chronic carriers of HBV. Obata et al. have performed such a study in Japan.[9] Seven of 30 HBsAg-positive patients with cirrhosis (23 percent) but only five of 85 HBsAg-negative patients with cirrhosis (6 percent) had PHC after about four years. These results are highly consistent with the prediction from the hypothesis.

7) In populations where HBV is endemic (sub-Saharan Africa, Asia, and Oceania), there is good evidence that many of the chronic carriers acquire HBV as a result of infection transmitted from their mothers early in life. (Although children of carrier mothers may be exposed in utero, at birth, or immediately afterwards, they do not become carriers until after about six weeks to three months.) That is, the mothers themselves are chronic carriers, and offspring born when the mothers are infectious are likely to become chronic carriers. Within a population, persons infected shortly after birth or during the first year of life will have been chronic carriers of HBV longer than persons of similar age who are infected later in life. Therefore, if the duration of being a chronic carrier is related to the likelihood of having PHC, one could predict that the mothers of patients with PHC would be more likely to be chronic carriers than the mothers of controls of similar age who do not have PHC. Studies in Senegal, West Africa, and in Korea are consistent with this prediction[10] (Table 3).

8) A further test of the HBV-PHC hypothesis is whether HBV-DNA is present in PHC tissue and whether such DNA is integrated into the tumor cell genome. Summers et al., using livers obtained at autopsy in Senegal, extracted HBV DNA base sequences from 9 of 11 primary liver cancers collected from patients with HBsAg in their serum and from one of four patients who were HBsAg negative but anti-HBs positive.[11,12] Several cell lines which produce HBsAg have been developed from human primary liver cancer. The first was produced by Alexander in South Africa (PLC/PRF/5) and has been studied in many laboratories.[13] This cell line produces large quantities of HBsAg 22 nm particles (1.3 mg/ml) but no Dane particles.[14] Marion and Robinson analyzed these cells and demonstrated 4 to 5 ng of HBV DNA per mg of cellular DNA.[15] Recently, Gray et al.[16] reported that at least six copies of HBV DNA are integrated into the cellular genomic DNA of the liver. Two of the six inserts are incomplete viral genomes, but all six contain the gene for HBsAg. They also isolated RNA transcripts for the HBsAg gene from the Alexander cell line. Brechot et al.[17] demonstrated integration of viral DNA in the cellular genomes of three primary liver cancers obtained at autopsy from HBsAg(+) men who lived in Ivory Coast, West Africa. Because only a few bands of integrated DNA were observed in each tumor extract, it is likely that the integration sites were the same within each cell of a given tumor. A third cell line that produces HBsAg has been derived from a human PHC by Aden and Knowles.[18] Recently, Shafritz et al.,[19] studied percutaneous liver biopsies and post mortem tissue specimens from patients with chronic liver disease associated with persistent HBV infection, and patients with PHC. In 12 patients with hepatocellular carcinoma who had persistent HBV in their serum, integrated HBV DNA was found in host liver cells. It was also found integrated in some patients who had PHC with anti-HBs. In addition, integration was found in the non-tumorous tissue. In carriers of HBV without PHC, integration was seen in two patients who were carriers for more than 8 years, but it was not integrated in individuals who were carriers for less than two years. From this it can be inferred that increasing time of infection increases the probability of integration.

9) In 1971,[20] based on the unusual clinical and epidemiologic characteristics of the hepatitis B virus, we had proposed that it was different from other viruses and that it represented the first of a series of viruses we termed Icrons. (The name is an acronym of the Institute for Cancer Research, ICR, with a neuter Greek ending.) The unique characteristics of the molecular biology of HBV (see below) have supported the notion that HBV is an unusual virus. Recent discoveries of other viruses which conform to the expectations

of the Icron model provide additional support for the hypothesis, and these
will be briefly described here.

Persistent infection with a virus similar to HBV is associated with a
naturally occurring primary carcinoma of the liver in Marmota monax, the woodchuck or groundhog.[21] Robert Snyder has trapped Pennsylvania woodchucks in the
wild and maintained a colony at the Philadelphia Zoological Garden for the past
20 years. Post-mortem examinations were performed in more than 100 woodchucks,
and about 25 percent of the animals had primary liver cancers. The tumors in
the animals were usually associated with chronic hepatitis.[22] Summers, at the
Institute for Cancer Research, examined serum samples from these animals for
evidence of infection with a virus similar to HBV. He based his investigation
on the hypothesis that viruses in the same class as HBV would have a similar
nucleic acid structure and similar DNA polymerase. HBV was known to have
unique characteristics: it contains a circular, double-stranded DNA genome with
a single-stranded region and a DNA polymerase capable of filling in the single-
stranded region to make a fully double-stranded, circular DNA. Summers found
that about 15 percent of the woodchuck serum samples had particles containing a
DNA polymerase and a DNA genome that were similar in size and structure to
those of HBV.[23] Examination of pellets from these serum specimens with an
electron microscope showed the three types of particles associated with HBV.
Later, Werner et al.[24] showed cross-reactivity of the core and surface antigens
of the virus in woodchucks (WHV) with the comparable antigens of HBV. A close
association between persistent WHV infection and PHC has also been found; DNA
from WHV hybridized to the cellular DNA in five woodchuck livers containing PHC
but did not hybridize to the DNA in nine livers without tumors. Finally,
Summers and his colleagues have demonstrated integration of one or two WHV
genomes into tumor-cell DNA in two woodchuck primary liver cancers. Integration appeared to occur at the same unique site in each cell of the tumor.
Thus, each tumor was a clone with respect to the integrated viral DNA, a
finding similar to that in the humans.

Liver cancer in the woodchuck is not what is generally regarded as a laboratory model of a human disease, that is, it was not designed or "created" by an
investigator for research purposes; rather, it is a naturally occurring disease
related to a naturally occurring virus, both of which have remarkable features
in common with their human counterparts. It provides impressive support for
the hypothesis and also an opportunity to perform observations and studies with
an other-than-human species.

Additional viruses with similarities to HBV have been found in Chinese
domestic ducks (in which there is a high frequency of liver cancer) as well as
domestic Pekin ducks in the United States. They have also been found in
California ground squirrels (Spermophilus beecheyi).

Our interpretation of these nine lines of evidence is that, taken together,
they strongly support the hypothesis that persistent infection with HBV is
required for the development of most cases of PHC, and therefore that the next
step is warranted: testing of the hypothesis that decreasing the frequency of
HBV infection will in due course decrease the frequency of PHC. The availability of the hepatitis B vaccine produced from HBsAg in human blood[3] and
increasing knowledge of the mechanisms of transmission of HBV will make such a
study feasible. Since the incidence of cancer is high in HBV carriers, it may
be possible to measure the effect of the program within a reasonable time. In
any case, the control of HBV infection is clearly justified as a public health
measure for the prevention of acute and chronic hepatitis and post-necrotic
cirrhosis, diseases of major importance in the same regions where PHC is
common.

Strategies for primary prevention

The exact strategies to be used in the forthcoming public health programs
will be determined as more experience is gained with the hepatitis B vaccine
and the knowledge of the methods of transmission and the natural history of HBV
increases. The vaccine appears to be effective in producing antibodies in very
young children including newborns. Even though children may be exposed to the
virus in utero and in early childhood when their mothers (or, less commonly,
other family members) are carriers, they do not become persistently infected
until about six weeks to two months after birth. In countries of high endemicity a very large percentage of carriers are a consequence of maternal transmission. A program in which vaccine is administered before one to two months
might, therefore, in a single generation considerably decrease the frequency of
carriers. Infection at an early age is associated with a higher probability of
becoming a carrier, while infection in later life is more likely to result in
the development of anti-HBs. Hence, even if the vaccination program is not
able to completely eliminate infection, if it can be delayed beyond childhood
and early growth, it could still have a marked effect on decreasing the frequency of carriers and increasing immunity in the population.

Intrafamily transmission

In areas of high HBV endemicity, transmission within the family group is extremely important and is likely to lead to the carrier state. We have started a series of family studies, including ethological observations on newborn children and their carrier mothers, to observe behaviors which might increase the probability of infection. The initial family observations have been made in West Africa and in the New Hebrides, areas with a high frequency of hepatitis infection and where traditional living patterns are still followed to a large extent. This may allow us to identify personal sanitation and health practices within the context of the culture which increase the probability of infection. From this, recommendations for simple preventive measures acceptable by the community may be made.

Insect transmission

There is considerable evidence that mosquitoes and bedbugs can transmit hepatitis. Several species of mosquitoes collected in areas where hepatitis is common in human populations carry the virus. Over 60% of bedbugs captured in beds whose main occupants are hepatitis carriers also carry the virus. The virus may persist in the infected bedbug for up to about five weeks after a single feeding on blood containing hepatitis virus. HBsAg can also be found in the feces of the bedbug up to five weeks after a feeding. The long-term persistence of the virus in an environment, the bed, in which transmission can occur from one person to another, may provide an important mechanism for the maintenance of the infection within families.

Bedbugs and mosquitoes can be controlled by the use of appropriate insecticides and also by traditional and environmental methods not requiring chemicals. Insect-borne infection may be a major mechanism for transmission of virus from a carrier mother (or other family member) to a young child; and, as already said, this is a particularly vulnerable period when carriers may develop. Control of virus-carrying insects, therefore, may have a particularly important impact on the control of chronic liver disease and PHC. There is an additional curious aspect of insect transmission. They may provide a mechanism for transmitting viruses from domestic and wild animals that are close to humans, and since these may contain genetic and other characteristics of their hosts, it may provide a means for the transmission of genetic information between species that are phylogenetically distant but physically proximate.

There are many methods by which hepatitis may be transmitted, which also means that there are many methods by which control can be effected. The use of the vaccine as well as other preventive measures may markedly decrease the high incidence of carriers. If this is so, it can be predicted that, in due course, the incidence of PHC will decrease.

A cellular model for primary hepatocellular carcinoma

The relation between HBV and PHC now allows the study of the role of a virus in the pathogenesis of a human tumor. Sufficient information is now available to propose a working model for the virus-cancer relation. A model developed for heuristic purposes should explain all the known data about the phenomenon it is designed to image and have an interesting character that will generate exciting experiments. (Copernicus also added that it should be elegant.) The model starts with the assumption that all (or nearly all) cases of PHC have been infected with HBV; and this was the conclusion arrived at from the hypothesis testing described in the first part of this paper. The clinical, epidemiologic, cellular and other features of HBV, the development of PHC, and other interactions with its host which have to be accounted for in the model include the following.

1) There is a long incubation period ($\sim$ 20 to 40 years) between the time of infection with HBV and the development of PHC.

2) More males than females develop PHC.

3) HBV is required for the development of diseases in addition to PHC (i.e. acute hepatitis, chronic liver diseases, the carrier state, etc.).

4) Whole virus, HBsAg and HBcAg appear to occur more commonly and in larger amounts in the cells which have not undergone malignant transformation than in the cells which have.

The model should also explain several other features of HBV infection not directly associated with cancer.

5) The fetus and newborn children (say within the first six weeks) of carrier mothers do not become persistently infected even though exposed to virus in utero, at the time of birth, and immediately thereafter.

6) Very young children (after about two months and before 10 years) are more likely to become chronic carriers if infected than adults, who are more likely to develop acute hepatitis.

The classical model of viral carcinogenesis indicates that the nucleic acid of the viral agent is integrated into the genome of the host target cell. This genetic integration results in an alteration of cell characteristics and malignant transformation occurs. Recent observations have resulted in a modified model in which viral DNA integrates at a site adjacent to a host gene which then directs the process of transformation (promoter insertion).

These models explain the process by which a cell becomes a cancer cell, but they do not deal in detail with the emergence of clinical cancer nor with the characteristics listed at the beginning of this section which pertain, in particular to cancer of the liver.

The model we propose posits the existence of two kinds of liver cells. 1) The S cell, which is susceptible to persistent productive (i.e. it produces whole virus, HBsAg particles, etc.) infection with the expression of viral characteristics within the cell and on its surface. 2) The R cell, which is resistant to persistent productive infection.

This notion had been discussed in our laboratory for several years when in 1980 London introduced the concept that the R cells are immature and undifferentiated cells and S cells are fully differentiated, i.e. a characteristic of liver cell maturation is its increased susceptibility to persistent productive infection with HBV. R cells are more likely to divide and when they do so can produce 1) two R cells, 2) one S and one R cell or 3) two S cells. The more differentiated and mature S cells, when they do divide, produce only other S cells (Figure 1). The fetus and newborns have mostly R cells; at about six weeks to three months there are more S cells and in adulthood nearly all S cells (Figure 2). We will return to the significance of this later.

Productive chronic infection of S cells leads to slow death of the cells both as a consequence of the response of the host's cellular and serological immune system to the expression of HBV on the surface of the infected cell and the interference with the S cell's metabolism as a consequence of massive viral infection. In the liver, the stimulus for cells to divide is the death of other cells, in contrast to, say, the skin where there is constant division and formation of new cells. Hence, in a liver chronically infected with HBV there is continuous cell death and cell regeneration. The death is primarily of S cells, while the R cells, stimulated by the deaths around them, continue to divide producing both R and S cells; the selective balance is tipped in favor of the R cells (Figure 3).

If the HBV DNA is integrated into host S cell DNA, and/or if another carcinogenic event occurs in an S cell, it will not be of long lasting consequence because, in due course, the S cells are likely to die. If, however, integration occurs in R cells and/or another carcinogen (i.e. aflatoxin, nitrosamines) causes transformation (Figure 4), there will be important consequences. Their cells are at a selective advantage relative to the S cells; the numbers of transformed R cells will increase and a clinically perceived cancer will develop.

Since the R cells are continually dividing in response to continuing S cell death, the probability of a transformation event is high. If the death of S cells is slowed or stopped by the control of the HBV infection, then the spread of the cancer will be halted and regression of small cancers may occur since the R cells are no longer at a selective advantage.

This model can explain phenomena not directly related to cancer (items 5 and 6 above). In a fetus or newborn there are very few S cells; hence, if the rare S cells are infected they will die and the infection will quickly terminate since there are few additional susceptible cells (Figure 5). Later in life (after about six weeks) there are a larger number of S cells in which infection may be perpetuated after the death of the initially infected cells. There are also sufficient R cells which can divide to provide additional S cells, and a persistent carrier state or chronic hepatitis can ensue. The nature of the liver damage will depend on the extent and nature of the host response to the infected cells. The cycles of dying, scarring and regenerating of new cells result in the pathological features of post-hepatic cirrhosis. If an adult is infected with HBV, the S cells will die, but there will not be sufficient R cells to generate new S cells to replace those that were killed. Hence, acute infections are more common in adults.

Several studies have shown that males, when infected, are more likely to become chronic carriers and females more likely to develop antibody. We have postulated that there are characteristics on many of the liver cells of males which allow chronic infection but that these characteristics are less common in females.

As long as there are sufficient numbers of R cells from which new liver cells are rejuvenated, liver function will be maintained. In heavy infection, with the death of many S cells, the R cells may be the main supplier of liver function. This may explain the clinical observation that cancer of the liver is often seen in patients with only minimal or moderate liver dysfunction. This results in an apparent anachronism; the R cells, including the transformed R cells, provide liver function until they become so numerous as to destroy the host.

Consequences of the model

We are now testing this model and in due course we will know if it is supported or rejected. There are several very interesting consequences of the model which can be acted upon if it is supported. The model is based on cellular development and explains phenomena of maturation, benign infection with hepatitis virus (the carrier state), acute and chronic hepatitis, and cancer. There is no factor that is found uniquely in the cancer cases that cannot be found in conditions without clinical cancer.

The model also suggests an approach to cancer therapy different from that usually used. Most conventional therapies are directed towards the total destruction of cancer cells, even though in the process normal tissues may be damaged or killed and this often limits the application of the treatment. The model just described suggests that an effort should be made to enhance the selective advantage of the S cells, i.e. to foster the viability of the non-cancerous cells so that they may increase their numbers and prevent the continued growth of tumors.

During the next few years, we plan to continue testing this model and its consequences. If these continue to be supported, it would encourage the investigation of similar models for other human cancers.

Prevention

The information now available allows us to proceed to test the feasibility of two of the three forms of prevention described in the introduction. The availability of the vaccine and our growing knowledge of transmission and epidemiology of HBV allow the design and execution of strategies for primary prevention by diminishing or eliminating infection, particularly in early childhood.

There are now large populations of southeast Asians in the United States, and many of them are in Philadelphia. We are developing plans to screen volunteers, identify HBV carriers and follow the latter to determine if any develop increases in their alpha fetoproteins (AFP). Chinese investigators, using only AFP testing, have reported that early tumors can be detected in this manner and that their removal increases survival.[25] We will try to determine if this approach is improved by the use of both HBV and AFP screening.

The model, if supported, could lead to an understanding of how prevention by delay might be effected. Methods for delaying integration or for decreasing the deadly infection of S cells might result in a sufficient delay to spare the carriers from cancer during their lifetime, and studies on this problem are now in progress.

TABLE 1

	PHC		CONTROLS	
		Hepatitis B surface antigen		
Country	No. tested	% Positive	No. tested	% Positive
Greece	189	55.0	106	4.7
Spain	31	19.3	101	2.0
U.S.A.	34	14.7	56	0
Senegal	291	51.9	100	12.0
Mozambique	29	62.1	35	14.3
Uganda	47	47.0	50	6.0
Zambia	19	63.1	40	7.5
S. Africa	138	59.5	200	9.0
Taiwan	84	54.8	278	12.2
Singapore	156	35.3	1516	4.1
Japan	260	37.3	4387	2.6
Vietnam	61	80.3	94	24.5
		Antibody to hepatitis B core antigen		
Greece	80	70.0	160	31.9
Spain	31	87.0	101	14.8
U.S.A.	33	48.5	56	0
Senegal	291	87.3	100	26.0
S. Africa	76	86.0	103	31.7
Hong Kong	37	70.3	58	36.2

Frequency of hepatitis B surface antigen (HBsAg) and antibody against hepatitis B core (anti-HBc) in patients with PHC and controls. Only studies using radioimmunoassay or a test of equivalent sensitivity for HBsAg and in which controls were included are used. These data have not been corrected for age.

TABLE 2

HEPATITIS B INFECTION IN CASES OF CHRONIC LIVER DISEASE
AND CONTROLS IN KOREA AND MALI, WEST AFRICA

Korea	n	% HBsAg(+)	% anti-HBc(+)	% anti-HBs(+)
Chronic active hepatitis	50	76	94	14
Cirrhosis	35	94	100	6
Controls[a]	104	6	75	54
Mali				
Chronic liver disease[b]	42	46	59	26
Controls	80	5	16	35

a - Controls are males greater than age 20 in the general population.
b - Not separated by diagnosis, but most are cases of advanced cirrhosis.

TABLE 3

PREVALENCE OF HBsAG AND ANTI-HBc IN MOTHERS OF PHC PATIENTS
AND CONTROLS

	n	HBsAg(+)	anti-HBc(+)
Senegal			
Mothers of PHC cases	28	20 (71.4%)	20 (70.4%)
Mothers of Controls[a]	28	4 (14.3%)	9 (32.1%)
Korea			
Mothers of PHC cases	10	4 (40.0%)	10 (100%)
Controls[b]	34	0	25 (73.5%)

a - In Senegal controls were mothers of individuals matched by sex, age and
neighborhood with the PHC cases.
b - Controls in Korea were women randomly selected from a pool of controls
such that the mean age and variance were equal to those for the mothers
of the PHC cases.

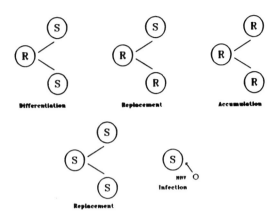

Fig. 1. R cells are resistant and S cells susceptible to productive infection with HBV. R cells are less differentiated than S cells. When R cells divide they can produce additional R cells and/or S cells, but S cells can produce only other S cells.

R and S Cells in Liver

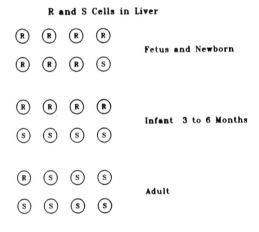

Fig. 2. There are few S cells in the undifferentiated fetus and newborn infants, but these increase with time. Adults have mostly S cells.

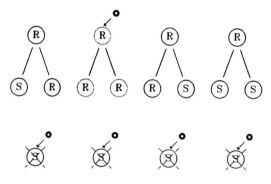

Chronic Infection

Fig. 3. Chronic infection of S cells results in death, which may be slow. The R cells are not killed and their numbers increase relative to the S cells. The HBV DNA may integrate into R cell host DNA and transformation may occur (dotted circles). Transformation may also be related to other carcinogens (i.e. aflatoxin, nitrosamines).

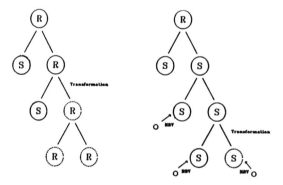

Fig. 4. Transformation of R cells can lead to tumors. Normal and transformed S cells will die if infected by HBV.

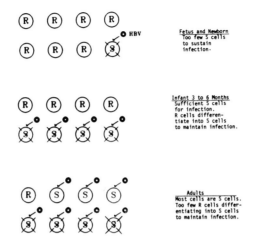

Fig. 5. Infection in fetus and newborn infants and adults.

306

ACKNOWLEDGMENTS

This work was supported by USPHS grants CA-06551, RR-05539, CA-22780 and CA-06927 from the National Institutes of Health and by an appropriation from the Commonwealth of Pennsylvania. Reprinted with the permission of the General Motors Research Foundation.

REFERENCES

1. London, W. T. (1981) Human Pathol. 12, 1085.
2. Blumberg, B. S., Larouze, B., London, W. T., Werner, B., Hesser, J. E., Millman, I., Saimot, G. and Payet, M. (1975) Am. J. Pathol. 81, 669.
3. Blumberg, B. S. and Millman, I. Vaccine against viral hepatitis and process. Serial No. 864,788 filed 10/8/69, Patent 36 36 191 issued 1/18/72, U.S. Patent Office.
4. Blumberg, B. S. and London, W. T. (1980) in Viruses in Naturally Occurring Cancers, Cold Spring Harbor Conferences on Cell Proliferation, Vol. 7. M. Essex, G. Todaro and H. zur Hausen, eds., Cold Spring Harbor Laboratory, p. 401.
5. Prince, A. M. (1980) in Virus and the Liver, Lancaster, England, MTP Press, Ltd., p. 399.
6. Nayak, N. C., Dhark, A., Sachdeva, R., Mittal, A., Seth, H. N., Sudarsanam, D., Reddy, B. Wagholikar, U. L. and Reddy, C. R. R. M. (1977) Int. J. Cancer 20, 643.
7. Omata, M., Ashcavi, M., Liew, C-T. and Peters, R. L. (1979) Gastroenterology 76, 279.
8. Beasley, R. P. and Lin, C. C. (1978) Am. J. Epidemiol. 108, 247.
9. Obata, H., Hayashi, N., Motoike, Y., Hisamits, T., Okuda, H., Kubayash, S. and Nishioka, K. (1980) Int. J. Cancer 25, 741.
10. Larouze, B., London, W. T., Saimot, G., Werner, B. G., Lustbader, E. D., Payet, M. and Blumberg, B. S. (1976) Lancet 2, 534.
11. Summers, J., O'Connell, A., Maupas, P., Goudeau, A., Coursaget, P. and Drucker, J. (1978) J. Med. Virol. 2, 207.
12. London, W. T. (1978) in Viral Hepatitis, G. N. Vyas, S. N. Cohen and R. Schmid, eds., Franklin Institute Press, Philadelphia, p. 455.
13. Macnab, G. M., Alexander, J. J., Lecatsas, G., Bey, E. M. and Urbanowicz, J. M. (1976) Br. J. Cancer 34, 509.
14. Skelley, J., Copeland, J. A., Howard, C. R. and Zuckerman, A. J. (1979) Nature 282, 617.
15. Marion, P. L. and Robinson, W. S. (1980) in Viruses in Naturally Occurring Cancers, Cold Spring Harbor Conferences on Cell Proliferation, Vol. 7, Cold Spring Harbor Laboratory, M. Essex, G. Todaro and H. zur Hausen, eds., Cold Spring Harbor Laboratory, p. 423.
16. Gray, P., Edman, J. C., Valenzuela, P., Goodman, H. M. and Rutter, W. J. (1980) J. Supramolec. Struc. Suppl. 4, 245.
17. Brechot, C., Pourcel, C., Louise, A., Rain, B. and Tiollais, P. (1980) Nature 286, 533.
18. Knowles, B. B., Howe, C. C. and Aden, D. P. (1980) Science 209, 497.
19. Shafritz, D. A., Shouval, D., Sherman, H. I., Hadziyannis, S. J. and Kew, M. C. (1981) New Engl. J. Med. 305, 1067.
20. Blumberg, B. S., Millman, I., Sutnick, A. I. and London, W. T. (1971) J. Exp. Med. 134, 320.
21. Snyder, R. L. and Ratcliffe, H. L. (1969) Acta Zool. Path. Antv. 48, 265.

22. Snyder, R. L. and Summers, J. (1980) in Viruses in Naturally Occurring Cancers, Cold Spring Harbor Conferences on Cell Proliferation, Vol. 7, M. Essex, G. Todaro and H. zur Hausen, eds., Cold Spring Harbor Laboratory, p. 447.

23. Summers, J., Smolec, J. M. and Snyder, R. (1978) Proc. Natl. Acad. Sci. (USA) 75, 4533.

24. Werner, B. G., Smolec, J. M., Snyder, R. and Summers, J. (1979) J. Virol. 32, 314.

25. Tang, Z., Yang, B., Tang, C., Yu, Y., Lin, Z. and Weng, H. (1980) Chinese Med. J. 93, 795.

BIOLOGICAL SIGNIFICANCE OF ANTIGENS SHARED BY LINE-10 HEPATOCARCINOMA CELLS AND <u>MYCOBACTERIUM BOVIS</u> (BCG).[+]

PERCY MINDEN, HERBERT L. MATHEWS[++] AND PETER J. KELLEHER.

[+]National Jewish Hospital and Research Center, Denver, CO 80206
[++]Department of Microbiology, Loyola University Medical School, Maywood, IL 60153.

INTRODUCTION

Antigenic components shared by <u>Mycobacterium bovis</u> (BCG) and certain experimental and human tumors have been demonstrated by a variety of methods.[1-7] The antigenic relationship was first noted between BCG antigens and the line-10 hepatocarcinoma of strain-2 guinea pigs.[1-3] This line of investigation was instigated by the fact that the line-10 tumor responded to therapy with BCG[8] and because this experimental tumor has been used as a model for the development of immunotherapy protocols for human tumors.[9,10] There is now evidence from several laboratories using different techniques that BCG shares antigens with line-10 cells.[1-3,5]

The occurrence of common antigens among bacteria and tumors resembles in some ways the known crossreactivity between mammalian tissue antigens and microorganisms. For example, components of streptococci crossreact with heart and kidney tissues[11,12] and antigens in human erythrocytes are shared by components of gram-negative organisms.[13] Some gram-negative bacteria are related to blood-group-active substances and so-called isoantibodies have their origin in the immunological response to crossreactive bacterial antigens.[14,15] Similar relationships exist between bacteria and histocompatibility antigens; e.g., streptococcal and staphylococcal organisms share antigenic specificities with some transplantation antigens.[16,17]

The mechanism(s)underlying bacterial immunotherapy of tumors is not completely understood but has been attributed to a "nonspecific" potentiation of immune mechanisms.[18,19] A more satisfactory understanding of the relationship between bacteria and tumors is needed because of the possibility that successful bacterial therapy may in part, be the result of "specific" stimulation due to shared or crossreacting antigenic stimuli. Perhaps of greater importance, this kind of antigenic relationship may be responsible for the observations that normal animals and humans frequently display immune responses to many kinds of tumor-associated antigens (TAAs).[20-23]

Although the evidence in favor of shared antigens between BCG and line-10 cells is substantial it is not entirely conclusive. The data derived from many experiments, although statistically significant, sometimes showed relatively small differences between experimental and control groups. The line-10 and BCG antigens by themselves consist of many components, only a few of which may be critical for the kind of binding and inhibition studies that have been described. Isolation of antigens and antibodies critical for the reactions reported above was therefore needed to evaluate further the significance of the antigenic relationships between BCG and line-10 cells.

Our studies were undertaken to provide information about the general biological importance of these shared antigens. Briefly, we isolated antigens shared by BCG and line-10 cells. When radiolabeled, they were found to bind in vitro to xenogeneic antibodies raised to both BCG and line-10 cells. These components were then tested for their ability to influence growth of the line-10 tumor in vivo.

ISOLATION OF SHARED ANTIGENIC COMPONENTS FROM LINE-10 ASCITES FLUID (AF).

AF from line-10-bearing animals has been shown to contain soluble line-10 tumor-derived antigens.[24] In one series of procedures we isolated antigenic components common to BCG and line-10 cells from AF. Forty milliliters of cell-free AF were passed through an immunoadsorbent to which a purified preparation of rabbit antibodies to BCG (anti-BCG-P) had been coupled. AF constituents that bound to these antibodies were then eluted.[25]

After passage of several samples of AF, the bound eluates were pooled and concentrated by Amicon filtration. When radiolabeled, the bound eluates consisted of AF components that bound to both anti-BCG and anti-10. The percentage of protein recovered in the eluates after affinity chromatography was very small, less than 0.1%. These "shared antigens" were designated Sh-ag-10. It was not certain whether Sh-ag-10 consisted exclusively of structures related to BCG and line-10 cells. Sh-ag-10 was then tested in vivo. Results of some of these experiments are summarized in Tables 1-3.

SUPPRESSION OF GROWTH OF THE LINE-10 HEPATOCARCINOMA BY SH-AG-10.

Strain-2 guinea pigs were injected intradermally (i.d.) into their left flanks with 10^6 line-10 cells suspended in various concentrations of Sh-ag-10. Injections were made within 30 min after the line-10 cells were mixed with Sh-ag-10, at which time viability by trypan blue dye exclusion was 90 to 95%.

In some animals erythema and induration developed at the injection sites but disappeared after 5 days. As shown in Table I, there was complete suppression of tumor growth in a considerable number of animals injected with 100 to 150 ug Sh-ag-10. Some animals that never developed tumors at the site of injection subsequently developed palpable lymph nodes in the neighboring axillary areas. These animals died after a course that was considerably longer than that for the untreated controls. All animals injected with line-10 cells alone succumbed to this tumor as they routinely do.[8] Approximately 60 days after the beginning of these experiments, animals that were tumor free were reinjected i.d. in their contralateral flanks with 10^6 line-10 cells alone. All of them demonstrated delayed cutaneous hypersensitivity (DCH) reactions to the line-10 cells, and 50% did not develop tumors. The remaining animals developed tumors and died after a prolonged course.

TABLE 1

Suppression of line-10 hepatocarcinoma by Sh-ag-10

Treatment (ug Protein)	No. Animals Tumor-free/No.Treated (%)	Rechallenge[a] No. Animals Tumor-Free/No Challenged (%)
Simultaneous injection of 10^6 line-10 cells together with different concentrations of Sh-ag-10[b]		
100	8/10	7/7
125	9/12	4/9
150	3/5	1/2
Total	20/27 (74.0)	9/18 (50)
Controls	0/28	

From Minden et al., (1980) (25), Courtesy of J. Immunol.
[a]Animals surviving initial treatment were rechallenged i.d. with line-10 cells alone on the opposite flank after about 2 mo, and observed for at least 60 days.
[b]Strain-2 guinea pigs were inoculated i.d. with 10^6 line-10 cells mixed with different concentrations of Sh-ag-10.

Suppression was dependent on the quantity of Sh-ag-10 employed. As shown in Table 2, tumors developed in most of the animals that were injected with 10, 30, or 50 ug of Sh-ag-10 together with 10^6 line-10 cells. In one experiment, six animals were injected i.d. with 10^6 cells suspended in 200 ug of unfractionated AF. There was no suppression of tumor growth in these animals.

TABLE 2

Ineffectiveness of other methods in suppressing growth of the line-10 tumor

Simultaneous injection of 10^6 line-10 cells together with:	
10 ug Sh-ag-10	0/5
30 ug Sh-ag-10	2/5
50 ug Sh-ag-10	1/5
200 ug unfractionated ascites fluid from tumor-bearing animals	0/6
170 ug of unbound effluent after ascites fluid was passed through anti-BCG immunoadsorbant	0/6
10^6 line-10 cells and 100 ug Sh-ag-10 injected separately in contralateral flanks[a]	0/6
Controls[b]	

From Minden et al., (1980) (25), Courtesy of J. Immunol.
[a]Animals received 10^6 line-10 cells i.d. in the right flanks and 100 ug Sh-ag-10 in the left flanks on the same day.
[b]Untreated controls were the same as those in Table I.

As noted earlier, Sh-ag-10 had been prepared by passing AF from tumor-bearing animals through an immunoadsorbent to which a purified preparation of anti-BCG had been coupled. Sh-ag-10 represented the eluate, or the components of AF that had bound to antibodies to BCG. The effluent, or unbound material, was similarly collected, concentrated, and passed again through an anti-BCG immunoadsorbent. This was repeated for a total of three passages. The effluent was then tested for its capacity to suppress tumor growth by injecting 170 ug of effluent suspended with 10^6 line-10 cells i.d. into a group of guinea pigs. Tumor growth was not retarded or suppressed, and all animals died with tumors at the same rate as the controls. These experiments indicated that only components of AF that bound to antibodies to BCG suppressed growth of the line-10 tumor. In another experiment, 100 ug of Sh-ag-10 were injected separately into the right flanks of a group of guinea pigs that received 10^6 line-10 cells into their contralateral left flanks. There was no tumor suppression, which indicated that close contact between tumor cells and Sh-ag-10 was important.

PROTECTIVE EFFECTS OF THE SH-AG-10:LINE-10 VACCINE.

Several groups of animals were given i.d. injections into their right flanks of Sh-ag-10 suspended with line-10 cells. This combination is called the Sh-ag-10 vaccine. In the following experiment, line-10 cells alone were injected i.d. into the opposite left flanks of groups of guinea pigs: a) 10 days before the vaccine; b) on the same day as the vaccine; c) 5 days after the vaccine; or d) 10 days after the vaccine. As shown in Table 3, growth of existing tumors was unaffected. However, tumor growth was suppressed at both injection sites of some of the animals that had received the vaccine 5 or 10 days before the challenge with line-10 cells alone. Animals that succumbed did so after a prolonged course. These experiments suggested that the vaccine initiated a systemic protective mechanism that in some animals was sufficient to completely prevent tumor growth. Sixty days after the beginning of the experiments, tumor-free animals were rechallenged with 10^6 line-10 cells alone and, as in the experiments shown in Table 1, approximately half the animals were resistant to the tumor.

TABLE 3

Protective effects of the Sh-ag-10:line-10 vaccine[a]

Time of Challenge with Line-10 Cells Alone	No. Animals Tumor-free/ No. Challenged	Rechallenge[c] No. of Animals Tumor-free/No. Challenged
a) 10 days before vaccine	0/5	
b) Exp. 1 - same day as vaccine	0/5	
Exp. 2. - same day[d] as vaccine	0/6	
c) 5 days after vaccine[d]	3/6	1/3
d) 10 days after vaccine	2/5	2/2
Controls[e]		

From Minden et al., (1980) (25), Courtesy of J. Immunol.
[a]Vaccine consisting of 100 ug Sh-ag-10 suspended with 10^6 viable line-10 cells was injected i.d. into right flanks.
[b]10^6 viable line-10 cells alone were injected i.d. into left flanks.
[c]Animals surviving initial treatment wer rechallenged i.d. with line-10 cells alone on the opposite flank after about 2 mo, and observed for at least 60 days.
[d]Vaccine and challenge each contained 5×10^5 line-10 cells.
[e]Untreated controls were the same as those in Table I.

314

Ten animals that had been rendered resistant to line-10 cells in the experiments described earlier were injected i.d. with 3×10^6 line-1 cells. The line-1 tumor is syngeneic with strain-2 animals and line-10 cells, but has distinct antigenic tumor-associated determinants. The line-1 tumor is not fatal when injected i.d., and in our study, the tumors grew over a period of 7 to 10 days, as they did in the normal controls, and regressed spontaneously as expected.[26] When rechallenged with line-1 cells about 30 days later, the line-1 cells were rejected within 72 hr. This experiment indicated that animals that had become resistant to line-10 cells were not resistant to line-1, a syngeneic but antigenically distinct tumor.

EXAMINATION OF SH-AG-10 BY ELECTROPHORESIS IN POLYACRYLAMIDE GELS.

Fifty-microgram samples of Sh-ag-10 were subjected to electrophoresis in polyacrylamide gels to obtain information regarding their physical-chemical characteristics. When stained by CBB, there were seven major and four minor protein staining bands. The latter were in the low molecular weight (m.w.) region of the gel (Fig. 1). By radioautography, all the bands, including those in the low m.w. areas, were readily visible. It was not certain from this analysis whether all the proteins noted were critical for the anti-tumor effects of Sh-ag-10.

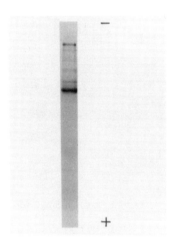

Fig. 1. Electrophoresis of 50 ug Sh-ag-10 in 10% SDS-polyacrylamide gel.

ISOLATION OF SHARED ANTIGENIC COMPONENTS FROM BCG.

Sh-ag-10 had been derived from antigens in line-10 cells. Dr. Herbert Mathews, in our laboratory carried out another approach this time to isolate such common antigens from BCG organisms.[27] In these experiments line-10 cellular immunoadsorbents were employed.[28] Briefly, line-10 cells treated with 1% formalinized saline were suspended in diethylaminoethyl cellulose (DE-52) that had been equilibrated with borate buffer, pH 7.4. Five x 10^8 line-10 cells were mixed with 50 ml DE-52 for one hour and transferred to a 25 mm glass column. Sera from rabbits that had been immunized with BCG (anti-BCG) were passed through this immunoadsorbent. The antibodies in anti-BCG that bound to line-10 cells were eluted and were designated anti-Sh-ag. Binding of anti-Sh-ag to line-10 cell surfaces was demonstrated by electron microscopy using hemocyanin as an immunospecific marker. Briefly, line-10 cells were incubated with anti-Sh-ag and then with goat anti-rabbit IgG. After washings, rabbit anti-hemocyanin was added and cells were incubated further with B. canniculatum hemolymph. When examined by electron microscopy, cells treated this way were shown to have anti-Sh-ag distributed over the entire cell surface, particularly upon the microvilli. See Fig. 2. In other experiments, anti-Sh-ag was also shown to bind to BCG antigens. Anti-Sh-ag was then itself coupled to Sepharose and a soluble BCG extract was passed through this immunoadsorbent. BCG components that bound to anti-Sh-ag on this immunoadsorbent were then eluted and were designated Sh-ag-BCG.[27] As shown below, components that were eluted were similarly found to be of biological importance since they were also capable of suppressing growth of the line-10 tumor in vivo.

316

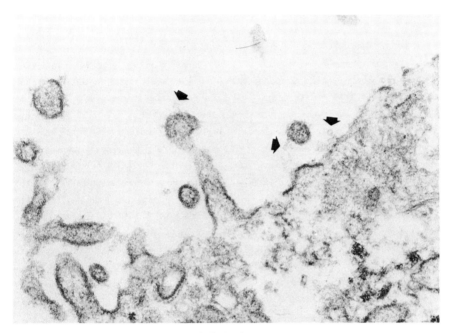

Fig. 2. From Mathews et al. (1982) (27) Courtesy of J. Biol. Resp. Modif.
Transmission electron microscopic appearance (X80.500) of line-10 cells
reacted with anti-Sh-ag and hemocyanin. Arrows indicate representative areas
of typical cell-associated hemocyanin.

SUPPRESSION OF GROWTH OF THE LINE-10 HEPATOCARCINOMA BY SH-AG-BCG.

Guinea pigs were injected i.d. into their left flanks with 10^6 line-10
cells suspended in various concentrations of Sh-ag-BCG. Injections were made
within 30 min after mixing Sh-ag-BCG with line-10 cells. Viability of line-10
was always greater than 95%. Results, as with Sh-ag-10, depended on the
amount of Sh-ag-BCG employed. As demonstrated in Figure 3A, injections of
line-10 cells alone caused tumors that grew quickly. When 10 ug of Sh-ag-BCG
were added to the line-10 cells the development of tumors was similar to that
after injections of line-10 cells alone, (3B). Injections of line-10 cells

together with 20 ug of Sh-ag-BCG (3C) resulted in a delay in tumor development in 3 of 4 animals tested, with two animals showing no measurable tumor growth until 16 d post injection.

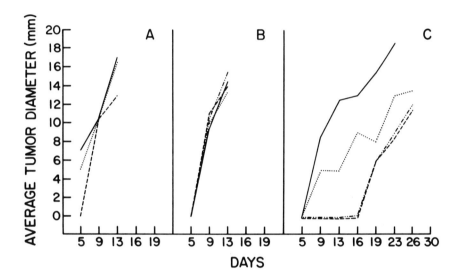

Fig. 3. From Mathews et al. (1982) (27) Courtesy of J. Biol. Resp. Modif. Increase in tumor diameters at the sites of injection of: A, 10^6 line-10 cells alone; B, 10^6 line-10 cells and 10 ug of Sh-ag-BCG; C, 10^6 line-10 tumor cells and 20 ug of Sh-ag-BCG. Each line represents a single animal.

There was complete suppression of tumor growth in one of four animals injected with line-10 cells and 50 ug of Sh-ag-BCG (4A) and in two of four animals injected with 100 ug of Sh-ag-BCG (4B). The other animals in these groups succumbed to the tumor after a course which was much longer than that of the untreated controls. Approximately sixty days after the initiation of these experiments, animals that were tumor free were reinjected i.d. into their opposite flanks with 10^6 line-10 cells alone. None of the rechallenged animals developed tumors indicating the development of systemic immunity. A separate group of animals was injected i.d. with 10^6 line-10 cells and with 50 ug Sh-ag-BCG at the same time in opposite flanks. There was no suppression of tumor growth with tumors increasing in size similar to those depicted in Figure 3A. As in previous experiments[25] direct contact between line-10 cells and Sh-ag-BCG was needed to induce immunity to the tumor.

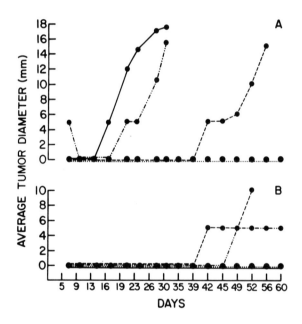

Fig. 4. From Mathews et al. (27) Courtesy J. Biol. Resp. Modif. Increase in tumor diameters at the site of injection of: A, 10^6 line-10 tumor cells and 50 ug of Sh-ag-BCG, B, 10^6 line-10 tumor cells and 100 ug of Sh-ag-BCG. Each line represents a single animal.

GENERAL CONCLUSIONS AND IMPLICATIONS

The experiments described above confirmed the existence of antigens shared by BCG and guinea pig line-10 hepatocarcinoma cells. They also demonstrated that by using immunochemical methods, components enriched with these shared antigens could be isolated from either line-10-associated antigens or from intact BCG. Of even greater importance, the shared antigens derived by both methods had significant anti-tumor properties *in vivo*. An understanding of the full relationship between bacterial and tumor-associated antigens therefore deserves serious continued consideration. Antigens shared by other tumors and microorganisms may be widespread. Antigens shared by human melanoma cells and BCG have also been demonstrated using procedures similar to the ones we described above.[29]

Immune responses are known to exist in normal humans to a wide variety of bacteria[30] and antibodies to many kinds of tumor-associated antigens have also been demonstrated in sera from normal humans[20-23]. These have been called "natural" antibodies. It is possible that because antigens are shared by bacteria and tumors that normal humans may develop an immune response to tumor-associated antigens as a result of natural exposure to bacteria in the environment. Whether the finding of natural killer (NK) cells in humans[31] has anything to do with stimulation by bacterial antigens has become another intriguing question. NK cells may possibly be the cellular counterpart of "natural" antibodies. In mouse experiments, pathogen-free animals have been reported to have little or no NK activity, whereas when they were moved to conventional quarters, they quickly developed considerable NK activity.[32] Immune responses by normal humans or animals to tumor-associated antigens are probably not "natural" or "nonspecific", but could be specific responses to direct stimulation by pathogenic or more likely, non-pathogenic microorganisms.

Accordingly, immune responses by patients to tumor-associated antigens may sometimes respresent an elevation of an "isoimmune" state, rather than a new actively acquired immune response. Such a response may conceivably influence the course of neoplastic disease. It is too early to tell whether shared antigens like the ones we have observed will eventually play an important role in the immunotherapy of cancer. Of great potential however is the possibility that immune reactions to TAAs by normal individuals may influence the initiation and course of spontaneously arising neoplasms. "Natural" antibodies and cellular activity initiated by antigens that are shared by bacteria and tumors may therefore constitute a low level of immunity that operates as an immune surveillance type of mechanism.

ACKNOWLEDGEMENTS

These studies were supported by grants CA-15446 and CA-30988 awarded by the National Cancer Institute. The advice and encouragement of Dr. Richard S. Farr is sincerely appreciated.

REFERENCES

1. Borsos, T. and Rapp, H.J. (1973) J. Natl. Cancer Inst. 51, 1085.

2. Minden, P., McClatchy, J.K., Wainberg, M., and Weiss, D.W. (1974) J. Natl. Cancer Inst. 53, 1325.

3. Bucana, C. and Hanna, M.G., Jr. (1974) J. Natl. Cancer Inst. 53, 1313.

4. Minden, P., Sharpton, T.R., and McClatchy, J.K. (1976) J. Immunol. 116, 1407.

5. McCoy, J.L., Bradhorst, J. and Hanna, M.G., Jr. (1978) J. Natl. Cancer Inst. 60, 693.

6. Kwapinski, G., Oliver, H., Kwapinski, E., and Stein, M. (1978) Oncology 35, 263.

7. Holan, V., Chutna, J., and Harsek, M. (1979) Cancer Res. 39, 593.

8. Rapp, H.J. (1973) Isr. J. Med. Sci. 9, 366.

9. Rapp, H.J. (1976) Ann. N.Y. Acad. Sci. 276, 550.

10. Zbar, B., Ribi, E., Kelly, M., Granger, D., Evans, C., and Rapp, H.J. (1976) Cancer Immunol. Immunother. 1, 127.

11. Kaplan, M.H. and Suchy, M.L. (1964) J. Exp. Med. 119, 643.

12. Kaplan, M.H. and Svec, K.H. (1964) J. Exp. Med. 119, 651.

13. Springer, G.F. (1967) in Cross-Reacting Antigens and Neo-Antigens, Trenton, J., ed., Williams and Wilkins, Baltimore, p. 29.

14. Goebel, W.F., Shedlovsky, T., Lavin, G.I., and Adams, M.H. (1943) J. Biol. Chem. 148, 1.

15. Muschel, L.H. and Osawa, E. (1959) Proc. Soc. Exp. Biol. Med. 101, 614.

16. Rapaport, F.T. (1972) in Tranplantation Antigens, Kahan, E.B. and Reisfeld, R.A., ed., p. 182.

17. Chase, R.M., Jr. and Rapaport, F.T. (1965) J. Exp. Med. 122, 721.

18. Old, L., Benacerraf, B., Clark, D.A., Carswell, E.A., and Stockert, E. (1961) Cancer Res. 21, 1281.

19. Weiss, D.W. (1972) Natl. Cancer Inst. Monogr. 35, 157.

20. Herberman, R.B. and Aoki, T. (1972) J. Exp. Med. 131, 94.

21. Minden, P., Gutterman, J.U., Hersh, E.M., Jarrett, C. and McClatchy, J.K. (1976) Nature (London) 263, 774.

22. Brunda, M.J. and Minden, P. (1977) J. Immunol. 119, 1374.

23. Bias, W.B., Santos, G.W., Burke, P.J., Mullins, G.M. and Humphrey, R.L. (1972) Science 178, 304.

24. Detrick-Hooks, B., Smith, H.G., Bast, R.C., Jr., Dunkel, V.C. and Borsos, T. (1976) J. Immunol. 116, 1324.

25. Minden, P., Mathews, H.L., and Kelleher, P.J. (1980) J. Immunol. 125, 2685.

26. Zbar, B., Wepsic, H.T., Rapp, H.J., Borsos, T., Kronman, B.S., and Churchill, W.H. (1969) J. Natl. Cancer Inst. 43, 833.

27. Mathews, H.L., Brenman, J., Kelleher, P.J., and Minden, P. (1982) In Press, J. Biol. Resp. Modif.

28. Mathews, H.L., Brunda, M.J., and Minden, P. (1980) J. Immunol., 124, 1141.

29. Minden, P., Kelleher, P., and Woods, L.K. (1982) Chapter 14, In Melanoma Antigens and Antibodies. Reisfeld, R.A., S. Ferrone (ed.), Plenum Press, NY.

30. Minden, P. and Farr, R.S. (1975) Chest, 68, 749.

31. Herberman, R.B. and Holden, H.T. (1979) J. Natl. Cancer Inst. 62, 441.

32. Clark, E.A., Russell, P.H., Egghart, M. and Horton, M.A. (1979) Int. J. Cancer 24, 688.

HOST RESPONSE TO GUINEA PIG TUMOR CELLS INFECTED WITH MURINE LEUKEMIA VIRUSES.

B. ZBAR, A. NAGAI, J. HOVIS, and N. TERATA.
Laboratory of Immunobiology, National Cancer Institute, NIH, Bethesda, Maryland.

INTRODUCTION

Recent experiments in experimental tumor immunology has focused attention on the lack of detectable tumor rejection antigens on naturally occurring tumors of mice and rats.[1,2] Superinfection of tumor cells with murine leukemia viruses has been suggested as one possible method for augmenting host response to "cryptic" intrinsic antigens of naturally occurring tumors.[3] This suggestion was based on the results of a series of experiments which demonstrated that immunization of syngeneic rats with viable, murine leukemia virus-infected cells produced potent specific immunity to challenge with uninfected tumor cells.[4] A conceptual framework for these observations was provided by Mitchison[5] who stressed that immune responses to weakly immunogeneic cell surface antigens could be amplified by incorporation of strongly immunogenic antigens into cell surfaces. Recent experiments by Bromberg and coworkers provide some support for this concept.[6,7] The humoral immune response of mice to the Thy 1.1 antigen was augmented by the presence of viral antigenic determinants in the immunizing thymocyte population; augmentation of the immune response to the Thy 1.1 antigen required priming of mice to viral antigens carried by the Thy 1.1 bearing thymocytes.

Investigators have usually studied the influence of MuLV infection on the immunogenicity of tumors that contained readily detectable tumor rejection antigens; consequently it has been difficult to determine whether immunization with virus-infected tumor cells would, in fact, produce immunity to weakly or nonimmunogenic tumor cells. In this report we present the results of our studies of the influence of MuLV superinfection on the growth characteristics and immunogenicity of two

Published 1983 by Elsevier Science Publishing Co., Inc.

Cancer: Etiology and Prevention, Ray G. Crispen, Editor

fibrosarcomas syngeneic to strain 2 guinea pigs. Information is also presented on experiments designed to determine whether it is feasible to modify tumor growth in vivo with retroviruses.

MATERIALS AND METHODS

Animals. Male Sewall Wright strain 2 guinea pigs 3-4 months old and weighing about 500 grams were obtained from the Laboratory Aids Branch, Division of Research Services, National Institutes of Health, Bethesda, Md. and from the Experimental Animal Breeding Facility of the National Cancer Institute, Frederick Cancer Research Facility, Frederick, Md.

Tumor lines. Fibrosarcomas were obtained from Dr. Charles Evans, Laboratory of Biology, National Cancer Institute, NIH. Tumor line 104C1 was induced by in vitro treatment of cells of a 43 day fetal carcass with benzo(a)pyrene; line 107C3 was induced by in vitro treatment of cells from the same fetal carcass with N-methyl-N′-nitro-N-nitrosoguanidine.[8] These cell lines lacked detectable tumor transplantation antigens and serologically detectable tumor associated antigens.[9] The biologic and immunologic characteristics of the line 10 hepatoma have been described in detail. [10]

Infection of guinea pig cultures. Cell cultures were infected 24 hours after the tumor cells were seeded by replacement of the existing nutrient medium with RPMI 1640 medium containing polybrene (2 ug/ml, Aldrich Biochemicals) and MuLV 4070A (10^5 infectious units). Infected cell lines were designated by the name of the cell line followed by the name of the virus used for infection.

Viruses and assays. An amphotropic MuLV, MULV 4070A, isolated by Dr. Janet Hartley, National Institute of Allergy and Infectious Diseases, NIH, was used to infect guinea pig tumor cells.[11] MuLV 4070A, present in supernatant fluids, was detected and quantitated by the mink S+L- assay.[12] Expression of MuLV antigens by infected guinea pig tumor cells was monitored with a direct immunofluorescence assay.

Drug treatment. Methotrexate (MTX sodium, Lederle Laboratories, Division
of American Cyanamide Co., Pearl River, New York) (5 mg) was injected i.p.
every 48 hours starting on the day of tumor cell injection. Fifteen injections
were given. Cyclophosphamide (CY, Mead Johnson, Evansville, Indiana) (10 mg)
was injected i.p. daily starting two days before injection of tumor cells.
Seven or 14 injections were given.

Evaluation of immunologic responsiveness. Guinea pigs were immunized with
a mixture of line 10 cells (10^6) and an oil-in-water emulsion of BCG cell
walls (212 ug).[13] Animals were skin tested with PPD (10 ug) and live line
10 cells 21 days after immunization. Delayed cutaneous hypersensitivity
reactions and tumor growth were measured. Sera from guinea pigs injected with
uninfected or virus-infected tumor cells was tested for antibody by the method
of Brown et al.[14]

Preparation of mixtures of uninfected and virus-infected tumor cells for
injection into guinea pigs. Virus-infected fibrosarcoma cells or fluids containing virus were added to uninfected line 10 hepatoma cells, mixed thoroughly
and injected i.d. in a volume of 0.1 ml. Equal volumes of infected and
uninfected tumor cells were mixed. When fluids containing virus were tested,
tumor cells were centrifuged, the supernatant fluid was removed and the tumor
cells were resuspended in virus-containing fluid.

RESULTS

Influence of MuLV 4070A infection of guinea pig fibrosarcomas on growth
in vivo and in vitro. Fibrosarcomas (104C1, 107C3) of strain 2 guinea
pigs were readily infected by the amphotropic MuLV, 4070A. Addition of
10^5 S+L- units of MuLV 4070A to flasks containing fibrosarcoma cells
led to infection of tumor cells as demonstrated by expression of MuLV
antigens as well as by release of infectious virus into supernatant fluids.
MuLV infection did not have any detectable cytopathic effect on the
fibrosarcoma cells. There were no differences in the yield or population

doubling times of infected or uninfected fibrosarcoma cells grown in RPMI 1640

medium containing fetal bovine serum. Growth in soft agar of virus-infected

and uninfected fibrosarcoma cells was measured to determine whether MuLV

infection had altered this characteristic of neoplastic cell lines. Both

virus-infected and uninfected tumor cells formed colonies in soft agar.

Injection of uninfected and virus-infected tumor cells into nude mice led to

the formation of progressively growing tumors.

Pronounced differences were observed in growth of uninfected and MuLV 4070A-

infected fibrosarcoma in syngeneic strain 2 guinea pigs. Intradermal injection

of 104C1 cells (10^4 to 10^6) or 107C3 cells (10^5 to 10^6) led to the formation

of progressively growing tumors which led to death of treated guinea pigs.

Intradermal injection of 104C1 MuLV 4070A (10^6) or 107C3 MuLV 4070A (10^6)

led to the formation of dermal tumor nodules which regressed. Dermal tumor

nodules, present at sites of injection of fibrosarcoma cells on days 5-10,

regressed by day 14. Animals injected with 104C1 MuLV 4070A (10^6 cells)

have remained tumor free. Animals injected with early passages of 107C3 MuLV

4070A have remained tumor free; some animals injected with late passages of

107C3 MuLV 4070A developed recurrences of tumor 50-60 days after injection.

Histology of skin nodules in guinea pigs receiving virus-infected or

uninfected tumor cells. Skin nodules were removed from guinea pigs 5 to 14

days after injection of 107C3 or 107C3 MuLV 4070A and prepared for histologic

examination. Examination by Dr. Stephen J. Galli of Epon embedded, Giemsa-

stained sections, 1 micron thick, revealed the presence of numerous basophils

at sites of rejection of virus-infected tumor cells.

Immune response of guinea pigs immunized with virus-infected fibrosarcoma

cells to uninfected or virus-infected fibrosarcoma cells. Sera from guinea

pigs immunized with virus-infected fibrosarcoma cells contained protein A-fixing

antibodies to virus-infected fibrosarcoma cells but not to uninfected fibro-

sarcoma cells. In tests performed by Dr. Harry Ohanian, sera containing virus-

specific protein A-fixing antibodies did not produce complement dependent
cytotoxicity of virus-infected fibrosarcoma cells as measured by a trypan
blue dye exclusion test. Spleen cells from unimmunized or immunized strain
2 guinea pigs were tested for the presence of cytotoxic effector cells using a
4 and 18 hour [51]chromium release method. Cells, with the ability to cause
release of radiolabel from uninfected or MuLV 4070A-infected fibrosarcoma
cells, were present in the spleens of immunized or unimmunized guinea pigs.
Spleen cells from immunized or unimmunized animals did not differ in ability
to injure tumor target cells. Animals previously injected with virus-infected
tumor cells rejected a second i.d. inoculum of virus-infected cells in an
accelerated fashion.

Three experiments were performed to determine whether guinea pigs immunized
with MuLV 4070A-infected line 104C1 or 107C3 had resistance to challenge with
the corresponding, uninfected tumor cell line. There were no significant
differences in tumor incidence in immunized animals compared to unimmunized
control animals in response to challenge with uninfected tumor cells (10^3-10^6).
This results was observed in animals immunized and challenged with cells grown
in medium containing fetal bovine serum and also in animals immunized with
tumor cells grown in medium containing fetal bovine serum and challenged with
tumor cells grown in guinea pig serum. While normal guinea pigs were able to
reject greater than 10^6 virus-infected tumor cells, immunized animals failed
to reject 100 fold fewer uninfected tumor cells.

Influence of immunosuppression with methotrexate or cyclophosphamide on
growth and regression of virus-infected tumor cells. Studies of the basis of
rejection of MuLV-infected guinea pig fibrosarcoma cells would be facilitated
if conditions could be identified that permit progressive growth of virus-
infected tumor cells in syngeneic animals. Studies of Moloney sarcoma virus-
induced tumors of BALB/c mice have shown that tumor rejection in adult mice
could be prevented by cyclophosphamide treatment.[15] Regression of a MuLV-

328

infected embryonal tumor of inbred rats was abolished by treatment of animals
with antilymphocyte serum.[16] Methotrexate was given according to regimens
shown to inhibit development of delayed cutaneous hypersensitivity to the line
10 hepatoma and to PPD and to inhibit the development of ability to reject the
line 10 hepatoma.[17] Injection of MuLV 4070A-infected 104Cl cells into control
guinea pigs led to the formation of dermal tumor nodules which regressed by
day 14. In methotrexate-treated guinea pigs there was a slight delay in
regression of virus-infected tumor cells. A significant difference in tumor
incidence in animals that received virus-infected tumor cells and MTX compared
to animals that received noninfected tumor cells and MTX was present on day 21
but not on day 14. Cyclophosphamide was given according to schedules shown to
inhibit antibody formation in the guinea pig.[18] The results of the experiment
with cyclophosphamide can be summarized as follows: a) virus-infected 104Cl
cells grew and regressed in normal strain 2 guinea pigs; b) uninfected tumor
cells grew progressively in normal guinea pigs; c) virus-infected tumor cells
grew and regressed in drug-treated animals; some delay in the rate of regression
was observed in drug treated animals. A significant difference in tumor
incidence in animals that received CY and virus-infected tumor cells compared
to animals that received CY and uninfected tumor cells was present on day 35
but not at day 28; d) cyclophosphamide treatment retarded the growth of
uninfected tumor cells. Treatment with methotrexate or cyclophosphamide did
not lead to progressive growth of MuLV 4070A-infected 104Cl cells in syngeneic
guinea pigs.

Attempts to modify tumor growth in vivo by infection with MuLV 4070A.
The results presented above indicated that immunization with MuLV 4070A-
infected 104Cl or 107C3 cells did not increase resistance to challenge
with the corresponding, uninfected tumor cell line. This result suggested
that immunization of animals with MuLV-infected tumor cells might not be
effective therapy for tumors which lack readily detectable tumor rejection

antigens. Consequently attempts were made to modify growth of tumors in vivo with MuLV. The line 10 hepatoma, a tumor which metastasizes through the lymphatic system, was used as the tumor target for these studies. Initial experiments were performed by preparing mixtures of MuLV 4070A-infected 107C3 cells and uninfected line 10 cells and injecting these mixtures into the skin of syngeneic animals. The results indicated that virus-infected 107C3 cells suppressed the growth of admixed, uninfected line 10 hepatoma cells. The response to injection depended on the ratio of infected to uninfected tumor cells. When mixtures contained 10 infected fibrosarcoma cells per hepatoma cell, the response could be divided into 4 stages: formation of small intra-dermal tumor nodules at sites of injection between days 0 and 7; regression of nodules between days 7 and 14; a tumor free interval of varying duration; and recurrence of tumors at sites of injection or in regional lymph nodes in some of the tested animals.

Suppression of line 10 growth by MuLV 4070A-infected fibrosarcoma cells required close contact between viable virus-infected cells and uninfected hepatoma cells. Injection of virus-infected fibrosarcoma cells contralateral to the line 10 tumor cells injection did not lead to inhibition of tumor growth. Injection of line 10 cells admixed with fluids containing infectious MuLV did not lead to inhibition of line 10 tumor growth.

Factors influencing the suppression of line 10 growth by MuLV 4070A-infected fibrosarcoma cells. We previously described examples of bystander suppression of tumor growth.[19,20] Two characteristics of this reaction were: a) the process occurred in nonimmune, control animals and was abrogated in animals immunized to line 1; and b) the process required living line 1 tumor cells; irradiation of the line 1 cells abolished suppression of growth of the admixed tumor target. Experiments were performed to determine whether irradiation would modify the ability of virus-infected tumor cells to suppress the growth of admixed line 10 cells. The results indicated that irradiated

MuLV 4070A-infected tumor cells had an inhibitory effect on line 10 cell growth but were significantly less effective in inhibiting tumor growth that non-irradiated, virus-infected tumor cells. An experiment was performed designed to determine whether established immunity to MuLV 4070A-infected 107C3 cells influenced the ability of virus-infected tumor cells to suppress the growth of admixed, uninfected line 10 cells. Suppression of growth of line 10 cells by admixed MuLV 4070A-infected cells was _less_ effective in animals with established viral immunity.

DISCUSSION

Our interest in superinfection of experimental tumors was stimulated by observations that immunization by injection of living MuLV-infected tumor cells produced potent specific transplantation immunity to uninfected tumor cells.[4] Immunization with living MuLV-infected tumor cells might provide a method for induction of immunity to weak or cryptic rejection antigens of naturally occurring tumors. We superinfected two fibrosarcomas syngeneic to strain 2 guinea pigs with amphotropic MuLV, 4070A. Immunization with MuLV 4070A-infected 104C1 cells or 107C3 cells did not increase resistance to uninfected tumor cells. These results resemble those of Stephenson and Aaronson[21] and Sobis et al.[16] who studied the host response to tumors transformed by Moloney sarcoma virus, but not releasing MuLV. Superinfection of these nonproducer tumors led to the acquisition of MuLV antigens; however immunization with virus-infected transformed cells did not produce resistance to challenge with uninfected tumor cells. Possibly, other murine retroviruses would be more suitable for the induction of immunity to rejection antigens than MuLV 4070A; eradication of tumor cells infected with MuLV 4070A may be too rapid to permit development of immunity to intrinsic tumor antigens. Our results, to date, suggest that augmentation of immunity to uninfected tumor cells by superinfection with murine leukemia viruses requires the presence of "intrinsic" tumor rejection antigens. Certain tumors may lack these antigens.

Rejection of virus-infected tumor cells appeared to be a host mediated event. Although MuLV 4070A-infected fibrosarcoma cells were indistinguishable from uninfected fibrosarcoma cells in growth in vitro or in nude mice, MuLV 4070A-infected fibrosarcoma cells grew and regressed in syngeneic guinea pigs. To study the basis of rejection of virus-infected tumor cells, immunosuppressive drugs were given in an attempt to abrogate tumor rejection. The process of rejection of virus-infected tumor cells in strain 2 guinea pigs was not reversed by treatment with cyclophosphamide or methotrexate. Analysis of the basis of rejection of virus-infected tumor cells may be facilitated by studies in thymectomized, lethally irradiated, bone marrow reconstituted, "B" guinea pigs.[22]

A series of experiments was performed to determine the conditions required for in vivo suppression of uninfected tumor cells mediated by murine retroviruses. Previous reports indicated that intralesional injection of MuLV into established tumors of mice or rats could promote tumor regression.[23,24] In our studies, suppression of growth of a transplantable hepatocarcinoma required close contact between viable, virus-infected and uninfected tumor cells. Growth of the line 10 hepatoma was not suppressed by MuLV 4070A alone or by an injection of MuLV 4070A-infected tumor cells at sites distant from the uninfected tumor cells.

The "bystander" reaction described in this report shared characteristics in common with the previously described bystander suppression of line 10 growth at sites of rejection of the line 1 tumor.[19,20] Both reactions were impaired by irradiation of the tumor cells eliciting the response and also by immunization to the tumor cells eliciting the response. In the case of the tumor line 1, the tumor cells that elicited the bystander reaction were cells of a chemically-induced tumor that grew and regressed in syngeneic animals. In the case described in this report, the cells were a chemically-transformed fibrosarcoma superinfected with MuLV that grew and regressed after injection in syngeneic

332

animals. Although these bystander reactions share characteristics in common, the basis of the reactions may differ. Histopathologic observations indicated that rejection of line 1 in nonimmune animals was accompanied by microvascular injury and tissue infarction; these changes were not seen in animals immune to line 1. Microvascular injury was not observed in preliminary histopathologic observations of sites of rejection of virus-infected fibrosarcoma cells. We favor the concept that bystander killing described in this report is a consequence of superinfection of line 10 in vivo mediated by close contact with virus-infected tumor cells. One explanation for the attenuation of tumor growth suppression by irradiation of MuLV 4070A-infected tumor cells and by established viral immunity is that both served to limit exposure of the line 10 cells to infectious MuLV. Protracted exposure of line 10 cells to MuLV appears to be required for antigenic conversion of line 10.

REFERENCES

1. Hewitt, H. B., Blake, E. R., and Walder, A. S. (1976) Br. J. Cancer, 33, 241-259.
2. Middle, J. G., and Embleton, M. J. (1981) J. Natl. Cancer Inst., 67, 637-643.
3. Klein, G., and Klein, E. (1977) Proc. Natl. Acad. Sci. USA, 74, 2121-2125.
4. Kobayashi, H., Kodama, T., and Gotohda, E. (1977) Xenogenization of Tumor Cells. Sapporo, Hokkaido, Japan: Hokkaido University School of Medicine.
5. Mitchison, N. A. (1970) Trans. Proc., II, 92-103.
6. Bromberg, J. S., Lake, P., and Brunswick, M. (1982) J. Immunol., 129, 683-688.
7. Bromberg, J., Brenan, M., Clark, E.A., Lake, P., Mitchison, N.A., Nakashima, I., and Sainis, K. B. (1979) GANN Monograph on Cancer Research, 23, 185-192.
8. Evans, C. H., and DiPaolo, J. A. (1975) Cancer Res., 35, 1035-1044.
9. Ohanian, S. H., McCabe, R. P. and Evans, C. H. (1981) J. Natl. Cancer Inst., 67, 1363-1368.
10. Zbar, B., Bernstein, I. D., and Rapp, H. J. (1971) J. Natl. Cancer Inst., 46, 831-839.
11. Hartley, J. W., and Rowe, W. P. (1976) Journal of Virology, 19, 19-25.
12. Peebles, P. T. (1975) Virology 67, 288-291.
13. Ashley, M. P., Zbar, B., Hunter, J. T., Rapp, H. J. and Sugimoto, T. (1980) Cancer Res. 40: 4197-4203.
14. Brown, J. P., Klitzman, J. M., and Hellstrom, K. E. (1977) J. Immunol. Methods, 15, 57-66.
15. Fefer, A. (1969) Cancer Res. 29: 2177-2183.
16. Sobis, H., Van Hove, L., Heremans, H., De Ley, M., Billiau, A., and Vandeputte, M. (1980) Int. J. Cancer, 26, 93-99.

17. Shu, S., Fonseca, L. S., Hunter, J. T., and Rapp, H. J. Transplantation, in press.

18. Maibach, R. I. and Maguire, H. C. (1963) Nature, 197, 82-83.

19. Bast, R. C., Jr., Zbar, B., and Rapp, H. J. (1975) J. Natl. Cancer Inst. 55: 989-994.

20. Galli, S. J., Bast, R. C., Jr., Bast, B. S., Isomura, T., Zbar, B., Rapp, H.J., and Dvorak, H.F. (1982) J. Immunol, 129, 1790-1799.

21. Stephenson, J. R., and Aaronson, S. A. (1972) J. Exp. Med., 135, 503-515.

22. Campos-Neto, A., Levine, H., and Schlossman, S. F. (1978) J. Immunol. 121, 2235-2240.

23. Greenberger, J. S. and Aaronson, S. A. (1973) J. Natl. Cancer Inst., 51, 1935-1938.

24. Kodama, T., Kato, H., Gotohda, E., Kobayashi, H., and Sendo, F. (1978) J. Natl. Cancer Inst., 61, 403-406.

HERPES SIMPLEX VIRAL ETIOLOGY OF HEAD AND NECK SQUAMOUS CARCINOMA: RELEVANCE TO
TREATMENT AND PREVENTION

PAUL B. CHRETIEN, M.D.
Dept. of Surgery, University of Maryland School of Maryland, Baltimore, Maryland
21201

This review presents the major accumulated experimental evidence for an
etiologic role of the Herpes simplex virus (HSV) in the genesis of head and neck
squamous carcinomas (HNSCa) and delineates potential utilizations of these data
for the treatment and prevention of the malignancies. The seroepidemiological
investigations reviewed were prompted, in part, by associations of squamous
carcinomas at the site of recurrent herpes labialis[1] and demonstrations of
oncogenic effects of HSV in experimental studies.[2] The studies presented and
discussed in this review are organized into: 1) The relation between cigarette
consumption and serum IgA antibodies specific for HSV in normal subjects and
patients with HNSCa; 2) The incidence of antibodies to HSV related non-virion
antigens (NVA) in the sera of patients with HNSCa and other malignancies; 3)
Recent investigations of the characteristics of HSV-induced tumor associated
antigens (TAA); and 4) The potential clinical uses of these antigens in clinical
investigations of the treatment and prevention of HNSCa.

RELATION OF SERUM ANTIBODIES TO HSV-INDUCED ANTIGENS (HSVIA) AND CIGARETTE
CONSUMPTION

In a search for a relationship between cigarette smoking, HSV and HNSCa, we
elected first to compare antibody responses to HSV in nonsmokers and normals
with varying levels of cigarette consumption. Our previous report of high
incidences of serum complement-fixing antibodies to HSV-TAA in patients with
HNSCa[3] and the finding of elevation of salivary IgA in patients with HNSCa[4]
provided the rationale for quantitation of immunoglobulin specific (IgA,IgG and
IgM) complement-fixing antibodies to HSVIA in patients at high risk for HNSCa.[5]

Study Populations. The study group consisted of 93 healthy volunteers, 35
men and 58 women, who smoked cigarettes on a daily basis and who had a mean age
of 41.8 years. Data regarding tobacco and alcohol consumption were obtained by
personal interview and questionnaire. Ninety-four nonsmoking and nondrinking
healthy volunteers, 37 men and 57 women with a mean age of 41.8 years, formed a
control group. The smoking-drinking group and the nonsmoking, nondrinking group

were both composed of volunteers. The smoking group was unselected, in that all available volunteers were used. To form the control group, nonsmoking, nondrinking volunteers were matched for age and sex to individuals in the smoking group.

Indirect Immunofluorescent Assay. Confluent monolayers of monkey kidney cells (Vero) were infected with a high input multiplicity of HSV-type 1. At 18 hours after infection, the cells were washed, centrifuged and kept at 0° until use. A suspension of uninfected Vero cells was prepared in a similar manner. Serial dilutions of human sera to be tested were placed in a microtitration plate and HSV-infected cells added.

The cells and human sera were incubated for 1 hour at 4° C. Excess serum was removed by washing, fluorescein-conjugated goat anti-human immunoglobulin serum (heavy-chain specific for gamma, alpha, or mu chains) was added and the cells were examined for membrane immunofluorescence.

Results. In the smoking group, 46.2% (43/93) of volunteers had detectable serum IgA antibody to HSVIA, whereas only 7.4% (7/94) of the nonsmokers had such antibodies. In contrast, 68.8% (64/93) of smokers and 73.4% (69/94) of nonsmokers had detectable IgG anti-HSVIA. IgM anti-HSVIA was detected in 61.5% (16/26) of smokers and in 64.7% (44/68) of nonsmokers. There were no significant differences in the frequencies of detectable IgG and IgM anti-HSVIA in the smoking group compared with the nonsmoking group. Testing of 26 randomly selected smokers and 68 randomly selected nonsmokers showed no significant differences between the patterns of humoral immunity to HSVIA in the IgM immunoglobulin class and the IgG class. Routine assay for IgM antibodies to HSVIA was therefore stopped to permit testing of a larger number of sera for IgG and IgA HSVIA antibodies.

Subjects with a smoking history of 10-19 pack-years had a significantly greater frequency of detectable IgA anti-HSVIA compared with the 1-9 pack-year smokers or matched nonsmokers. All groups with 20 or greater pack-year cigarette exposure had a significantly higher frequency of serum IgA anti-HSVIA compared with their matched control groups. There was no significant increase in the frequency of IgA anti-HSVIA in groups with a 20 or greater pack-year smoking history compared with the 10-19 pack-year smokers.

The drinking group had a significantly higher IgA anti-HSVIA mean titer compared with the nondrinking group. There were no significant differences in IgA anti-HSVIA frequencies or IgG anti-HSVIA frequencies and mean antibody titers between the drinking and nondrinking groups.

Comment. This study[5] demonstrates a relationship between tobacco and alcohol
use and changes in the pattern of humoral immunity to HSV-induced antigens.
Smokers had an increased frequency of detectable serum IgA anti-HSVIA. Although
smokers and nonsmokers had comparable frequencies of detectable IgG and IgM
anti-HSVIA, the smokers had higher titers of IgG and IgM anti-HSVIA than the
nonsmokers. The increased frequency and titers of IgA anti-HSVIA occurred
independent of elevation of IgG anti-HSVIA titer in individual smokers. Smokers
had a higher frequency of detectrable IgA anti-HSVIA than nonsmokers after a
10-19 pack-year smoking experience. Additional cigarette use was not associated
with increases in the frequency of detectable IgA anti-HSVIA. Smokers who
imbibed alcoholic beverages had a higher mean IgA anti-HSVIA titer than
nondrinking smokers, but there were no significant changes in the pattern of
humoral immunity to HSVIA with graded alcohol consumption. The results of the
study suggest an association between exposure to cigarette smoke, alcohol, and
altered humoral immunity to HSV in a population with an increased risk of
developing head and neck squamous cell cancers.

SERUM ANTIBODIES TO HSVIA IN PATIENTS WITH HEAD AND NECK SQUAMOUS CARCINOMAS

To define the relation between antibody responses to HSV-induced antigens and
head and neck squamous carcinoma[6], we used the indirect immunofluorescent assay
described in the preceeding section. Serum antibodies to HSV-induced antigens
in IgA, IgG, and IgM classes were quantitated in patients with head and neck
squamous carcinoma before and after treatment, in patients with nonsquamous
malignancies, and in smoking and nonsmoking normal volunteers.

Study Populations. Patients with head and neck squamous carcinomas: A total
of 122 tumor-bearing patients with histologically proved squamous carcinoma of
the head and neck region (HNSCa-TB) were studied. Among these, 110 had not been
treated and 12 had local recurrence after previous therapy. A group of 93
patients clinically free of tumor six months to sixteen years after treatment of
head and neck squamous carcinomas (HNSCa-TF) was studied. For controls,
twenty-seven patients with nonsquamous malignancies were studied. A group of
thirty healthy volunteers who consumed cigarettes on a daily basis formed a
second control group. Thirty-six healthy volunteers who did not use tobacco or
alcohol formed another control group. For the smokers, an additional criterion
was cigarette consumption that matched that of the HNSCa patients.

Results. A total of 61% of patients with HNSCa had IgA anti-HSVIA antibodies
compared with 11% of patients with nonsquamous malignant tumors. This

difference is significant (p 0.0005). The percentages of each group with IgG and IgM anti-HSVIA antibodies were similar in the 79 to 92% range, indicating that a majority of subjects in both groups had been infected by the virus. The percentages of HNSCa-TF patients with serum IgA anti-HSVIA antibodies (56%) as well as IgG and IgM anti-HSVIA antibodies did not differ from the percentages of TB patients with these antibodies.

The percentage of heavy smokers with sera positive for IgA anti-HSVIA antibodies (57%) did not differ significantly from the percentage of sera positive in HNSCa-TB patients (61%), in HNSCa patients TF three years or less after treatment (62%), or in the HNSCa patients TF more than three years after treatment (44%). Also, all groups had similar percentages of sera positive for IgG anti-HSVIA. By contrast, the mean titer of IgA anti-HSVIA antibodies in smokers was significantly less than that in HNSCa-TB patients and HNSCa-TF patients assayed three years or less after treatment but did not differ significantly from the titer in HNSCa-TF patients assayed more than three years after treatment or the titer in healthy nonsmokers.

In sera with detectable IgA HSVIA antibodies, titers of IgA anti-HSVIA were significantly higher in patients TF three years or less after treatment than in smokers, whereas the titers of IgA anti-HSVIA in HNSCa patients TF more than three years after treatment did not differ from that of smokers. The titers of both IgA and IgG anti-HSVIA in the patients three years or less after treatment were significantly higher than those in TB patients, patients TF more than three years after treatment, and the smokers. The titers of IgA anti-HSVIA antibodies in patients TF more than three years after treatment were similar to those of TB patients. However, the percentages of patients TF more than three years after treatment with sera positive for IgA anti-HSVIA were significantly lower than those in TB patients or patients TF three years or less after treatment, and did not differ from those of smokers. The titers of IgG anti-HSVIA antibodies in patients TF more than three years after treatment were comparable to those in TB patient and smokers.

Comments. The data show that TB patients had significantly higher titers of IgA anti-HSVIA than did smokers; patients TF three years or less after treatment had higher titers of IgA and IgG anti-HSVIA antibodies than did TB patients; and patients TF more than three years after treatment had a significantly lower percentage of sera positive for IgA antibodies to HSVIA than did TB patients or patients TF three years or less and was similar to that of smokers.

The persisting elevations of serum IgA anti-HSVIA antibodies after tumor treatment in patients with head and neck squamous carcinoma suggests a remaining stimulus to synthesis of the antibody in these patients. The site of this stimulus could be in the dysplastic mucosal cells that are commonly found in patients with head and neck squamous carcinoma even after treatment.

The major finding in this study[6] is that heavy smokers and patients with HNSCa had a five to eightfold higher percentage of IgA antibodies specific for HSV-induced antigens than did patients with nonsquamous cancer or nonsmokers, and the titer of these antibodies was higher in patients with squamous carcinoma than in smokers. The frequencies of IgG and IgM anti-HSVIA antibodies were uniformly high in all the groups of normal subjects and cancer patients studied, which shows that the majority in each group had been exposed to HSV. The data thus evidence a humoral immune reaction (with production of immunoglobulins in the IgA class to neoantigens serologically indistinguishable from those induced in primate cells in vitro by infection with HSV) that was detected in high frequency only in heavy smokers and in patients with HNSCa. This study confirms the findings described in the preceeding section of a high frequency of antibodies to HSV-induced antigens confined to subjects at high risk of developing HNSCa and demonstrates for the first time a similar finding in patients with these malignancies, as well as a correlation between the levels of these antibodies and clinical course after treatment. These findings are evidence for an association between the herpes simplex virus, heavy cigarette consumption, and head and neck squamous carcinoma.

SERUM ANTIBODIES TO HSV-NVA IN PATIENTS WITH HEAD AND NECK SQUAMOUS CARCINOMAS.

In 1970, Tarro and Sabin[7] reported complement-fixing antibodies in the sera of patients with carcinomas of the urogenital tract that had specificity for NVA isolated from cultures of cells infected with HSV. Their finding provided rationale for an investigation of sera from patients with HNSCa for the presence of HSV-NVA. In this study[3], we screened sera from patients with HNSCa and uterine cervical SCa that was obtained prior to treatment and also from patients who were treated for the same types of tumors 5 or more years prior to study and who were considered cured.

Cultured human fetal kidney cells infected with HSV were harvested at 24 hours, disrupted with sonication, and centrifuged. The pellets were sequentially sonicated, centrifuged, pooled and concentrated by ultrafiltration. The antigens were separated by polyacrylamide gel electrophoresis (PAGE) into three gel regions. Previous studies showed that region 3, near the anodal end of the gels, is positive for complement-fixing (CF) reactivity with the antisera specific for HSV-NVA.

Antibodies to HSV-NVA were found in 36 of 38 (95%) patients with laryngeal cancer and 2 of 36 (5%) controls. However,there were no differences between the patients and controls in frequency or titers of antibodies to HSV, as assayed by complement-fixation assay or by a microneutralization technique. Thus, the presence of antibodies to the HSV-NVA is tumor associated and is not solely due to past infection with HSV.

Among patients with squamous malignancies, there was no difference in incidence of sera positive for HSV-NVA from tumor-bearing patients and those clinically cured of cancer; sera from 48 of 57 (84%) tumor-bearing and 20 of 28 (71%) cured patients were positive for HSV-NVA. Antibodies were present in the sera of 21 of 24 (87%) women with carcinoma of the cervix and in 15 of 24 (62%) patients with HNSCa other than larynx. Only 2 of 24 sera (8%) from patients with nonsquamous cell cancers were positive.

Comment. In this study, the high incidence of antibodies to HSV-NVA among patients with squamous cell carcinomas but not among normal subjects or patients with nonsquamous cell cancers suggests an association between the HSV and squamous cell malignancies. The results obtained in untreated patients with carcinoma of the cervix confirms previous reports.[8] The continued presence of antibodies to the NVA after successful treatment of the malignancy paralleled the finding in our study of IgA antibodies to HSV in patients previously treated for HNSCa discussed in the preceeding section. If the antibodies were produced to antigens in the tumors, eradication of the tumor should lead to disappearance of the antibodies. However, removal of the malignancy may not eliminate all cells producing the antigens; clinically normal adjacent mucosa may, nevertheless, contain transformed cells, or cells in the premalignant stage of the disease might remain, or nonmalignant cells lytically infected with virus during recurrent infection might provide an antigen source for continued antibody stimulation. This may explain the well-documented, repeated development of new primary squamous cell carcinomas in these patients. This study[3] is the first report of antibodies to HSV-NVA isolated from HSV infected cells in patients with HNSCa as well as in patients clinically cured of these malignancies. Further studies[9,10] of the serum antibodies of patients with head and neck and other squamous carcinomas which have specificity for NVA isolated from HSV-infected cells present evidence that these antigens are tumor associated (TAA).

Notter and Docherty[11] confirmed our observations, using, in part, the serum panel we studied. From HSV-infected cultures, these authors isolated both NVA-TAA[3] and the AG-4 antigen described by Aurelian.[8] Both antigens reacted with sera from patients with squamous carcinomas of the head and neck region and cervix in similar high incidences (63 to 81%). Paralleling our finding, sera from patients with other histologic types of malignancies and from normal subjects yielded low incidences of antigen-antibody reactions. In a subsequent study[12], the authors found a similar incidence of complement-fixing antibodies in the same patient groups with the use of antigen isolated from HSV-transformed cells.

RECENT INVESTIGATIONS OF HSV-TAA IN HEAD AND NECK SQUAMOUS CARCINOMAS

To obtain HSV-TAA free of contaminants, investigators in Tarro's laboratory extracted the antigen from human kidney carcinoma[13]. The HSV-TAA isolated is a glycoprotein with a molecular weight of about 70,000 Daltons. To increase the sensitivity and specificity over that obtained with complement-fixation, the investigators developed an enzyme-linked immunoabsorbent assay (ELISA) for detection of antibodies to the HSV-TAA in serum specimens[14]. Using TAA isolated from HSV-infected cells, the results with the ELISA correlated with those obtained with complement-fixation and offered the advantages of smaller amounts of antigen required for the tests and greater reproducibility of the results. In a screen of cancer sera, Tarro[15,16] found that, among patients with HNSCa, 78% were positive, while only 8% of sera from controls and 6% from patients with other malignancies were positive. In a subsequent study[17], they obtained similar results with the ELISA in an assay of coded sera provided by the NCI. The sera consisted primarily of specimens from patients with urologic and gynecologic malignancies and included only 9 patients with HNSCa, the purpose of the study being to reassess the results obtained with malignancies other than HNSCa obtained in previous studies. The investigators have also presented a study of antibodies to HSV-TAA in patients with urologic tumors[18], that confirms the data they reported previously. Recently, they have developed a monoclonal antibody to HSV-TAA[19] that is currently being investigated for specificity and sensitivity using tumor specimens from which HSV-TAA have been isolated in previous studies.

RELEVANCE OF HSV-TAA TO THE TREATMENT AND PREVENTION OF HEAD AND NECK SQUAMOUS
CARCINOMAS

During the past 12 years, investigators have demonstrated and confirmed that
patients with HNSCa have high incidences of antibodies with specificity for
antigens isolated from HSV infected and transformed cells and from non-HNSCa
tumors associated with high incidences of serum antibodies to HSV-TAA. The data
warrant the conclusion that these are TAA and provide justification for the
evaluation of the usefulness of the antigens in treatment and prevention of
HNSCa.

For immunotherapy of human malignancies, current concepts give priority to
antigens that elicit cellular responses. Preliminary studies would determine
the effects of HSV-TAA innoculations on cellular immunity in patients with
advanced HNSCa. The patients would be monitored for improvement of the
depressed cellular responses[20], as well as diminution of serum levels of immune
depressive factors[21], elevated acute phase proteins[22,23], elevated circulating
immune complexes[24] and HSV-TAA. Changes in the levels of HSV specific IgA[6]
should be studied for evidence of the function of these antibodies, since it is
possible that they form immune complexes which depress cellular kill of tumor
cells. Improvements in these factors that influence systemic cellular immunity
would provide rationale for the use of the HSV-TAA as adjuvants with standard
treatment for the tumors.

The use of HSV-TAA derived from HSV-infected cultures for immunotherapy
offers a unique advantage not available for similar treatment of non-HSV related
tumors. Conventional preparations of tumor vaccines are derived from
malignancies excised from cancer patients. As a result, the quantities of tumor
antigen available are limited compared to the amount needed for large-scale
trials. Also, preparations of the vaccines from tumors entail the challenge of
reproducible isolation of TAA from contaminations such as histocompatibility and
developmental antigens. By contrast, HSV-TAA can be prepared in limitless
quantities from infected cultures, using reproducible techniques.

Attempts at prevention of malignancies that current data suggest are HSV
induced is a reasonable and timely goal. The study populations would not have
previously experienced primary HSV infections. Thus the appropriate age groups
for the studies would be adolescent and young adult. With such groups, the
first goal would be vaccination against primary HSV infection. Prophylaxis
against HNSCa as well as urogenital and gynecologic malignancies would be

secondary goals of the program. Vaccine preparations of subunit proteins that
are devoid of HSV DNA have been evaluated experimentally[25,26,27] for use in
prophylaxis against HSV and no adverse experiences have been encountered thus
far. The current increasing morbidity from HSV infections supports vaccination
for protection against the acute and recurrent disease. For persons who do not
have evidence of exposure to HSV, the vaccines may consist only of virion
subunit proteins. But, those with antibodies to HSV would require TAA derived
from HSV-infected cells, with the hypothesis that vaccination with NVA-TAA may
prevent the survival of HSV-transformed cells in subjects who were exposed to
HSV prior to vaccination with HSV-TAA. Expansion of the goals of vaccination
programs to prevent not only HSV infection but also for protection against a
significant proportion of human malignancies gives high priority to such
investigations.

REFERENCES

1. Kvasnicha, A. (1965) Neoplasma, 12, 61.
2. Nahmias, A.J., Naib, Z.M., Josey, W.E., Murphy, F.A., and Luce, C.F. (1970) Proc. Soc. Exp. Biol. Med., 134, 1065.
3. Hollinshead, A.C., Lee. O., Chretien, P.B., Tarpley, J.L., Rawls, W.E., and Adam, E. (1973) Science, 182, 713.
4. Brown, A.M., Lally, E.T., Frankel, A., et.al. (1975) Cancer, 35, 1154.
5. Smith, H.G., Horowitz, N., Silverman, N.A., Henson, D.E., and Chretien, P.B. (1976) Cancer, 38, 1155.
6. Smith, H.G., Chretien, P.B., Henson, D.E., Silverman, N.A., and Alexander, J.C.Jr. (1976) Am. J. Surg., 132, 541.
7. Tarro, G. and Sabin, A. (1970) Proc. Nat. Acad. Sci. U.S.A., 65, 753.
8. Aurelian, L., Schuman, B., Marcus, R.I., and Davis, H.J. (1973) Science, 181, 161.
9. Silverman, N.A., Alexander, J.C. Jr., Hollinshead, A.C., and Chretien, P.B. (1976) Cancer, 37, 135.
10. Hollinshead, A.C., Chretien, P.B., Lee, O.B., Tarpley, J.L., Kerney, S.E., Silverman, N.A., and Alexander, J.C. (1976) Cancer Res., 36, 821.
11. Notter, M.F.D. and Docherty, J.J. (1976) J. Natl. Cancer Inst., 57, 483.
12. Notter, M.F.D. and Docherty, J.J. (1976) Cancer Res., 36, 4394.
13. Cocchiara, R., Tarro, G., Flaminio, G., DiGioia, M., Smeraglia, R., and Geraci, D. (1980) Cancer, 46, 1594.
14. Cocchiara, R., Tarro, G., Flaminio, G., DiGioia, M., and Geraci, D. (1980) Cancer, 45, 938.
15. Tarro, G., Flaminio, G., Cocchiara, R., DiGioia, M., and Geraci, D. (1980) Cellular and Molecular Biology, 25, 329.
16. Tarro, G., D'Alessandro, G., Esposito, C., Flaminio, G., Mascolo, A., and Maturo, S. (1981) Cancer Detection and Prevention, 4, 47.
17. Tarro, G., Flaminio, G., Maturo, S., Esposito, C., and Cocchiara, R. (1982) Clin. Immunol. and Immunopath., 25, 126.
18. Siracusano, F., Tarro, G., Biviano, D., Flaminio, G., Saladino, I., and Piccolo, A. (1982) Cancer, 50, 2215.

19. Karpas, A., Wheeler, T., and Tarro, G. (1981) International Workshop on Herpesviruses, Session VII, 232.
20. Browder, J.P. and Chretien, P.B. (1977) Semin. Oncol., 4, 431.
21. Sample, W.F., Gertner, H.R. Jr., and Chretien, P.B. (1971) J. Natl. Cancer Inst., 46, 1291.
22. Wolf, G.T., Chretien, P.B., Elias, E.G., Makuch, R.W., Baskies, A.M., Spiegel, H.E., and Weiss, J.F. (1979) Am. J. Surg., 138, 489.
23. Baskies, A.M., Chretien, P.B., Weiss, J.F., Makuch, R.W., Beveridge, R.A., Sample, W.F., Catalona, W.J., and Spiegel, H.E. (1980) Cancer, 45, 3050.
24. Baskies, A.M., Chretien, P.B., Maxim, P.E., Veltri, R.W., and Wolf, G.T. (1980) Surg. Forum, 31, 526.
25. Zaia, J.A., Palmer, E.L., and Feorino, P.M. (1975) J. Infect. Dis., 132, 660.
26. Kitces, E.N., Morahan, P.S., and Tew, J.G. (1977) Infect. Immun., 16, 955.
27. Skinner, G.R.B., Williams, D.R., Buchan, A., Whitney, J., Harding, M., and Bodfish, K. (1978) Med. Microbiol. Immunol., 166, 119.

1982 RESULTS OF TUMOR IMMUNOPHARMACOLOGY

GEORGES MATHE[+], IRENE FLORENTIN[+], MARTINE BRULEY-ROSSET[+], AND
PETER REIZENSTEIN[++], [+]Service des Maladies Sanguines et Tumorales et I.C.I.G.,
Hôpital Paul-Brousse, 94804 Villejuif Cédex, France; [++]Present address:
Karolinska Institute, Stockholm, Sweden.

INTRODUCTION

While oncologists had expected chemotherapy to solve rapidly the cancer
problems, a) the discovery of second neoplasias in patients cured by chemo-
(± radio-) therapy and of chromosomal and chromatid abnormalities in pharma-
cists and nurses working with oncostatic agents on one hand, b) the risk of
Kaposi sarcoma in immunodepressed subjects, iterative pneumonia victims and
male homosexuals confirming Ehrlich's theory on immunity tumor surveillance,
restored a major interest in cancer immunotherapy. Furthermore, the present
significant results of adjuvant active immunotherapy which concern many more
tumors than adjuvant chemotherapy, the new approaches of passive and adoptive
immunotherapy and of the use for biological response modifiers other than
immunity modifiers are new data.

The availability of molecules which exert an immunomodulating (such as
azimexon) or an immunorestorating effect (such as bestatin), the availability
of tests for clinical immunity monitoring (based on the use of monoclonal
antibodies) will add to the promotion of immunobiotherapy.

PRESENT RESULTS

Although immunopharmacology was introduced in 1967[1,2], while chemotherapy
was born in 1946[3], today however adjuvant immunotherapy controlled trials are
more frequently reported to be favorable than adjuvant chemotherapy studies[2-31]
(table I).

NEW EXPERIMENTAL RESULTS

The hybrid mice F1 (C57Bl/6 x DBA2) have all the C57Bl/6 controlling immunological reactions. At the age of 24 months these mice become immunosuppressed
and 30-40% of them die from leukemia or lymphoma[32]. Immunorestorators like
bestatin[33], and tuftsin[34,35] can prevent these tumors.

IMMUNODEPRESSION IN MAN

In 1976[36], immunodeficiency in man was discussed, but at this time few

Cancer: Etiology and Prevention, Ray G. Crispen, Editor

TABLE I

ADJUVANT[a] IMMUNOTHERAPY AND ADJUVANT CHEMOTHERAPY RANDOMIZED TRIALS
FROM WHICH ACTUARIAL FAVORABLE RESULTS WERE RECENTLY PUBLISHED

	IMMUNOTHERAPY	CHEMOTHERAPY
ACUTE LYMPHOID LEUKEMIA	- CELLS + BCG[2,4] [b] - LEVAMISOLE [6]	
ACUTE MYELOID LEUKEMIA	- CELLS + BCG[7] - LEVAMISOLE[8] - NEURAMINIDASE TREATED CELLS[9]	
HODGKIN DISEASE		- MOPP[10]
NON HODGKIN LYMPHOMA	- BCG[11] - BCG[12]	
MYELOMA	- LEVAMISOLE[13]	
MELANOMA	- BCG[14] - BCG[15]	
BRONCHIAL CARCINOMA	- ANTIGENS[16] - BCG[17] - NR, CWS[c] [18]	
BREAST CANCER	- POLY A-POLY U[19]	- CYCLOPHOSPHAMIDE[20] - MELPHALAN[21] - CMF[22] - AVCF[23]
GASTRIC CANCER	- BCG,CWS[d] [24] - PDP [e] [26] - PSK [f] [26] - LENTINAN[27]	
COLORECTAL CARCINOMA	- LENTINAN[27] - MER[28]	- RAZOXANE [29]
OSTEROSARCOMA	- INTERFERON[g] [30]	- N.S.
OVARIAN CARCINOMA	- BCG[31]	

[a]Adjuvant here means postoperative or postremission chemotherapy.
[b]The surviving patients belong predominantly to HLA A33 and B17[5].
[c]*Nocardia Rubra*, cell wall skeleton.
[d]BCG cell wall skeleton
[e]Plant derived polysaccharide
[f]Krestin = polysaccharide - protein (of *Coriolus versicolor*).
[g]Geographic non-randomized controls.
N.S. = no studies found.

immunological tests were available. Recently[37], immunosuppression has become a recognized entity in patients with cured Hodgkin's disease[38], and in homosexual sujects with herpes infection, and amyl nitrite consumption[40]. In these patients, the risk of Kaposi's sarcoma is increased[41].

IMMUNORESTORATORS

Azimexon seems to stimulate immunological reactions in young mice with normal immune reactions, but not in old immunodepressed mice[35]. Bestatin[33] restores the immunological reactivity only in immunosuppressed animals. Tuftsin and its analogs[34,35] act both in young and old mice. We are presently conducting a trial with the comparative study project of Onco-France, comparing azimexon and bestatin[42] as melanoma adjuvant therapy according to the modalities of adjuvant therapy indications and phase III studies[43].

TUMOR-ASSOCIATED ANTIGENS

Virus-induced tumors were initially shown to have group-antigens[44,45] whereas chemically induced tumors were thought to have private ones[46,47]. Some of these spontaneous tumors appeared weak or not antigenic[48]. Since antigens are studied with monoclonal antibodies, most animal and and human tumors appear to carry associated antigens[49,50].

It is probable that specific antigens are not required for immunotherapy, since macrophages[51], NK-cells[52], and autoreactive cells[53] seem to have non-specific cytotoxic activity.

This non-specific cytotoxicity may be necessary since tumor cells are heterogeneous[54,55] and since antigenic modulation occurs[56].

PASSIVE IMMUNOTHERAPY

Immunomodulation was seen in patients with acute lymphoid leukemia treated in remission with a monoclonal antibody, J5, against the so-called common acute lymphoid leukemia (cALLA) antigen[56].

Non specific cytotoxic activity may also be required for resistance against tumors since metastases are less antigenic than primary tumors[55]. In the absence of non-specific cytotoxicity, no less than 3 different monoclonal antibodies were required to cure at least 50% of mice with leukemia[54].

Transportation of cytostatics with the help of monoclonal antibody may also be considered a form of passive immunotherapy, a method which we first used in 1958[57].

ADOPTIVE IMMUNOTHERAPY

It seems now to be confirmed that patients with a graft versus host reaction after a bone marrow transplant also have a graft versus leukemia reaction, improving their survival[58], as we experimentally showed in 1960[59,60], and this was confirmed by Bortin[61].

BIO-IMMUNOLOGICAL RESPONSE MODIFIERS

Interferon seems to act as a NK-cell activator, as a cytostatic, as a differentiating and retro-transforming agent[62]. In myeloma and chronic lymphatic leukemia[63,64], its therapeutic activity was found and one case of meningeal leukemia presented a complete remission[65]. In non-Hodgkin lymphoma, breast cancer and melanoma, partial regressions have been described[66]. In kidney and partial bladder tumors, complete regression has been induced (67).

Retinoids also seem to act as differentiating agents and anti-oncogenic agents. We observed, in an uncontrolled study, a significant reduction in the bronchial epithelial metaplasia in smokers [68,69,70].

REFERENCES

1. Mathé, G., et al. (1968) Revue Française d'Etudes Cliniques et Biologiques, 13, 881.
2. Mathé, G.,et al. (1969) Lancet 1, 697.
3. Haddow, A., and Sexton, W.A. (1946) Nature (London) 157, 500.
4. Mathé, G. et al.(1979) in Adjuvant Therapy of Cancer II, Jones, S.E., and Salmon,S.E., eds., Grune & Stratton, New York, p. 191.
5. Tursz, T. et al. (1982) in Adjuvant Therapies of Cancer, Mathé, G., Bonadonna, G., and Salmon, S., eds., Springer Verlag, Heidelberg-New York, pp. 26.
6. Pavlovsky, S., et al. (1980) Proc. Amer. Soc. Clin. Oncol., 21, 436 (abstract N°C-462).
7. Reizenstein, P., Anderson, B., and Beran, M. (1982) in Adjuvant Therapies of Cancer, Mathé, G., Bonadonna, G., and Salmon, S., eds., Springer Verlag, Heidelberg-New York, pp.64.
8. Lehtinen, M., et al. (1982) in Adjuvant Therapies of Cancer, Mathé, G., Bonadonna, G., and Salmon, S., eds., Springer Verlag, Heidelberg-New York, pp. 70.
9. Bekesi, J.G., and Holland, J.F. (1982) in Adjuvant Therapies of Cancer, Mathé, G., Bonadonna, G., and Salmon, S., eds., Springer Verlag, Heidelberg New York, pp. 42.
10. Rosenberg, S.A., Kaplan, H.S., and Brown, B.W. jr (1979) in Adjuvant Therapies of Cancer II, Jones, S.E., and Salmon, S.E., eds., Grune & Stratton, New York, pp. 109.
11. Hoerni, B., et al. (1982) in Adjuvant Therapies of Cancer, Mathé, G., Bonadonna, G., and Salmon, S., eds., Springer Verlag, Heidelberg-New York, pp. 92.
12. Jones, S.E., Salmon, S.E., and Fisher, R. (1979) in Adjuvant Therapy of Cancer II, Jones, S.E., and Salmon, S.E., eds., Grune & Stratton, New York, pp. 163.

13. Salmon, S.E. Personal communication.
14. Morton, D. (1982) in International Symposium on Basic Mechanisms and Clinical Treatment of Tumor Metastasis. December 6-8, Fukuoka, Japan.
15. Mathé, G. et al. (1982) in International Symposium on Basic Mechanisms and Clinical Treatment of Tumor Metastasis. December 6-8, Fukuoka, Japan.
16. Stewart, T.H.M.et al.(1982) in Adjuvant Therapies of Cancer, Mathé, G., Bonadonna, G., and Salmon, S., eds., Springer Verlag, Heidelberg-New York, pp. 232.
17. Maver, C. et al.(1982) in Adjuvant Therapies of Cancer, Mathé, G., Bonadonna, G., and Salmon, S., eds. Springer Verlag, Heidelberg-New York, pp.227.
18. Yasumoto, K. (1982) in International Symposium on Basic Mechanisms and Clinical Treatments of Tumor Metastasis. December 6-8, Fukuoka, Japan.
19. Lacour, F. et al. (1982) in Adjuvant Therapies of Cancer, Mathé, G., Bonadonna, G., and Salmon, S., eds, Springer Verlag, Heidelberg-New York, pp. 200.
20. Nissen-Meyer, R. (1979) in Adjuvant Therapy of Cancer II, Jones, S.E., and Salmon, S.E., eds., Grune & Stratton, New York, pp. 207.
21. Fisher, B., and Redmond, C. (1979) in Adjuvant Therapy of Cancer II, Jones, S.E., and Salmon, S.E., eds., Grune & Stratton, pp. 215-226.
22. Bonadonna, G. et al. (1979) in Adjuvant Therapy of Cancer II, Jones, S.E., and Salmon, S.E., eds., Grune & Stratton, New York, pp. 227.
23. Mathé, G. et al. (1982) in International Symposium on Basic Mechanisms and Clinical Treatments of Tumor Metastasis. December 6-8, Fukuoka, Japan.
24. Ochiai, T. (1982) in International Symposium on Basic Mechanisms and Clinical Treatments of Tumor Metastasis. December 6-8, Fukuoka, Japan.
25. Kondon, M. (1982) in International Symposium on Basic Mechanisms and Clinical Treatments of Tumor Metastasis. December 6-8, Fukuoka, Japan.
26. Kumashiro, R. (1982) in International Symposium on Basic Mechanisms and Clinical Treatments of Tumor Metastasis. December 6-8, Fukuoka, Japan.
27. Taguchi, T. (1982) in International Symposium on Basic Mechanisms and Clinical Treatments of Tumor Metastasis. December 6-8, Fukuoka, Japan.
28. Robinson, E. et al. (1979) Biomedicine, 31, 8.
29. Hellman, K. (1982) in 1982 Tumor Pharmacotherapy, Mathé, G., and Mihich, E., Masson, New York, in press.
30. Strander, H. et al. (1982) in Adjuvant Therapies of Cancer, Mathé, G., Bonadonna, G., and Salmon, S., eds. Springer Verlag, Heidelberg-New York, pp. 103.
31. Alberts, D. et al. (1979) in Adjuvant Therapy of Cancer II, Jones, S.E., and Salmon, S.E., eds., Grune & Stratton, New York, pp. 483.
32. Bruley-Rosset, M. et al. (1980) Proc. Amer. Assoc. Cancer Res., 21, 250 (abstract 1004).
33. Bruley-Rosset, M. et al. (1979) Immunology, 38, 75.
34. Bruley-Rosset, M. (1981) J. Nat. Cancer Inst., 66, 113.
35. Florentin, I. et al. (1980) in Cancer Chemo- and Immunopharmacology. 2. Immunopharmacology, Relations and General Problems, Mathé, G., and Muggia, F.M., eds., Springer Verlag, Heidelberg New York, pp. 153.
36. Mathé, G. (1976) Immunothérapie Active des Cancers: Immunoprévention et Immunorestauration. Une Introduction. Expansion Scientifique, Paris.
37. Masur, H. et al. (1981) New England J. Med., 305, 1431-1438.
38. Fisher, R.I., et al. (1980) Ann. Intorn. Med, 92, 595-599.
39. Siegal, F.P. et al. (1981) New England J. Med., 305; 1439-1444.
40. Marmor, M., et al. (1982) Lancet 1, 1083-1087.
41. Gottlieb, G.J. and Ackerman, A.B. (1982) Human Pathol.,13, 882-892.

42. GI2C. Clinical phase I study with bestatine (1982) in Cancer Pharmaco-
    therapy, Mathé, G., Mihich, E., and Reizenstein, P., eds., Masson Publ.,
    New York (in press).
43. Reizenstein, P. et al. (1983) Cancer Treat. Reviews (submitted).
44. Kein, G. (1966) Israel J. Med., 2, 135.
45. Law, L.W. (1970) Transplant. Proc., 2, 117.
46. Klein, G. et al. (1960) Cancer Res., 20, 1561.
47. Prehn, R.T.,and Main, J.M. (1957) J. Nat. Cancer Inst., 18, 769.
48. Hewitt, H.B., Blake, E.R., and Walder, A.S. (1976) Brit. J. Cancer, 33,241.
49. Canon, C. et al. (in preparation) The common acute lymphatic leukemia
    antigen in blood, bone marrow and lymph nodes in lymphatic malignancies at
    diagnosis and in remission.
50. Irie, R. (1982) in International Symposium on Basic Mechanisms and Clinical
    Treatments of Tumor Metastasis, December 6-8, Fukuoka, Japan.
51. Keller, R. (1976) in Immunobiology of the Macrophage, Nelson, D.S., ed.,
    Academic Press, New York, pp. 487.
52. Stutman, O., Lattime, E.C., and Figarella, E.F. (1981) Fed. Proc., 40,
    2669.
53. Olsson, L., Kiger, N., and Kronstrom, H. (1981) Cancer Res., 41, 4706.
54. Olsson, L., and Mathé, G. (1981) Blood Cells, 7, 281-286.
55. Kiger, N., and Olsson, L. (1982) Réunion Commune de la Belgian Society of
    Immunology, de la Société Française d'Immunologie, et de la Société Suisse
    d'Allergologie et d'Immunologie. March 25-26, Strasbourg, France (abstract
    V-07).
56. Ritz, J. et al. (1981) Blodd, 58, 141-152.
57. Mathé, G., Tran Ba L., and Bernard, J. (1958) C.R. Acad. Sci. Paris, 246,
    1626-1628.
58. Sullivan, K. et al. (1981) Proc. Amer. Soc. Clin. Oncol., 22, 477 (abs-
    tract C-563).
59. Mathé, G., Amiel, J.L., and Bernard, J. (1960) Bull. Cancer, 47, 331.
60. Mathé, G., Amiel, J.L., and Friend, C. (1962) Bull. Cancer, 49, 416.
61. Bortin, M.M. et al. (1979) Nature, 281, 490-491.
62. Brouty-Boyé, D., and Gresser, I. (1982) in Cancer Pharmacotherapy, Mathé,
    G., Mihich, E., and Reizenstein, P., eds., vol. 1, Masson Publ., New York
    (in press).
63. Misset, J.L. et al. (1982) Biomed. Pharmacother., 36, 55-59.
64. Misset, J.L. et al. (1982) Biomed. Pharmacother., 36, 112-116.
65. Misset, J.L., Mathé, G., and Horoszewicz, J.S. (1981) New England J. Med.,
    301, 1544.
66. Sherwin, S. (1982) in Cancer Pharmacotherapy, Mathé, G., Mihich, E., and
    Reizenstein, P., eds., vol. 1, Masson Publ., New York (in press).
67. Braun, S. (1982) in 2nd International Conference on Immunopharmacology,
    July 5-10, Washington, D.C., USA.
68. Bollag, W. (1979) Cancer Chemother. Pharmacol., 3, 207-215.
69. Gouveia, J., et al. (1982) Lancet, 1, 710-712.
70. Mathé, G. et al. (1983) Cancer Detect. Prevent. (in press).

AN EVALUATION OF THE EPIDEMIOLOGIC EVIDENCE ABOUT BCG PROPHYLAXIS AGAINST
CANCER

JOHN D. CLEMENS† AND BONITA F. STANTON††
†Department of Medicine, Yale University School of Medicine, 333 Cedar Street,
New Haven, CT 06510; ††Hill Health Center, Department of Pediatrics, Yale
University School of Medicine

INTRODUCTION

An antagonism between tuberculosis and cancer was reported as early as 1929
in a famous autopsy study by Raymond Pearl.[1] Although it was later suggested
that the conclusions of this study were fallacious,[2] interest in the antagonism
between tuberculosis and cancer reawakened in the 1960's when the importance of
"immune surveillance"[3] was appreciated, and when the immune-stimulating properties of BCG were recognized.

Several studies evaluated the effect of BCG in animals and found that BCG
had a favorable effect upon leukemia and several other tumors.[4,5,6,7] This
work ultimately motivated epidemiologic studies to assess whether BCG vaccination could prevent cancer in humans. The first study, which evaluated the
effect of BCG in preventing fatal childhood leukemia, was published by Davignon
and colleagues.[8,9] Their data (Table 1) indicated that BCG proportionately reduced the occurrence of fatal childhood leukemia by 58%.

Since this initial report, 13 additional studies of BCG prophylaxis against
human cancer[10-25] have been published in article or letter form. Table 2 presents pertinent details of all 14 studies. The studies have been conducted in
diverse locations, including England, Scotland, Scandinavia, France, North
America, Puerto Rico, New Zealand, and Malaysia. Seven of the
studies[8-11,14,15,19,24] reported results describing the potency of BCG against
only leukemia, and seven[12,13,16-18,20-23,25] assessed BCG efficacy against a
wide range of cancers. As if to replicate the literature on the effect of BCG
against tuberculosis, the studies have produced markedly conflicting evidence
about BCG: three of the studies found BCG to be effective and 11 of the studies
found BCG to be ineffective. Augmenting the uncertainty about BCG are three
studies that not only found BCG to be ineffective, but also reported a greater
occurrence of certain hematologic neoplasms in BCG recipients, including
lymphosarcoma and Hodgkin's disease,[21] lymphoma and leukemia,[13] and non-Hodgkin
lymphoma.[23]

TABLE 1

RATE OF DEATHS DUE TO LEUKEMIA AMONG QUEBEC CHILDREN AGED ⩽ 14 YEARS, BY BCG
STATUS, FOR THE INTERVAL 1960 - 1963†

Vaccine Status	Leukemia Death Rate (per 100,000 at Risk)
Vaccinated	2.3
Non-Vaccinated	5.6

†After Davignon, et al (8,9)

Simple rearrangements of the studies do not resolve the conflicting data.
For example, of the 12 studies providing specific assessments of BCG prophylaxis against leukemia,[8-15,17-24] three studies found BCG to be effective and nine
studies did not. Conversely among the seven studies evaluating BCG against a
variety of non-leukemic cancers,[12,13,16-18,20-23,25] one study reported high
BCG efficacy while six found no efficacy. Although the neonatal period has
been cited as the optimal time for BCG vaccination,[26] only two[8,9,17,18] of the
five studies evaluating neonatal vaccination[8,9,10,17,18,22,25] found BCG to be
effective.

Since only three of the 14 studies found BCG to be effective, and since only
three studies described a neoplastic risk conferred by BCG, it might be concluded that the weight of evidence supports neither BCG efficacy nor BCG toxicity. However, because various study designs differ in their capacities to
establish causal relationships, it is important to contemplate the designs used
by these studies before accepting this sort of simple assessment.

Evaluation of the Evidence by the Potential Strength of the Study Designs

The 14 studies employed four basic study designs. Probably the intrinsical-
ly weakest epidemiologic design to study BCG prophylaxis is the ecologic
association study, used in six of the investigations.[10,11,14,15,23,25] In this
type of study, the investigator compares BCG vaccination rates and cancer
occurrence rates in populations from different geographic areas, or in populations from different secular periods within a given geographic area. For
example, in the study by Nilsson and Widstrøm[25] malignant tumor rates in
Swedish children were compared during two sequential secular periods. In the
first period, neonatal BCG vaccination was practiced routinely, and in the
second period, vaccination had largely been discontinued. Major weaknesses of

TABLE 2

BASIC FEATURES OF STUDIES EVALUATING BCG PROPHYLAXIS AGAINST HUMAN CANCER

First Author and References	Vaccinated Population	Cancer Outcome Studied	Conclusion About BCG	
			BCG Effective?*	BCG Harmful?†
Davignon[8,9]	Quebec neonates and children	Fatal leukemia	Yes	No
Waaler[10]	Swedish neonates Danish children, Norwegian adolescents	Fatal leukemia	No	No
Berkeley[11]	Scottish infants	Fatal leukemia	No	No
Comstock[12,13]	Georgia-Alabama general population	All cancers	No	Yes
Hems[14]	English adolescents	Fatal leukemia	Yes	No
Kinlen[15]	Canadian and Scottish infants	Fatal leukemia	No	No
Nilsson[25]	Swedish neonates	All cancers	No	No
British Medical Research Council[16]	English adolescents	Fatal hematologic and non-hematologic cancers	No	No
Rosenthal[17,18]	Chicago neonates	Fatal leukemic and non-leukemic cancers	Yes	No
Mathé[19]	French children	Leukemia	No	No
Comstock[20,21]	Puerto Rican children and adolescents	All cancers	No	Yes
Salonen[22]	Finnish neonates	All cancers	No	No
Skegg[23]	New Zealand adolescents	Fatal and non-fatal hematologic cancer	No	Yes
Sinniah[24]	Malaysian children	Leukemia	No	No

*Refers to a reduction in cancer occurrence by BCG
†Refers to an increased risk of cancer in BCG recipients

this type of study result from the fact that the unit of analysis for the study is a group, not an individual (giving rise to the so-called "ecologic fallacy"[27]), and that secondary data sources of uncertain comparability and reliability, such as routine population vital statistics, are used to derive the associations.

Another design used in several of the studies[8,9,17,18,24] is the contrived control study. In a contrived control study, the investigator compares one group in which BCG vaccination and cancer occurrence are directly ascertained for each individual, with another, "contrived", control group in which vaccination rates and/or cancer occurrence rates are indirectly ascertained from population vital statistics. The word "contrived" is used to describe the control group, since it is not an actual group of individuals directly assembled and individually inspected by the investigator. An example of this type of study was published by Sinniah et al.[24] These authors assembled a group of children hospitalized with acute leukemia in Kuala Lumpur and directly ascertained their antecedent BCG vaccination histories. The proportion of BCG-vaccinated individuals in this group was then compared to the vaccination rate for a contrived control group, consisting of published figures for the proportion of Malaysian children given BCG. The use of secondary data sources of this type for the control group provides little assurance of the comparability of data used to contrast the groups, and hence creates uncertainty about the validity of the assessment.

A somewhat stronger design than those already mentioned is the case-control study, employed by two of the BCG studies.[19,22] In a case-control study, vaccine efficacy is assessed by comparing the prevalence of antecedent BCG vaccination in a group of cancer "cases", with the prevalence of antecedent vaccination in non-cancer "controls". For example, Salonen[22] used the Finnish cancer registry to identify all cases of childhood malignancy occurring between 1959-1968. The prevalence of neonatal BCG vaccination among cancer cases was then compared with the prevalence of BCG vaccination among non-cancer controls, who were the immediately preceding parturients at the same maternal health center. This design is superior to the previous designs primarily because information about BCG vaccination and cancer status is directly determined for each subject in the compared groups. The weaknesses of this type of study result from the cross-sectional fashion in which this information is obtained.

The final design employed by the BCG studies is the clinical trial, in which the investigator allocates subjects to receive or not to receive BCG, and then follows the BCG and control groups forward in time to assess the comparative incidence of cancer. This design, which was used in three of the studies,[12,13,16,20,21] is potentially the most powerful design available, since investigator control over vaccine allocation offers the potential to assign BCG in a non-preferential fashion, and since prospective follow-up provides the opportunity to ensure equal follow-up and detection of cancer in the compared groups.

Table 3 lists the study designs in order of potential strength, from most powerful (clinical trials) to least powerful (ecologic association studies), according to a ranking system proposed by Feinstein.[28]

TABLE 3

RESULTS OF THE 14 STUDIES OF BCG PROPHYLAXIS AGAINST CANCER, ACCORDING TO STUDY DESIGN

Design of Study†	References*	Studies Showing High BCG Efficacy
Clinical Trial	12,13,16,20,21	0
Case Control	19,22	0
Contrived Control	8,9,17,18,24	2
Ecologic Association	10,11,14,15,23,25	1

†Arranged in decreasing order of potential methodological strength, in accordance with the ranking system proposed by Feinstein.[28]
*Denotes references of all studies employing the cited study designs.

Strikingly, all three studies that found substantial BCG efficacy employed designs with the least potential strength, and all studies in the two categories with the greatest potential strength failed to find a significant prophylactic effect. Although, it might be concluded on this basis that the weight of credible evidence suggests that BCG is ineffective, a more detailed evaluation of the fashion in which each study was actually executed yields a somewhat different assessment.

Methodologic Evaluation of Study Execution

Several standards of study execution are necessary to ensure the scientific validity of results evaluating the effect of BCG, regardless of the particular study design employed. First, the study should include a suitable control group. Accordingly, as a minimal requirement, the study should choose a control group from the same population and from the same secular period as the comparison group,[29] and the study should provide controls that enable a direct assessment of cancer occurrence in persons actually receiving BCG, vs. persons not receiving BCG. Second, the study should assure equal baseline susceptibility to cancer in groups compared to assess BCG. In studies that allocate BCG in an effectively random fashion, reasonable assurance about this equality can be provided by the demonstration that at least several important risk factors for cancer are equidistributed in the compared groups, or are unequally distributed in a way that does not affect the study results. In studies for which random BCG assignment is not possible, a more comprehensive examination of the distributions of all recognized risk factors for the cancer, with suitable analytic attention to any unequally distributed risk factors in the compared groups, is necessary. A further requirement to ensure equal baseline susceptibility in studies that do not randomly allocate BCG is the specific exclusion of subjects given BCG because of early manifestations of cancer. Observational studies that do not exclude such subjects are vulnerable to a systematic overestimation of the association between BCG and cancer (so-called "protopathic bias"), and to an underestimation of BCG efficacy.

Third, histories of BCG vaccination should be ascertained in the same fashion for each subject. Fourth, the study should arrange for suitable management of patient migration and follow-up. To safeguard against biases resulting from selective emigration of subjects from the study population, the study should demonstrate that the compared groups had equal and extensive (e.g., $\geq 70\%$) levels of follow-up, or at least that cases of cancer detected among emigrants from the study population have no substantial influence upon the study results. Biases can also result from the selective immigration of certain types of patients into the study population; to avoid these biases, all such immigrants should be excluded from the analyses. Furthermore, to circumvent biases that can result from disparate periods of risk in the compared groups, the study should report results at comparable periods of risk.

Fifth, to avoid bias from unequal surveillance for cancer in groups compared to assess BCG, the study should demonstrate consistency of results by the mode of cancer detection (e.g., screening of asymptomatic subjects, evaluation of patients presenting with symptoms, and autopsy detection), and should identify all cancer cases in the compared groups with the same reporting mechanisms (e.g., by the same tumor registry). Sixth, the study should ensure accurate and unbiased diagnostic ascertainment of cancer cases in the compared groups by performing an objective review of the diagnostic evidence for cancer in all cases and suspects.

TABLE 4

ASSESSMENT OF THE 14 STUDIES OF BCG PROPHYLAXIS AGAINST CANCER FOR FULFILLMENT OF SIX METHODOLOGIC STANDARDS

Study†	Suitable Control Group	Equal Prognostic Susceptibil-ity	Equal BCG Ascertain-ment	Suitable Management of Migration and Follow-Up	Equal Cancer Surveil-lance	Accurate and Unbiased Ascertainment of Cancer
Davignon	+	−	−	−	−	−
Waaler	−	−	−	−	−	−
Berkeley	−	−	−	−	−	−
Comstock*	+	+	+	−	−	−
Hems	−	−	−	−	−	−
Kinlen	−	−	..	−	−	−
Nilsson	−	−	−	−	−	−
MRC**	+	+	+	−	−	..
Rosenthal	+	−	−	±	−	−
Mathé	+	−	−	−	−	+
Comstock	+	+	+	−	−	−
Salonen	+	−	−	−	−	−
Skegg	−	−	−	−	−	−
Sinniah	−	−	−	−	−	+

† Denoted by first author
* References 12-13
§ References 20-21
**British Medical Research Council

In Table 4, each of the 14 studies is rated for fulfillment (indicated by a "+") or lack of fulfillment (indicated by a "-") of these standards. When authors provided too few details to ascertain fulfillment of a standard, the study was rated as "-"; and when details were provided, but the fulfillment of the standard was equivocal, a "±" was noted. No study was found to be adequate with respect to more than four of the seven standards for study validity. There was a tendency for studies with greater potential methodologic strength to fulfill more of the standards than the studies with less potential strength. For example, no ecologic association study satisfied the criteria for even one of the standards, whereas each of the clinical trials satisfied four of the standards. Despite this gradient in methodologic quality, however, none of the studies was carried out in a way that yielded convincing evidence about BCG efficacy.

Evaluation of Evidence Citing BCG as a Risk Factor for Cancer

As mentioned earlier, three studies[13,21,23] reported evidence suggesting that BCG vaccination confers an increased risk for the development of various hematologic neoplasms. Because the methodologic weaknesses shared by all 14 studies impair the assessment of both BCG efficacy and BCG toxicity, none of these studies can be regarded as having provided cogent evidence that BCG is a cancer risk factor. Furthermore, three additional considerations weaken the alleged risk of cancer in BCG recipients.

The first problem, exhibited in the study by Skegg,[23] involves the use of mortality data to assess the risk. This study found a statistically significant risk of non-Hodgkin lymphoma in BCG recipients only when non-Hodgkin lymphoma mortality data were examined. In contrast, a significant excess of this type of cancer was not evident in BCG vaccinees when incident cases were analyzed. Conceivably, the significant risk shown only by mortality data, but not in incidence data, could have reflected different patterns of death certification, different prognoses of diagnosed cases, or different qualities of antineoplastic care -- and not a different risk of non-Hodgkin lymphomas -- in the populations compared to assess BCG efficacy. These uncertainties weaken the conclusion that BCG is a significant risk factor for non-Hodgkin lymphomas.

A second problem, evident in all three studies citing BCG as a potential risk factor for cancer, involves a statistical consideration. Each of the three studies found only a marginally significant ($P < .05$) cancer risk in BCG recipients, and this statistical significance was discovered in the context of multiple therapeutic comparisons of BCG against various cancer outcomes, and in several patient subgroups. The number of therapeutic comparisons of BCG in these studies range from seven, in the study by Skegg,[23] to 61 in the study reported by Kendrick.[13] Because multiple therapeutic comparisons may substantially increase the probability of finding a significant therapeutic association when none really exists, the nominal significance level of $P < .05$ for each of the BCG risks was probably inadequate to protect against false-positive conclusions about BCG toxicity.

The third problem, shared by two[13,21] of the three studies, concerns the method of data analysis used to find the BCG-cancer association. These two studies were able to demonstrate a statistically significant risk of hematological neoplasms only by creating new cancer outcome categories after inspection of the original data analyses. For example, in the clinical trial of BCG conducted in Puerto Rico,[21] analyses of overall and type-specific cancer risks showed no statistically significant excesses of cancer among BCG recipients. It was only after the authors created a new category, consisting of lymphosarcoma and Hodgkin's disease, that the risk became significant at P < .05. Although such post hoc data analyses are useful as exploratory exercises, they make a study very vulnerable to the discovery of false-positive associations, and therefore cannot be regarded as suitable for testing etiologic hypotheses.

COMMENT

Our methodologic evaluation indicates that none of the 14 studies of BCG prophylaxis against cancer exhibited sufficient methodologic strength to permit conclusions about BCG efficacy or BCG toxicity. Furthermore, statistical problems created by multiple therapeutic comparisons of BCG, and by data analyses performed upon new outcomes created after inspection of the data, make the "statistical significance" of cancer risk in BCG recipients quite questionable.

In addition, the analysis illustrates an important methodologic point. Although various study designs can be ranked according to their potential strength, this useful heuristic is inadequate by itself to evaluate the strength of an individual study, or to assess the comparative strengths of a collection of studies. Thus, in the present series of 14 studies, a simple rank display of the studies by the potential strength of their designs appeared to resolve the conflicting data: studies finding BCG to be effective employed the weakest study designs, and all studies using the strongest designs found BCG to be ineffective. Moreover, when the actual execution of the studies was examined in detail, studies with the highest potential methodologic strength (clinical trials) satisfied more methodologic standards than studies with the lowest methodologic strength (ecologic association studies). Despite this gradient in quality, however, no study in this series demonstrated enough methodologic strength to provide convincing evidence about the role of BCG in the prevention of cancer.

In this regard, it is of interest to consider why the clinical trials of BCG faired relatively poorly in the detailed methodologic evaluations. Each of these trials was designed to evaluate BCG efficacy against tuberculosis, not against cancer. BCG prophylaxis against cancer was assessed in the trial populations either retrospectively or as a secondary outcome. As a result, none of the trials exhibited adequate protection against various biases in the surveillance and detection of cancer. In contrast, when the same trials were evaluated according to similar criteria in their evaluations of BCG prophylaxis against tuberculosis, they exhibited considerably greater methodologic strength.[30]

Our exclusive use of published data, and our practice of giving negative ratings to studies that omitted methodologic details, constitute potential limitations of this analysis. These considerations are particularly applicable to studies published only as letters in medical journals.[10,11,14,25] However, although several studies might have faired better in the analysis had they been published in greater detail, no study would have approached satisfying all six of the standards, even if credit had been given to all errors of omission.

Finally, in the absence of convincing evidence about BCG prophylaxis against cancer, it is reasonable to consider what sort of studies should be undertaken to resolve the current uncertainty. As pointed out in an earlier review of this subject by Hoover,[26] a clinical trial specifically mounted to evaluate BCG prophylaxis against cancer would require an enormous sample size and a prohibitively long period of follow-up to ensure an adequate evaluation of BCG efficacy and toxicity. The paucity of populations that have not received BCG -- or that have not rejected the use of BCG -- creates the additional problem of finding a location for a trial, even if these logistical obstacles were surmountable. In view of these considerations, non-experimental studies probably constitute the only feasible way of clarifying the role of BCG prophylaxis against cancer. Regardless of whether they are conducted in a prospective or in a retrospective manner, such studies will have to be designed with exacting attention to the basic methodologic prerequisites for scientifically credible evidence. Interest in the non-experimental evaluation of clinical therapy is currently increasing,[31] and the evaluation of BCG prophylaxis against cancer may provide an exciting opportunity for the development of rigorous observational methods of therapeutic assessment.

REFERENCES

1. Pearl, R. (1929) Cancer and Tuberculosis. Am. J. Hygiene 9, 97-159.
2. Wilson, E.B., Maher, H.C. (1932) Cancer and Tuberculosis, with Some Comments on Cancer and Other Diseases. Am. J. Cancer 16, 227-250.
3. Burnet, F.M. (1967) Immunological Aspects of Malignant Disease. Lancet 1, 1171-1174.
4. Old, L.J., Clarke, D.A., Benacerraf, B. (1959) Effect of Bacillus Calmette-Guerin Infection on Transplanted Tumours in the Mouse. Nature (London) 184, 291-292.
5. Weiss, D.W., Bonhag, R.S., DeOme, K.B. (1961) Protective Activity of Fractions of Tubercle Bacilli Against Isologous Tumours in Mice. Nature (London) 190, 889-891.
6. Lemonde, P., Clode, M. (1962) Effect of BCG Infection on Leukemia and Polyoma in Mice and Hamsters. Proc. Soc. Exp. Biol. Med. 111, 739-742.
7. Zbar, B. (1972) Tumor Regression Mediated by Mycobacterium Boyis (Strain BCG). Natl. Cancer Inst. Monogr. 35, 341-344.

8. Davignon, L., Robillard, P., Lemonde, P., Frappier, A. (1970) BCG Vaccination and Leukemia Mortality. Lancet 2, 638.
9. Davignon, L., Lemonde, P., St. -Pierre, J., Frappier, A. (1971) BCG Vaccination and Leukemia Mortality. Lancet 1, 80-81.
10. Waaler, H. (1970) BCG and Leukemia Mortality. Lancet 2, 1314.
11. Berkeley, J.S., (1971) BCG Vaccination and Leukemia Mortality. Lancet 1, 241.
12. Comstock, G.W., Livesay, V.T., Webster, R.G. (1971) Leukemia and BCG. Lancet 2, 1062-1063.
13. Kendrick, M.A., Comstock, G.W. (1981) BCG Vaccination and the Subsequent Development of Cancer in Humans. J. Natl. Cancer Inst. 66, 431-437.
14. Hems, G., Stewart, A. (1971) BCG and Leukemia. Lancet 1, 183.
15. Kinlen, L.J., Pike, M.C. (1971) BCG Vaccination and Leukemia. Lancet 2, 398-402.
16. Great Britain, Medical Research Council. (1972) BCG and Vole Bacillus Vaccines in the Prevention of Tuberculosis in Adolescence and Early Adult Life. Bull. Wld. Hlth. Org. 46, 371-385.
17. Rosenthal, S., Crispen, R., Thorne, M., Piekarski, N., Raisys, N., Rettig, P. BCG and Leukemia Mortality 222, 1543-1544.
18. Crispen, R.G., Rosenthal, S.R. (1976) BCG Vaccination and Cancer Mortality. Cancer Immun. of Immunother. 1, 139-142.
19. Mathé, G., Facy, F., Hatton, F., Halle-Pannenko, O. (1974) BCG Vaccination and Acute Leukemia. Biomedicine 21, 132-134.
20. Comstock, G., Martinez, I., Livesay, V. (1975) Efficacy of BCG Vaccination in Prevention of Cancer. J. Natl. Cancer Inst. 54, 835-839.
21. Snider, D.E., Comstock, G.W., Martinez, I., Caras, G. (1978) Efficacy of BCG Vaccination in Prevention of Cancer: An Update. J. Natl. Cancer Inst. 60, 785-788.
22. Salonen, T., (1976) Prenatal and Perinatal Factors in Childhood Cancer. Ann. Clin. Res. 7, 27-42.
23. Skegg, D.C.G. (1978) BCG Vaccination and the Incidence of Lymphomas and Leukemia. Int. J. Cancer 21, 18-21.
24. Sinniah, D., White, J.C., Omar, A., Chua, C.P. (1978) Acute Leukemia in Malaysian Children. Cancer 42, 1970-1975.
25. Nilsson, B.S., Widstrøm, O. (1979) Neonatal BCG Vaccination and Childhood Cancer. Lancet 1, 222.
26. Hoover, R.N. (1976) Bacillus Calmette-Guerin Vaccination and Cancer Prevention: A Critical Review of the Human Experience. Cancer Res. 36, 652-654.
27. Susser, M. (1973) Causal Thinking in the Health Sciences, Oxford. Oxford University Press.
28. Feinstein, A.R. (1979) Efficacy of Different Research Structures in Preventing Bias in the Analysis of Causation. Clin. Pharmacol. Ther. 26, 129-141.
29. Gifford, R.H., Feinstein, A.R. (1969) A Critique of Methodology in Studies of Anticoagulant Therapy for Acute Myocardial Infarction. New Engl. J. Med. 280, 351-357.
30. Clemens, J., Chuong, J., Feinstein, A. The BCG Controversy: A Methodologic and Statistical Reappraisal. Unpublished Manuscript.
31. Horwitz, R.I., Feinstein, A.R. (1981) An Improved Observational Method for Studying Therapeutic Efficacy, with Evidence Suggesting that Lidocaine Prophylaxis Prevents Death in Acute Myocardial Infarction. J. Amer. Med. Assn. 246, 2455-2459.

CANCER RISK IN TUBERCULOSIS PATIENTS: A PROSPECTIVE STUDY

KIYOHIKO MABUCHI AND IRVING I. KESSLER
Department of Epidemiology & Preventive Medicine
University of Maryland
655 W. Baltimore Street
Baltimore, Maryland 21201, USA

INTRODUCTION

Over a century ago, pathologists referred to an "antagonism" between florid, active tuberculosis and cancer. Rokitansky, for example, believed that lung cancer rarely occurred at sites commonly infected by pulmonary tuberculosis.[1] In 1929, Pearl reviewed the then existing literature and concluded that the decline in tuberculosis mortality had been accompanied by a marked increase in lung cancer.[2] Such views led to some laboratory experiments in which mice resistant to the tubercle bacillus were injected with mixtures of cancer cells and living myocobacteria, without the production of tumors.[3] There is even an anecdotal report of a therapeutic trial involving the injection of bovine tubercle bacilli into cancer patients.[4]

Somewhat later, pathologists began to consider the possibility that the two diseases were positively related. In particular, they speculated on an etiologic relationship between bronchial carcinoma and antecedent tuberculosis with its associated scarring of lung tissue, calcification of lymph nodes, etc. The notion of "Narbenkarzinom" thus came into existence[5], and it was during the same period that epidemiologic evidence on chronic bronchitis as a risk factor for lung cancer was compiled.[6]

Unfortunately, there have been very few systematic epidemiologic assessments of the relationship between tuberculosis and cancer. Pearl investigated the association in 7,500 autopsies performed at the Johns Hopkins Hospital and noted that tuberculosis lesions were significantly less frequent among 816 cases with cancer than among 816 age-, sex-, and race-matched controls without cancer.[2] Regrettably, the control group in this study appears to have provided a biased estimate of the prevalence of tuberculosis owing to the disproportionate number of such patients who died of this disease.

© 1983 Elsevier Science Publishing Co., Inc.
Cancer: Etiology and Prevention, Ray G. Crispen, Editor

In a British investigation of 1,465 patients with lung cancer and 853 other cancer patients, fewer than expected of the former reported a prior history of pulmonary tuberculosis, though the difference was not statistically significant.[7] An actuarial analysis of the mortality experience of 6,502 ex-servicemen in Australia showed a statistically significantly excess mortality from lung cancer among subjects with a prior history of tuberculosis.[8] A record linkage study of the cancer and tuberculosis registries in Israel also revealed that tuberculosis patients, as compared with the general population, stood a 5 to 10-fold greater risk of developing pulmonary cancer, a risk similar in magnitude to that of heavy smokers.[5]

The significance of the association between tuberculosis and cancer in man has been enhanced in recent years by several new findings. Growing evidence on the possible role of cell-mediated immunity in cancer and the rediscovery of Freund's observation that living mycobacteria are excellent stimulants of a delayed hypersensitivity response[9] have led to an increasing interest on the value of BCG in the prevention and treatment of cancer. An early investigation suggested a possible relationship between prior BCG vaccination and reduced leukemia mortality.[10] Current epidemiologic evidence on this issue is reviewed elsewhere in this Symposium.[11]

MATERIALS AND METHODS

The approach in the present study was to determine cancer risk prospectively over a period of time in a cohort of confirmed tuberculosis patients. During the period 1946-1960, a total of 18,006 tuberculosis patients were registered in the Central Tuberculosis Registry of Baltimore City. Of these, 17,701 were identified though a review of the registry records. These comprised the study subjects.

The registry record review also yielded information on patient identity, race, sex, date of birth, site of tuberculosis and its activity and stage at the time of registration. Some of the information which was missing on the registry records was supplemented by a review of other records available from such sources as sanatoria, chest clinics and hospitals.

The follow-up of the 17,701 tuberculosis patients was begun in 1977 and is still underway. The methods used to trace the patients include: (1) search of death certificates in Maryland vital statistics offices; (2) search of Social Security Administration mortality files; (3) search of State motor vehicle registration records; (4) search of Board of Elections files in Baltimore City and surrounding counties; (5) contact with family physicians mentioned on registry records; (6) review of records at sanatoria and selected hospitals in Maryland; and (7) search of U.S. Postal Service records.

At the present time, the highest percentage of patients traced (either to death or survival) are the white males of the study population. Of all white males, 19% have been found alive at some time between 1977 and 1982 and 40% have been found to be deceased. The present analysis was focused on the white male cohort.

For each deceased person, a copy of the death certificates was obtained, and the underlying cause of death and year at death were determined from information on the death certificate. Underlying causes were coded using the 8th revision of the International Classification of Diseases.

In the analysis of mortality data, the observed numbers of deaths from all or selected causes were compared with the numbers expected on the basis of the U.S. white mortality experience. The expected numbers were computed by the indirect method with adjustment for age and calendar year. In computing person-years, persons (tuberculosis patients) were entered into observation in the year of their registration. Persons whose vital status was unknown were withdrawn from the study at the time of the last contact. This is based on the assumption that those who have not been located have a mortality experience similar to that of those who have been traced.

The Standardized Mortality Ratio (SMR) is the ratio of the observed to the expected number of deaths. Computations and tabulations of SMRs were generated by a computer program provided by Monson.[12]

RESULTS

The distribution of all tuberculosis patients registered during the period of 1946-1960 by sex and race is presented (Table 1). Excluded are a small number of patients whose sex or race information was not available.

TABLE 1

SEX AND RACE DISTRIBUTION OF
REGISTERED TUBERCULOSIS PATIENTS
BALTIMORE, 1946 - 1960

SEX	RACE		TOTAL
	WHITE	NON-WHITE	
MALE	5,984	4,991	10,975
FEMALE	3,135	3,575	6,710
TOTAL	9,119	8,566	17,685

The follow-up of the tuberculosis patients proved to be a difficult task because of the limited available information on their location or residence. For reasons alluded to earlier, the present analysis is based on data for white males alone. The discussion will solely refer to this particular subgroup of tuberculosis patients.

In Table 2 is presented the distribution of white male tuberculosis patients by age at registration. It is not clear how closely age at registration approximates age at first diagnosis.

TABLE 2

AGE DISTRIBUTION OF TUBERCULOSIS PATIENTS
WHITE MALES

AGE (YEARS)	PATIENTS*	
	NUMBER	PERCENT
< 20	282	5.8
20-29	580	12.0
30-39	810	16.8
40-49	1,031	21.4
50-59	1,034	21.4
60-69	823	17.1
70+	264	5.5
Total	4,824	100.0

*Excludes patients of unknown age

The data reveal that a substantial proportion of the tuberculosis patients had active and advanced lesions at the time of registration, suggesting a considerable lapse between onset of disease and time of registration (Table 3).

TABLE 3

ACTIVITY AND STAGE OF TUBERCULOSIS AT REGISTRATION
WHITE MALES

Characteristic	Detail	PATIENTS	
		NUMBER	PERCENT
ACTIVITY:	Active	1,925	39.6
	Inactive	466	9.6
	Unspecified/Unknown	2,465	50.8
	Total	4,856	100.0
STAGE:	Advanced	2,894	59.6
	Minimal	1,475	30.4
	Unspecified/Unknown	487	10.0
	Total	4,856	100.0

The majority of the tuberculosis patients had pulmonary lesions with neglible proportions suffering from lesions of bone or joint, or tuberculous peritonitis (Table 4).

TABLE 4

SITE OF TUBERCULOSIS AT REGISTRATION
WHITE MALES

SITE	PATIENTS	
	NUMBER	PERCENT
PULMONARY	4,216	86.8
MEDIASTINAL	65	1.3
PLEURAL EFFUSION (ONLY)	49	1.0
PRIMARY	46	0.9
BONES/JOINTS	10	0.2
PERITONITIS	4	0.1
UNSPECIFIED	463	9.5
Total	4,856	100.0

At the time of registration, a secondary tuberculous lesion was absent in the majority of the patients (Table 5).

TABLE 5

SECONDARY SITE OF TUBERCULOSIS AT REGISTRATION
WHITE MALES

SECONDARY SITE		PATIENTS	
		NUMBER	PERCENT
ABSENT		4,746	97.6
PRESENT:	TOTAL	110	2.3
	MEDIASTINAL	8	0.2
	BONES/JOINTS	7	0.1
	GENITO-URINARY	2	0.0
	UNSPECIFIED SITE	93	1.9
	Total	4,856	100.0

The SMRs for all causes, all malignant neoplasms combined, and selected
non-malignant causes are summarized in Table 6. Overall, there was a 41%
excess mortality risk among the white male tuberculosis patients as compared
with U.S. white males in general. The excess mortality was largely due to
deaths from tuberculosis per se. Thus, the SMR for tuberculosis exhibited the
highest ratio, 48.98. A significant excess mortality among tuberculosis
patients was also observed for malignant neoplasms, diseases of the
respiratory system (especially pneumonia and emphysema), and diseases of the
digestive system (especially cirrhosis of the liver). A significant mortality
deficit was found for diseases of the circulatory system (especially vascular
lesions of the central nervous system), diseases of the genito-urinary system
and external causes (especially accidents).

TABLE 6

AGE AND TIME STANDARDIZED MORTALITY RATIOS FOR ALL & SELECTED
CAUSES OF DEATH AMONG TUBERCULOSIS PATIENTS
WHITE MALES

CAUSES OF DEATH	NUMBER OF DEATHS		
	OBS.	EXP.	SMR (O/E)
All Causes	1,702	1,203.0	1.41***
All Infective & Parasitic Diseases	493	16.7	29.50***
Tuberculosis	485	9.9	48.98***
All Malignant Neoplasms	294	207.7	1.42***
Allergic Endocr. Metabol., & Nutr. Diseases	22	19.0	1.16
Diseases of Blood & Blood Forming Organs	3	3.0	0.99
Mental Disorders	4	3.5	1.15
Diseases of Nervous System & Sense Organs	4	7.8	0.51
Diseases of Circulatory System	593	709.1	0.84***
Arterioscl. Heart Disease	452	454.3	0.99
Vascular Lesions of CNS	59	119.0	0.50***
Respiratory Diseases	143	72.9	1.96***
Pneumonia	54	31.7	1.71***
Emphysema	37	17.5	2.12***
Diseases of Digestive System	67	48.4	1.39**
Liver Cirrhosis	40	18.6	2.15***
Diseases of Genito-Urinary System	12	22.7	0.53*
Diseases of Musculo-Skeletal System	4	1.8	2.27
All External Causes	49	71.1	0.69*
Accidents	36	51.0	0.71*
All Other Causes	14	20.8	0.67

* α = .05   ** α = .01   *** α = .005

By specific cancer site, cancer of the respiratory system (including the
lung and larynx) and cancer of the buccal cavity and pharynx showed a
statistically significantly increased mortality. No significantly decreased
mortality was observed for any specific cancer site. Of special interest was
the mortality from leukemia and other malignancies of the blood and
hematopoietic tissue. Although mortality from all malignancies of the blood
and blood-forming organs among the tuberculosis patients was somewhat
decreased, the difference was not statistically significant (Table 7).

TABLE 7

AGE AND TIME STANDARDIZED MORTALITY RATIOS FOR ALL & SELECTED
CANCER SITES AMONG TUBERCULOSIS PATIENTS
WHITE MALES

CAUSES OF DEATH	NUMBER OF DEATHS		
	OBS.	EXP.	SMR (O/E)
All Malignant Neoplasms	294	207.7	1.42***
Cancer of Buccal Cavity & Pharynx	17	6.6	2.57***
Cancer of Esophagus	4	5.0	0.80
Cancer of Stomach	17	16.2	1.05
Cancer of Large Intestine	27	20.7	1.30
Cancer of Rectum	6	8.6	0.70
Cancer of Liver	8	5.4	1.49
Cancer of Pancreas	10	11.8	0.85
Cancer of Lung	124	52.6	2.36***
Cancer of Larynx	13	3.1	4.17
Cancer of Bone	2	1.2	1.69
Cancer of Prostate	12	21.4	0.56
Cancer of Bladder	4	8.3	0.48
Cancer of Kidney	5	4.7	1.07
Cancer of Blood and Blood-Forming Organs	13	18.6	0.70
Cancer of Other Tissues and Organs	32	21.4	1.50

* α = .05   ** α = .01   *** α = .005

The SMRs for specific types of cancer of the blood and blood-forming organs
are shown in Table 8; none of the differences between the observed and
expected numbers were statistically significant.

TABLE 8

AGE AND TIME STANDARDIZED MORTALITY RATIOS FOR SPECIFIC CANCERS
OF BLOOD AND BLOOD FORMING ORGANS AMONG TUBERCULOSIS PATIENTS
WHITE MALES

CAUSES OF DEATH	NUMBER OF DEATHS		
	OBS.	EXP.	SMR (O/E)
All Cancers of Blood & Blood-Forming Organs	13	18.6	0.70
Lymphosarcoma & Reticulosarcoma	2	4.2	0.48
Hodgkin's Disease	2	2.0	1.01
Leukemia & Aleukemia	3	8.5	0.35
Cancer of Other Lymphatic Tissues	6	3.8	1.57

Further analysis was undertaken to examine the effect of age at registration on the risk of cancer and the temporal relationship between tuberculosis and cancer. As stated earlier, age at registration can only be regarded as a crude measure of age at onset of tuberculosis. The SMRs cross-tabulated by age at registration and years after registration were presented for all malignancies (Table 9) as well as for respiratory cancer (Table 10). Because of the small numbers of deaths, such analyses could not be undertaken for other specific causes.

TABLE 9

STANDARDIZED MORTALITY RATIOS FOR ALL CANCERS
BY AGE AT REGISTRATION AND YEARS AFTER ENTRY
WHITE MALES

YEARS AFTER ENTRY		AGE AT REGISTRATION				
		<40	40-49	50-59	60-69	70+
0-4	OBS.	1	3	20	50	17
	EXP.	1.6	4.5	12.6	20.0	9.4
	SMR	0.63	0.66	1.58	2.50	1.81
5-9	OBS.	2	7	19	28	8
	EXP.	1.9	5.8	12.8	15.6	4.7
	SMR	1.08	1.21	1.49	1.80	1.69
10-14	OBS.	2	11	31	18	2
	EXP.	3.0	7.8	12.8	12.0	2.5
	SMR	0.68	1.41	2.43	1.50	0.82
15-19	OBS.	3	18	14	13	1
	EXP.	4.9	9.2	11.5	8.8	1.4
	SMR	0.61	1.95	1.21	1.48	0.74
20-24	OBS.	4	6	5	5	1
	EXP.	5.9	7.7	7.9	5.9	.3
	SMR	0.68	0.78	0.63	0.85	3.13
TOTAL*	OBS.	13	46	93	116	29
	EXP.	22.1	39.6	61.9	65.8	18.3
	SMR	0.59	1.16	1.50	1.76	1.59

*Also includes patients followed 25 years or longer

TABLE 10

STANDARDIZED MORTALITY RATIOS FOR RESPIRATORY CANCERS
BY AGE AT REGISTRATION AND YEARS AFTER ENTRY
WHITE MALES

YEARS AFTER ENTRY		AGE AT REGISTRATION				
		< 40	40-49	50-59	60-69	70+
0-4	OBS.	0	1	11	29	10
	EXP.	0.2	1.2	3.7	4.7	1.2
	SMR	0.00	0.70	3.00	6.17	8.26
5-9	OBS.	0	2	9	17	0
	EXP.	0.4	1.9	4.0	3.6	0.6
	SMR	0.00	1.04	2.24	4.74	0.00
10-14	OBS.	0	7	9	8	1
	EXP.	0.9	2.8	4.1	2.6	0.3
	SMR	0.00	2.46	2.21	3.03	3.33
15-19	OBS.	1	8	9	4	1
	EXP.	1.8	3.5	3.6	1.68	0.2
	SMR	0.56	2.28	2.51	2.38	6.25
20-24	OBS.	2	3	4	1	0
	EXP.	2.3	2.8	2.22	0.9	0.1
	SMR	0.85	1.06	1.80	1.08	0.0
TOTAL*	OBS.	3	21	43	60	12
	EXP.	7.7	13.9	18.5	14.1	2.3
	SMR	0.39	1.52	2.32	4.27	5.19

*Also includes patients followed 25 years or longer

The data on all malignancies (Table 9) seem to suggest that cancer risk
among younger tuberculosis patients may be reduced and remain reduced, for up
to 25 years, while cancer risk is higher among patients aged 50 and up even
shortly after tuberculosis onset. A similar pattern is observed for
respiratory cancer (Table 10). However, because the SMRs for young age groups
are based on small numbers of deaths, these findings must be regarded as
tentative. No clear pattern was apparent on the relationship between the
diagnosis of tuberculosis (as estimated by time of registration) and cancer
development (as estimated by death from cancer).

DISCUSSION

It should be noted that follow-up of the tuberculosis patients is still underway and incomplete at this time. Compilation of data on the remaining patients may result in findings modified from those presented here. Certainly however, some of the current findings appear worthy of further consideration.

As reported by previous investigators, an excess risk of respiratory cancer was observed among the tuberculosis patients. Whether this is due to such extraneous factors as smoking and occupational exposures cannot be resolved at this time because of the absence of relevant data. However, there is little reason to suspect that smoking is substantially more common among the tuberculous than in the general population. One may even suppose that such patients are likely to refrain from smoking. The excess mortality due to non-malignant respiratory diseases may also suggest a high prevalence of smoking in this population, but may also be due to the direct effects of tuberculosis. Further studies, perhaps utilizing the case-control technique, are required to answer the question.

An excess mortality from cancers of the buccal cavity and pharynx was also noted in the tuberculosis patients. This could be related to alcohol ingestion or even smoking. The possibly high alcohol consumption in this patient group is supported by their elevated mortality ratio for liver cirrhosis.

The reduced risk of leukemia and other malignancies of the blood and hematopoietic tissues has been associated with BCG vaccination in some earlier studies.[11] Mortality from cancers of the blood and blood-forming organs in tuberculosis patients was decreased, though not statistically significantly so, in the present investigation.

The data also suggest that age at diagnosis of tuberculosis may be an important determinant of cancer risk, and that, if tuberculosis infection acts in some way to reduce cancer risk, the effect may be limited to patients who contract tuberculosis at young ages.

Although our data on age at registration may not accurately reflect age at onset of tuberculosis, one may reasonably assume that patients who were young in age at the time of registration, were also young at the onset of their tuberculosis. Many of the patients whose tuberculosis was registered at older ages (e.g. 50 years or more) must actually have contracted their tuberculosis at much younger ages. Thus, the pattern of SMR's seen in Tables 9 and 10 suggests that the protective effect of tuberculosis against cancer, if any, may be greatest in the year immediately following the mycobacterial infection and may become attenuated with the passage of time thereafter. Further studies on this issue are urgently needed.

Follow-up studies of all tuberculosis patients in the present study, including all sex and race groups are continuing. Findings will be reported subsequently.

REFERENCES

1. Rokitansky, C. (1855). Lehrbuch der Pathologischen Anatomie. Wilhelm Braumuller, Wien, p. 303.
2. Pearl, R. (1929). Am. J. Hygiene, 9:97-159.
3. Centanni, E. and Rezzesi, Fr. (1926). Rif. Med (Napels) 42:195-200.
4. Loeffler, F. (1901). Deutsche Med. Wochenschr. 27:725-726.
5. Steinitz, R. (1965) Am. Rev. Resp. Dis., 92:758-766.
6. Case, R.A.M. and Lea, A.J. (1955). Br. J. Prev. Soc. Med., 9:62-72.
7. Doll, R. and Hill, A.B. (1952). Br. Med. J., 2:1271-1286.
8. Campbell, A.H. (1961) Australas Ann. Med. 10:129-136.
9. Levy, N.L., et al. (1972) Int. J. Cancer 10:244-248.
10. Davignon, L., et al (1970) Lancet 2:638.
11. Clemens, J.D. (1982). The 7th Chicago Cancer Symposium. Oct. 4-6.
12. Monson, R. (1974). Comput. Biomed. Res. 7:325-332

STUDY OF THE POSSIBLE PREVENTIVE EFFECT OF BCG AGAINST CANCER IN ADULTS[++]

LISE FRAPPIER-DAVIGNON[+], BERTHE LAVERGNE[+], MARIE DÉSY[+], and JEAN PELLERIN[+]
[+]Institut Armand-Frappier,P.O.Box 100,Laval-des-Rapides,Quebec, Canada, H7V 1B7
[++]This project has been supported by a grant of the National Health Research and Development Program, Ottawa, Canada

INTRODUCTION

Following the work of Lemonde et al.[1] on the preventive effect of BCG (Bacille Calmette-Guérin) against leukemia in mice, Davignon et al. published in 1970 results of the first study on the preventive effect of BCG against leukemia in humans[2,3]. The methodology was later criticized because of the retrospective nature of the study in which the administration of the vaccine had not been randomized. It was suggested that a true prospective study should be planned to assess more definitively the protective effect of BCG against leukemia[4].

In 1972, the Great Britain Medical Research Council published the fourth report of its anti-tuberculous vaccine clinical trials[5]. This paper reported the 15-year results of a controlled clinical trial of BCG and Vole bacillus vaccines in the prevention of tuberculosis as well as findings with respect to non-tuberculous diseases; 54,239 children aged 14 participated in this prospective study. They were randomly assigned to either the vaccinated or non-vaccinated group. The authors reported that "...the mortality from neoplasms of lymphatic and hematopoietic tissues between the ages of 15 and 30 years was 2.4/100,000 per year in the two vaccinated groups combined and 4.1/100,000 per year in the tuberculin negative unvaccinated group. The difference is of the same order of magnitude as that found by Davignon et al. but is not statistically significant. Hence the figures from that trial, although small, support the findings in Quebec." The small number of cases is explained by the low incidence of leukemia in the 15 to 30 years age group and also by the relatively small population in each group. These various findings and those of Rosenthal et al.[6] raised the need for evaluating the possible protective effect of BCG against cancer in adults. The present study was designed for that purpose.

METHODS

A cohort study was carried out among the nurses of the Province of Quebec. This particular population was chosen because it satisfied several conditions. The population needed to be large enough and fairly equally balanced between vaccinated

Cancer: Etiology and Prevention, Ray G. Crispen, Editor

and non-vaccinated subjects so as to provide optimal statistical power. The population had to be old enough to allow the accumulation of a sufficient number of cancer cases. Since the intensive BCG vaccination programme started only in 1949 in the province of Quebec, it was not easy to find a large number of vaccinated subjects over 40 years of age. The age at vaccination had to be similar for all subjects. Vaccinated and non-vaccinated subjects had to be comparable with respect to age, sex, socio-economic levels and duration of exposure.

Between 1952 and 1967, over 21,000 nurses had graduated from the various nursing schools in the province. The Quebec Order of Nurses provided us with their names, that of their school, their year of graduation and the address of those working in the province. BCG vaccination had started around 1950 in the nursing schools, but had not been applied systematically in all schools. Vaccination was not given on a voluntary basis. The choice was left to the schools to use BCG or not among their students. This reduces the risk of self-selection bias in this study.

A questionnaire was sent to each nurse to ascertain the following: 1) The information required to verify her BCG vaccination status in the BCG Central Record, namely: date of birth, place and date where vaccination had been given and father's name; 2) dates of occurrence of diseases and operations that had taken place since graduation; 3) names of classmates who had died since graduation with cause and date of death if known. The Order of Nurses and the schools' alumni also gave us names of persons they knew to be deceased.

Causes of death were verified in vital statistics departments of different Canadian provinces and, for some, of different American states. Reported cancers were confirmed by hospitals' pathologists.

Vaccination status. The BCG vaccination status was ascertained by searching through the BCG Central Record of the province of Quebec where files of all vaccinated persons in the province have been kept since 1926. No record is kept of people who never received either a tuberculin test or the vaccine. Those for whom no record was found were classified as non-vaccinated not confirmed. The non-vaccinated confirmed were those for whom only a tuberculin test was registered.

As the computerized list sent to us by the Order of Nurses did not include the age or date of birth of nurses, it was not possible to verify the vaccination status for non-respondents, except for the graduates of 1965 and 1966 for whom the information was provided. In those years the proportion of vaccinated and non vaccinated were similar among respondents and non-respondents.

Statistical analysis. We have used cohort life-table analysis to evaluate differences between BCG vaccinated and unvaccinated. The 5-year age groups mortality rates of the total cohort was established between 1952 and 1974 by a three-year period from 1952 to 1954 and then by 5-year periods through 1974. To obtain expected deaths in each sub-group, the total cohort's rates were applied to the person-years accumulated for vaccinated and non-vaccinated subjects for each period in each age group from the year of graduation through the first of June 1974 or through the time of death if before this date. The ratio of observed over expected deaths gives the standardized mortality ratio (SMR). The ratio of the SMR of the unvaccinated over the SMR of the vaccinated gives the relative risk (RR). Confidence limits at 95% were calculated following the method described by Ederer and Mantel[7].

RESULTS

We received from the Order of Nurses 21,476 names of nurses graduated in the province of Quebec between 1952 and 1966. Among those, 6,816 were not practicing and the Order could not give us their addresses. We were unable to locate the addresses for 2,239 of those persons. They are considered as "lost to sight".

Of the 19,237 persons remaining, 13,711 completed our questionnaire, 233 were deceased, and 5,275 did not answer (table 1). The response rate was similar for each year of graduation (table 2).

TABLE 1

POPULATION STATUS AS OF JUNE 1st, 1974

	No. nurses with known addresses	No. nurses without any known address	Total	
Total population	14 660	6 816	21 476	
Deceased	18	215	233	
Responses	10 651	3 060	13 711	
Refusal or incomplete questionnaires	11	7	18)	
Non responses	3 980	1 295	5 275)	35%
Untraced	–	2 239	2 239)	

TABLE 2

RESPONSE RATE BY YEAR OF GRADUATION

Year of graduation	Number of graduates	Response Number	Response %
1952	870	578	66
1953	975	620	64
1954	1 145	749	65
1955	1 070	706	66
1956	1 026	666	65
1957	1 133	717	63
1958	1 133	716	63
1959	1 294	866	67
1960	1 199	766	64
1961	1 308	825	63
1962	1 562	997	64
1963	1 966	1 235	63
1964	2 110	1 364	65
1965	2 630	1 751	67
1966	2 055	1 388	68
Total	21 476	13 944	65

In the total cohort, age at graduation varied from 18 to 50 years, age at vaccination also varied from birth to 30 years. As we intended to follow an homogeneous population, our analysis was restricted to the group of nurses having graduated between 20 to 24 years of age. This group represents 83% of those who answered or 11,341 nurses among whom 11,175 were still living and 166 were deceased. They were distributed in three groups: 1) non-vaccinated, confirmed or not; 2) vaccinated between 17 and 24 years of age; and 3) vaccinated at another age (table 3).

TABLE 3

CHARACTERISTICS OF VACCINATED AND NON VACCINATED NURSES
GRADUATED BETWEEN 20 AND 24 YEARS OF AGE

	no.	pers.-yrs	No. deaths	No. cancers deceased	No. cancers living
1) Non-vaccinated confirmed	1 813	20 976.31	40	10	14
Non-vaccinated non-confirmed	4 028	62 427.71	75	16	42
2) Vaccinated between 17 and 24 years of age	2 304	30 140.57	30	5	10
3) Vaccinated at another age	3 030	30 714.53	21	1	19

Mortality and morbidity. Vaccinated and non-vaccinated nurses with their BCG vaccination status confirmed or not were first compared for total mortality, total cancer mortality, and total cancer morbidity (table 4).

TABLE 4

MORTALITY AND MORBIDITY
NURSES WHO GRADUATED BETWEEN 20 AND 24 YEARS OF AGE
NON-VACCINATED VERSUS VACCINATED

	Non-vaccinated			Vaccinated			RR	95% confidence limits
	Obs.	Exp.	SMR	Obs.	Exp.	SMR		
Total mortality	115	104.0	1.11	51	61.9	0.82	1.35	(.69 - 3.34)
Cancer mortality	26	21.4	1.21	6	10.5	0.57	2.12	(.85 - 6.31)
Non-cancer mortality	89	82.6	1.08	45	51.4	0.88	1.23	(.58 - 3.19)
Cancer morbidity	56	54.1	1.03	29	31.1	0.93	1.11	(.69 - 1.79)

Obs.: observed; Exp.: expected; SMR: standard mortality ration; RR: relative risk.

Variations in length of time after vaccination should be reduced to a minimum when trying to determine the BCG protective effect. In order to do so, non-vaccinated confirmed were compared to vaccinated between 17 and 24 years of age (table 5).

TABLE 5

MORTALITY AND MORBIDITY
NURSES GRADUATED BETWEEN 20 AND 24 YEARS OF AGE
NON-VACCINATED CONFIRMED VERSUS VACCINATED BETWEEN 17 AND
24 YEARS OF AGE

	Non-vaccinated confirmed			Vaccinated 17-24 years			RR	95% confidence limits
	Obs.	Exp.	SMR	Obs.	Exp.	SMR		
Total mortality	40	33.0	1.21	30	37.0	0.81	1.49	(1.38 - 2.48)
Cancer mortality	10	6.9	1.45	5	8.1	0.62	2.33	(.73 - 8.73)
Non-cancer mortality	30	24.3	1.23	25	27.0	0.93	1.33	(.76 - 2.36)
Cancer morbidity	14	14.8	0.95	10	17.1	0.58	1.64	(.67 - 4.08)

Abbreviations as in table 4.

In both analyses, non-vaccinated nurses show higher risks than vaccinated and this risk is slightly increased when age at vaccination was known to be between 17 and 24. However, except for total mortality between non-vaccinated confirmed and vaccinated between 17 and 24 years of age, the relative risks are never beyond the limits which could reasonably be ascribed to sampling variability (at 0.05 level).

DISCUSSION

Many difficulties had to be overcome in this study. The first one was the large number of nurses without any known address. It took nearly a year to retrace two thirds of this group by working with school Alumni Associations when possible and with classmates who had already answered the questionnaire. The majority of deaths were in the group without addresses. Because of their large number and because we had no date of birth for most of them, the life status of the "lost to sight" was not verified at the Population Registry. We are probably missing a fair number of deaths in this group.

Mail strikes were also a major problem during the period of the study. Our first and second letters had just been sent when unexpected mail strikes occurred and it is likely that many nurses never received our letters or that their questionnaires never reached us. This could explain the large number of unanswered letters (24.5%). Fortunately, the response rate was similar for each year of graduation. There are good reasons to believe that most non-respondents were still living, as all nurses had to pay their annual dues in 1973 to be included in the list sent to us by the Order; furthermore, very few deaths were found in the group with addresses.

Vaccination status. The declaration of a subject on his vaccination status cannot be accepted as necessarily correct. Forty one per cent of those 7,729 nurses for whom it was possible to verify either did not know their status or were wrong about it.

Sex. In Lemonde's works, the incidence of spontaneous leukemia in AK mice was reduced 45% in males and only 20% in females after intravenous BCG vaccination at 10 weeks of age[8]. Turcotte and Potworowski[9] found that BCG stimulated the growth of Rous sarcoma in chickens and decreased the number of regressions, and this enhancing effect was more marked in females than in males. In humans, Gutterman[10] observed a difference in results between sexes in immunotherapy for melanoma. Women may not have been the best subjects to demonstrate any effect of BCG against cancer but they were the only group available to us for the study.

Protective effect of BCG. The apparent protective effect of BCG in total mortality analysis between confirmed non-vaccinated and vaccinated nurses between 17 and 24 years of age is due to the high mortality from cancer among non-vaccinated. If we take out deaths from cancer from total causes of death, the difference between vaccinated and non-vaccinated disappears.

In the analysis of mortality from cancer, the difference between vaccinated between 17 and 24 years of age and confirmed non-vaccinated is due not only to a decrease in mortality among vaccinated, as could be expected if BCG had a preventive effect, but also to an increase in mortality among non-vaccinated. The same phenomenon was observed in the BCG trial in Great Britain[5]. In the latter study, the mortality from neoplasms of lymphatic and hematopoietic tissues was less among vaccinated than among unvaccinated but the mortality for other neoplasms was significantly higher among the initially tuberculin-positive than among the initially tuberculin-negative. In our study most of the non-vaccinated confirmed are in this group because of their positivity to tuberculin test.

The British study also showed that protection offered by the vaccine against tuberculosis was in the order of 80% during the first 5 years after vaccination and then decreased gradually. The efficacy was still high (59%) between 10 to 15 years after vaccination. A better way of looking at the non-specific effect of BCG against cancer would be to compare the vaccinated with the unvaccinated subjects during successive five-year periods after vaccination. In this manner, it might be possible to show the gradual decrease of a protective effect present a few years after vaccination. This has been done but the number of cases in each category in our cohort is small, especially in the first 5-year period, as cancer is less frequent in a younger population. These small numbers do not permit statistical analysis.

While our study was in progress, Comstock[11] published results of a study done on young adults; it did not show any protective effect of BCG against cancer. The efficacy of BCG against tuberculosis in this cohort[12] was in the order of 30% which is very low compared to similar studies done elsewhere. Factors that were responsible for such a low specific protection could have also acted against a non-specific effect.

CONCLUSION
In all our analyses, the estimated risks were lower among the vaccinated. This does not necessarily imply that BCG vaccine had a protective effect against cancer.

382

There was a high non-response rate; the implications of this are unknown. Our population in 1974 was still a young one; therefore the number of cancers found and especially the number of deaths from cancer was not large enough to rule out variations due to chance. A longer follow-up of this cohort may help to correct these drawbacks. The unexpected finding of greater risk of dying from cancer among tuberculin-positive compared with tuberculin-negative vaccinees merits further study.

ACKNOWLEDGMENTS

The authors wish to acknowledge the help of Mr. Duncan Thomas, Ph.D., and Mr. Jack Siemiatycki, Ph.D., in the statistical analysis of the results and in the revision of the text.

REFERENCES

1. Lemonde, P. and Clode, P. (1962) Proc. Soc. Exp. Biol. Med. III: 739-742.
2. Davignon, L., Lemonde, P., Robillard, P. and Frappier, A. (1970) Lancet II: 638.
3. Davignon, L., Lemonde, P., St-Pierre, J. and Frappier, A. (1971) Lancet I: 80-81.
4. Bast, R.C. Jr., Zbar, B., Borsos, T. et al. (1974) New Engl. J. Med. 290: 1413-1420 and 1458-1469.
5. Medical Research Council (1972) Bull. World Health Organ. 46: 371-385.
6. Rosenthal, S.R., Crispen, R.G., Thorne, M.G., Piekarski, N., Roisys, N. and Rettig, P.G. (1972) J. Amer. Med. Assoc. 222: 1543-1544.
7. Ederer, F. and Mantel, N. (1974) Amer. J. Epidemiol. 100: 165-167.
8. Lemonde, P. (1966) Lancet II: 946-947.
9. Turcotte, R. and Potworowski, E. (personal communication).
10. Gutterman, J.U. (personal communication).
11. Comstock, G.W., Martinez, I. and Livesay, V.I. (1975) J. Nat. Cancer Inst. 54: 835-839.
12. Comstock, G.W., Livesay, V.T. and Waolpert, S.F. (1974) Amer. J. Public Health 64: 283-291.

BCG VACCINATION OF NEWBORNS AND INCIDENCE OF CHILDHOOD LEUKEMIA IN ISRAEL

LEAH KATZ AND R. STEINITZ
Israel Cancer Registry, Ministry of Health, Jerusalem, Israel

INTRODUCTION

The possibility, that the reported non-specific immunity conferred by BCG may prevent leukemia in children, is investigated. In Israel, routine BCG vaccination of newborns was introduced in December 1955 and discontinued in April 1982, in all, except the Jerusalem maternity wards. All children (including Jerusalem) are also tuberculin-tested and the non-reactors are BCG vaccinated at age 11-12. From 1955 on, practically all deliveries in Jewish women in Israel are in hospital. The percentage of BCG vaccinations in the vaccinating hospitals rose gradually from 60% of live births in 1956 to 91.5% in 1962 and has remained steady since in all vaccinating hospitals. In Jerusalem, however, BCG was given to newborns only exceptionally, when specifically indicated. In short, an "experimental" situation arose, in which children born in Jerusalem (roughly 10% of all Jewish children born) remained unvaccinated in the first decade of their life, whereas over 90% of those born elsewhere in the country were BCG vaccinated during their stay in the newborn ward. It was possible to examine the incidence of leukemia in these two populations from the Israel Cancer Register. The Israel Cancer Register was founded in 1960 by Dr. Ruth Steinitz. It registers all malignant neoplasms, (except Basal Cell Carcinoma and Squamous Cell Carcinoma of skin) diagnosed in Israel since 1960. The diagnosis and the date of diagnosis are invariably recorded and a printout by diagnosis, hospital and date of diagnosis facilitates access to special series of cases. Demographic data, such as country and date of birth, population group and residence are recorded from the outset. Lately, these can also be verified in the Population Register.

ⓒ1983 Elsevier Science Publishing Co., Inc.
Cancer: Etiology and Prevention, Ray G. Crispen, Editor

Approximately 15-20 new cases of leukemia in the first decade of life are diagnosed yearly in Israel-born Jewish children. The M/F ratio is 1.4. 55% of the cases occur in the 0-4 age group and 45% in the 5-9 age group.

MATERIALS AND METHODS

Study population

The study population consists of all cases of leukemia diagnosed since 1960 in Jewish children born in Israel since 1956, up to and including age 9. In the preliminary stage, 374 possible cases were collected. The Population Register was checked to verify exact date and place of birth, etc. (1 case only could not be located in the Population Register). A total of 27 cases was found not to fit the criteria: 15 were over the age of 10 at the time of diagnosis, 7 were born previous to 1956, 5 were born abroad. Subsequently, the case records were reviewed. 16 doubtful cases had to be excluded. 11 cases of congenital/perinatal leukemia were excluded from the study, since they occurred before BCG vaccination could be given. 5 cases of Down's Syndrome and 1 case with a history of irradiation were also excluded, because of their specific etiology, the numbers being too small for separate tabulation. A total of 314 verified cases was left in the study. 250=79.6% were fully documented, including hospital case summaries. 21 cases=6.7% were based on death certificate only.

Place of residence

The place of residence at the time of diagnosis was verified from the Population Register. (Former place of residence was also available from the same source for all those who moved within the country from 1971 on).

Hospital of birth

The hospital of birth was ascertained from the following sources (with some overlap of the information):

37 from hospital case summaries

16 from the Population Register (births from 1976 on)

95 from the original birth records, at the Ministry of Interior

Unfortunately, birth records from the period before 1967 were available only from ledgers of each of 18 District Offices of Registration, in batches accumulated by date of registration (not date of birth). Therefore, the attempt to locate all birth records had to be abandoned.

Hospital of birth was ascertained in 116, i.e. 36.9% of the cases. All cases born in Jerusalem were resident in Jerusalem at the time of diagnosis, and all cases born outside Jerusalem were resident outside Jerusalem. It was decided, therefore, to define place of birth as place of residence at the time of diagnosis.

Denominator

Since no yearly population figures by 5 year age-groups and place of residence were available, person-years of experience were calculated from the yearly number of births in Jerusalem, and in Israel minus Jerusalem. Deaths in the first year of life were subtracted from the number of births. The sum of the person-years of experience was as follows:

Place of birth/age	0-4	5-9	total
Jerusalem	504,791	348,561	853,352
Non-Jerusalem	4,671,976	3,292,310	7,964,286

Calculation of rates

Average annual incidence rates per 10^5 for the age groups 0-4 and 5-9, both sexes combined, were calculated from the sum of person-years of experience and the sum of cases for the whole period.

RESULTS

A total of 314 cases were studied: 178 M and 136 F. The M/F ratio was 1.3. 67.5% of cases were at ages 0-4 and 32.5% at ages 5-9.

Comparison of incidence rates:

Leukemia in Israel, 1960-78, Jews born in Israel, ages 0-4 and 5-9, both

sexes. Numbers and average annual incidence rates/10^5, by place of birth

and relative risk.

Place of birth/age	0-4		5-9	
	No	R	No	R
Jerusalem	30	5.94	14	4.02
Non-Jerusalem	182	3.90	88	2.36
Relative risk:				
Jerusalem /Non-Jerusalem	1.52		1.51	

CONCLUSIONS

The relative risk of childhood leukemia for the presumably unvaccinated children born in Jerusalem is approximately 1½ times that of the presumably vaccinated children born in other areas. This is true for both, the 0-4 and 5-9 age-groups. Three points of doubt may be raised as to the validity of the study methods and the results.

1) The substitution of place of residence for place of birth on the basis of a sample of approximately 1/3 of the cases. Possible bias may arise from the fact that place of birth could be ascertained readily for recent births, whereas locating place of birth before 1967 was hampered by discrepancy between the place of birth and place of residence.

2) The definition of vaccination status by hospital of birth may be wrong in some cases.

3) The small number of cases.

It is intended to enlarge the number of cases by continuing the study until all birth cohorts that can be included in the study will reach the age of 10. The feasibility of ascertaining vaccination status at least in a sample of cases is investigated.

BCG VACCINATION AND LEUKEMIA IN AUSTRIA
EPIDEMIOLOGICAL AND CLINICAL STUDIES

F. AMBROSCH[+], G. WIEDERMANN[+] AND P. KREPLER[++]
[+]Institute for Specific Prophylaxis and Tropical Medicine, University of Vienna, Kinderspitalgasse 15, A 1095 Vienna, Austria; [++]St. Anna Children's Hospital Vienna, Kinderspitalgasse 6, A 1095 Vienna, Austria

INTRODUCTION

During the last two decades tuberculosis morbidity and mortality decreased considerably in Austria as well as in many other countries. Therefore deliberations were made to stop BCG vaccination which has been offered to all newborns. Although the risk as well as the cost benefit balance were still in favour of vaccination, real benefits compared with previous years had diminished[1-2].

In this situation the eventual non-specific effect of BCG vaccination concerning certain neoplastic disorders such as leukemia became an important argument in the discussion. A protective effect of BCG vaccination against leukemia was reported in several studies[3-8], whereas other investigators could not detect any significant effect[9-13]. Also there were some interesting data resulting from epidemiological analyses that BCG vaccination might reduce leukemia mortality[14-17]. However, there were other critical comments raising various objections against these studies in which a protective effect was reported[18-22].

For these reasons we decided to investigate this problem again using statistical and clinical data from Austria. These studies were performed during the years 1978-81[23-25].

PREREQUISITES

Austria is a small country with an area of 83.852 km^2 and with a population of approximately 7.5 million. There are nine provinces with their own provincial health authorities and a Federal Ministry of Health located in Vienna.

The BCG vaccination program was started in 1949 and was extended gradually during the years following. A Copenhagen strain vaccine was manufactured in Austria. With the mother's signed consent BCG vaccination was offered to all newborns during the first week. Until 1975 vaccinations could be performed only on children born in hospitals.

The consent forms are used as the basis for the vaccination statistics. They are counted in the hospitals and the numbers reported to the district health departments. From there they are forwarded to the provincial health authorities and finally to the Ministry of Health. Therefore, reliable data on BCG vaccinations are available from most Austrian provinces. Similarly, the official death

©1983 Elsevier Science Publishing Co., Inc.
Cancer: Etiology and Prevention, Ray G. Crispen, Editor

388

certificates are the basis for the statistics on leukemia deaths. The death certificate is issued by hospitals or public health officers indicating the exact
cause of death. A copy is sent to the Central Statistical Office for evaluation.
Therefore the data on leukemia mortality can also be considered to be accurate.

EPIDEMIOLOGICAL STUDY

In our first epidemiological analysis we tried to find an association between BCG vaccination rate - this is the proportion of vaccinated children - and
leukemia mortality during the first five years of life. This period of time was
chosen for two reasons: 1. leukemia morbidity and mortality reach their peak
during the third and fourth year and 2. a protective effect of BCG vaccination
should be detectable more easily during the first five years after vaccination.

As a first step we analyzed the course of leukemia mortality in different
age groups (fig. 1). The overall mortality has increased steadily since 1946,
due to the increased longevity. The age group from 15 to 40 years shows a slight
decline probably due to improved therapeutic measures. However, the age group
0 - 5 years shows a remarkable decrease from nearly 7 to 2 deaths in 100.000
children per year beginning in 1955.

It was therefore very interesting to compare leukemia mortality in this age
group and BCG vaccination rates (fig. 2). It can be clearly demonstrated that
leukemia mortality started to decrease soon after the introduction of BCG
vaccination and a reciprocal course of these parameters resulted.

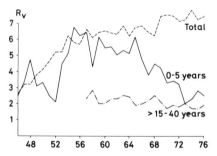
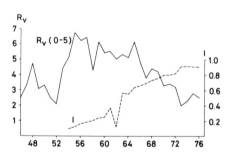

Fig. 1. Leukemia mortality in different
age groups in Austria

Fig. 2. Leukemia mortality in children
0 - 5 years (R_v) and BCG vaccination
rate (I) in Austria

Next we analysed the correlation between leukemia mortality and BCG vaccination
rate by means of a linear regression (fig. 3). This was done during the different 3-year periods from 1964 to 1975. We found a significant negative correlation with a coefficient of 0.98, suggesting a protective effect of BCG vacci-

nation. Objection could be raised against this interpretation stating that decrease of mortality might be due to more successful treatment only. It is highly
improbable, but not impossible, that therapeutic improvement developed parallel
with the increase of the vaccination rate. To exclude this possibility we compared the 10 year period leukemia mortality (1966-1975) in the age group 0 - 5
years and the vaccination rate of the 5 largest adjacent provinces of Austria
(fig. 4). Again, we found a significant correlation and an almost identical
regression line.

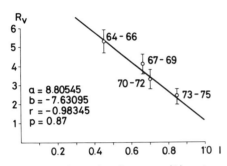

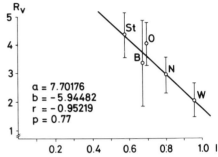

Fig. 3. BCG vaccination rate (I) and
leukemia mortality (R_V) in children
0 - 5 years in different 3-year
periods in Austria.

Fig. 4. BCG vaccination rate (I) and
leukemia mortality (R_V) in children
0 - 5 years in different Austrian
provinces 1966 - 1975.

From this regression line the protection rate of BCG vaccination regarding leukemia mortality can be calculated. The formula $R_V = R_0.(1-pI)$ gives the connection between the risk of leukemia mortality R, protection rate p and vaccination rate I. R_V is the risk in a partially vaccinated population and R_0 the
corresponding risk in a non-vaccinated population.

From that formula we can deduct $R_V = R - (R_0.p).I$, and this equation can be
considered as regression line $R_V = a - bI$. Then the intercept $a = R_0$, the slope
$b = R_0.p$. From that the protection rate p can be calculated as $p = \frac{b}{a}$ or slope
divided by intercept. Using this formula we were able to calculate a protection
rate for BCG vaccination with regard to leukemia mortality of 0.77.

Another statistical analysis was performed by means of Spearman rank correlation (table 1). Vaccination rate I and leukemia mortality R_V of these five
provinces were classified for the periods 1966 1970, 1971-1975 and 1966-1975.
The Spearman correlation coefficient is significant in each period, in the
period 1971-1975 even highly significant . In particular, it is very interesting that some provinces changed their positions of the vaccination rate as
well as leukemia mortality from one period to the other.

TABLE 1

LEUKEMIA MORTALITY (R_v) AND BCG VACCINATION RATE (I) IN DIFFERENT PROVINCES
OF AUSTRIA

SPEARMAN RANK CORRELATION

	1966 - 1970			
	I	Rank	R_v	Rank
W	0.945	1	2.20	1
B	0.663	3	3.58	3
N	0.796	2	3.18	2
O	0.595	4	5.14	4
St	0.438	5	5.15	5
	1971 - 1975			
	I	Rank	R_v	Rank
W	0.962	1	1.84	1
B	0.679	5	3.09	5
N	0.798	3	2.61	2
O	0.803	2	2.66	3
St	0.742	4	2.75	4
	1966 - 1975			
	I	Rank	R_v	Rank
W	0.953	1	2.03	1
B	0.670	4	3.35	3
N	0.797	2	2.92	2
O	0.690	3	4.01	4
St	0.572	5	4.31	5

Here too one might consider, that treatment could differ in its efficacy in various provinces and that leukemia mortality and BCG vaccination rate might be correlated by coincidence. This fact will be disproved in the second part of this study by showing that there are only minor differences in leukemia case fatality rates in the various Austrian provinces.

The final step was an attempt to calculate the annual number of leukemia deaths in Austria on the basis of births, vaccination rates, the protection rate p and the mortality risk in a non-vaccinated population R_o (fig. 5). The course of the expected deaths (interrupted line) is very similar to that of the reported deaths (solid line). Minor deviations as shown in the figure are only accidental.

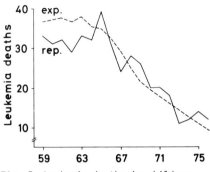

Fig. 5. Leukemia deaths in children 0 - 5 years in Austria 1959 - 1976. Comparison between expected and reported deaths.

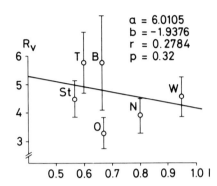

Fig. 6. Leukemia morbidity (R_V) in children 0 - 5 years and BCG vaccination rate (I) in different provinces of Austria 1967 - 1976.

RETROSPECTIVE CLINICAL STUDY

Although these findings seem to be quite convincing, there is a theoretical possibility that the associations between BCG vaccination rate and leukemia mortality, temporal and regional, occur by chance or by some unknown factor. It therefore became necessary to observe other leukemia parameters which also could be influenced by BCG vaccination. A hypothetical protective effect of BCG vaccination should in some way influence not only mortality but also morbidity, case fatality, 5-year survival, survival time, manifestation age and frequency of different kinds of leukemia. To clarify this question a retrospective clinical study was performed in 1980. A total number of 613 cases of leukemia in children was reported from 21 hospitals in answer to questionnaires which were sent to all paediatric hospitals and departments in Austria. The following data were collected for each child: date of birth, maternity hospital or other place of birth, BCG vaccination according to hospital records, BCG vaccination according to birth protocol, BCG vaccination according to central BCG record, diagnosis, date of diagnosis, date of death and hospital or clinic where the child received therapy.

Birth protocols of the leukemic children, as far as they were born in hospitals, were examined by our assistants. Similarly, the vaccination status was checked through the central BCG records in Vienna. In addition, subsequent deaths occurring after hospital dismissal were recorded with the help of the official registration offices.

From a total of 613 leukemic children, 269 were selected for further evaluation. These children became ill between 1967 and 1976 during the first five years of their life. This means that the observation time of the children in this group was at least three years. All these data were computerized for further evaluation.

To begin with we analyzed BCG vaccination rate and leukemia morbidity in different provinces of Austria (fig. 6). A slightly negative correlation with a calculated protection rate of 0,32 was found, but probably due to underreporting in some provinces this was not significant.

Furthermore, the case fatalities in different provinces were compared (table 2), considering the before mentioned objection that leukemia mortality and BCG vaccination rate might be correlated by coincidence due to differences in therapeutic efficacy in the various provinces. There were only slight differences in case fatality. The province of Vienna, which shows the lowest leukemia mortality, had a fatality rate of 60 %. This comparison disproves the theory, that the association between leukemia mortality and BCG vaccination might be due to differences in therapy.

TABLE 2

CASE FATALITY IN CHILDREN 0-5 YEARS IN DIFFERENT PROVINCES OF AUSTRIA 1967-1976

Province	Cases	Deaths	Case fatality
B	12	6	50 %
K	25	18	72 %
N	43	31	72 %
O	35	30	85 %
S	9	7	77 %
St	45	35	77 %
T	30	17	56 %
V	11	8	72 %
W	43	26	60 %
Total	269	186	69 %

One of the major goals of this study was to compare the BCG vaccination status with the course of the disease. Previous studies showed some difficulties in ascertaining whether or not a certain person had been vaccinated. In our study we used three different sources of information for the verification of a BCG vaccination: hospital record, birth protocol and central BCG record (table 3). None of these sources can be considered completely correct. To combine these data we used a score evaluating every objective and revisable information with +1 or -1, every subjective, uncertain or unknown information with 0 points (table 3).

TABLE 3
AVAILABLE INFORMATION ON BCG VACCINATION STATUS

Criterion	Cases	Score
Hospital report:		
Date of vacc. acc. to vacc. certificate	48	+1
yes	160	0
unknown acc. to mother's report	19	0
no	42	0
Birth protocol:		
BCG vacc. entered	108	+1
protocol missing	130	0
BCG vacc. not entered	31	-1
Central BCG record:		
listed	26	+1
recording system not established	231	0
not listed	12	0

The total score ranging from -1 to +3 points indicates the probability that the child had been vaccinated. If there are three positive informations on one child (+3), we can assume that BCG vaccination had actually been performed. If only a negative information is available (-1), it is highly improbable that the child had been vaccinated.

The children were divided into different groups according to the total score. For each group case fatality and mean manifestation age were calculated. This shows that case fatality (table 4) is decreasing with greater probability that children had been vaccinated. Furthermore we also calculated mean survival time and survival rate after 5 years, and obtained corresponding results.

Similarly, the mean manifestation age increased with higher total score

(table 5). In children with a score of +3 the disease occurred on an average of
more than one year later than in children with a score of -1, indicating a transient protective effect of some years following BCG vaccination.

TABLE 4
CASE FATALITY IN RELATION TO BCG VACCINATION SCORE

Total score	Cases / deaths	Case fatality
3	11 / 2	18,2 %
2	34 / 18	52,9 %
1	76 / 55	72,4 %
0	124 / 93	75,0 %
-1	25 / 19	76,0 %

TABLE 5
MANIFESTATION AGE IN RELATION TO BCG VACCINATION SCORE

Total score	Cases	Mean age of manifestation (days)
3	11	1379
2	34	1304
1	76	1354
0	124	1193
-1	25	971

Finally we tried to ascertain whether BCG vaccination influences the frequency of different kinds of leukemia. The ratio of lymphoblastic to myeloblastic leukemia shows considerable differences between vaccinated and non-
vaccinated children (table 6). Obviously, myeloblastic leukemia occurs less
frequently in vaccinated children.

Similarly, the frequency of chronic leukemia decreases with more intense
application of BCG vaccination (table 7).

TABLE 6

RATIO OF LYMPHOBLASTIC (LL) TO MYELOBLASTIC LEUKEMIA (ML) ACCORDING TO BCG
VACCINATION STATUS

	LL	:	ML
Hospital report:			
Date of vacc. acc. to vacc. certificate	1	:	0,2
yes, unknown, no acc. to mother's report	1	:	0,36
Birth protocol:			
BCG vacc. entered	1	:	0,25
BCG vacc. not entered	1	:	0,59

TABLE 7

RATIO OF ACUTE TO CHRONIC LEUKEMIA ACCORDING TO BCG VACCINATION

	Acute L.	:	Chronic L.
Hospital report:			
Date of vacc. acc. to vacc. certificate	1	:	0,036
yes, unknown, no acc. to mother's report	1	:	0,058
Birth protocol:			
BCG vacc. entered	1	:	0,033
BCG vacc. not entered	1	:	0,125

CONCLUSIONS

Summarizing the results of our studies we found that BCG vaccination of newborn babies is significantly correlated with the following effects on infantile
leukemia (table 8): reduction of mortality, reduction of case fatility, improvement of 5-year survival, prolongation of survival time, delay of manifestation, reduction of frequency of myeloblastic and chronic leukemia.

A significant reduction of morbidity was not revealed in our study.

396

TABLE 8
BCG VACCINATION AND LEUKEMIA IN AUSTRIA
RESULTS OF EPIDEMIOLOGICAL AND CLINICAL STUDIES

Effect	Statist. significance (p)
Reduction of mortality	< 0.01
Decrease of morbidity	n.s.
Reduction of case fatality	< 0.01
Improvement of 5-year survival	< 0.01
Prolongation of mean survival time	< 0.05
Delay of manifestation	< 0.05
Reduction of trequency of myeloic leukemia	< 0.05
Reduction of frequency of chronic leukemia	< 0.1

ACKNOWLEDGMENT

We gratefully acknowledge the support of our retrospective clinical study by the Austrian Federal Ministry of Health and Environmental Control and the excellent assistance of Dr. M. Kundi and Dr. P. Ambrosch in the statistical evaluation.

REFERENCES

1. Ambrosch, F. and Wiedermann, G.: Changes of risk and benefit in immunization against pertussis and tuberculosis. (1979) Develop. biolog. Standard., 43, 85-90.
2. Ambrosch, F., Klima, H. and Wiedermann, G.: Cost-benefit analysis of BCG-
   vaccination in Austria. (1979) Develop. biolog. Standard., 43, 121-126.
3. Davignon, L., Robillard, P., Lemonde, P. and Frappier, A.: B.C.G. vaccination and leukaemia mortality. (1970) Lancet, ii, 638.
4. Davignon, L., Lemonde, P., St. Pierre, J. and Frappier, A.: B.C.G. vaccination and leukaemia mortality. (1971) Lancet, i, 80-81.
5. BCG and vole bacillus vaccines in the prevention of tuberculosis in adolescence and early adult life. British Medical Council (1972), Bull. WHO,
   46, 371-385.
6. Rosenthal, S.L., Crispen, R.G., Thorne, M.G., Piekarski, N., Raisys, N.
   and Rettig, P.G.: BCG vaccination and leukemia mortality. (1972) JAMA,
   222, 1543-1544.
7. Crispen, R.G., Rosenthal, S.R.: BCG vaccination and cancer mortality.
   (1976) Cancer Immunol. Immunother., 1, 139-142.
8. Rosenthal, S.R.: BCG vaccination against cancer and leukemia: suggestions
   for retrospective studies. (1976) in: BCG in Cancer Immunotherapy, Gilles
   Lamoureux ed., Grune & Stratton, New York, San Francisco, London, 313-321.
9. Comstock, G.W., Livesay, V.T., Webster, R.G.: Leukaemia and B.C.G., a controlled trial. (1971) Lancet, ii, 1062-1063.
10. Comstock, G.W., Martinez, I. and Livesay, V.T.: Efficacy of BCG vaccination
    in prevention of cancer. (1975) Journal of the National Cancer Institute,
    54, 835-839.
11. Kinlen, L.J. and Pike, M.C.: B.C.G. vaccination and leukaemia, evidence of
    vital statistics. (1971), Lancet, ii, 398-402.
12. Salonen, T. and Saxén, L.: Risk indicators in childhood malignancies.
    (1975) Int. J. Cancer, 15, 941-946.
13. Skegg, D.C.G.: BCG vaccination and the incidence of lymphomas and leu-
    kaemia. (1978) Int. J. Cancer, 21, 18-21.
14. Waaler, H.T.: B.C.G. and leukaemia mortality. (1970) Lancet, ii, 1314.
15. Berkeley, J.S.: B.C.G. vaccination and leukaemia mortality. (1971),
    Lancet, i, 241.
16. Hems, G. and Stuart, A.: B.C.G. and leukaemia. (1971) Lancet, i, 183.

17. Neumann, G.: BCG - Impfung und bösartige Neubildungen. (1972) Bundesge-
    sundheitsblatt, 15, 129-133.
18. Pike, M.C. and Vessey, M.P.: Letter to the editor. (1970) Lancet, ii,
    983-984.
19. Stewart, A. and Draper, G.: B.C.G. vaccination and leukaemia mortality.
    (1971) Lancet, ii, 983.
20. Stewart, A. and Draper, G.: B.C.G. vaccination and leukaemia mortality.
    (1971), Lancet, i, 799.
21. Bast, R.C.Jr., Zbar, B., Borsos, T. and Rapp, H.J.: BCG and cancer (second
    of two parts). (1974) The New England Journal of Medicine, 1458-1469.
22. Hoover, R.N.: Bacillus Calmette-Guêrin vaccination and cancer prevention:
    A critical review of the human experience. (1976) Cancer Research, 36/II,
    652-654.
23. Ambrosch, F., Krepler, P. and Wiedermann, G.: Zur Frage des Einflusses der
    BCG-Neugeborenen-Impfung auf die Leukämie-Häufigkeit. (1978) Münch. Med.
    Wschr., 120, 243-246.
24. Ambrosch, F., Wiedermann, G., Krepler, P. and Kundi, M.: BCG-Impfung und
    Leukämie. Epidemiologische Untersuchungen zum Einfluß der BCG-Impfung auf
    die Leukämie. (1978) Fortschritte der Medizin, 96, 2231-2234.
25. Ambrosch, F., Wiedermann, G., Krepler, P., Kundi, M. and Ambrosch, P.:
    Einfluß der BCG-Neugeborenenimpfung auf Häufigkeit und Verlauf kindlicher
    Leukämien. (1981) Fortschritte der Medizin, 99, 1389-1393.

CAN BCG VACCINATION AT BIRTH PREVENT CANCER AND LEUKEMIA?

SOL ROY ROSENTHAL AND RAY G. CRISPEN
ITR, University of Illinois Health Sciences, Chicago, IL

From both experimental and clinical trials, one must conclude that a immuno-logical mechanism does play a role in host resistance to neoplasms. Burnett developed the concept that there is a constant immunological surveillance against natural somatic mutation.[1] This mechanism may account for the suppression of incipient neoplastic cell foci and thus prevent clinical manifestations of cancer. It is postulated that as long as the immunological mechanism of the body is properly functioning and is not overtaxed, tumor proliferation is suppressed.

BCG is a potent stimulator of the host's immunological mechanism through the lymphoreticuloendothelial system (RES). Many other substances also stim-ulate the RES.

BCG vaccination of mice,[2-8] rats,[33,34] hamsters,[9,10] and guinea pigs[11,12] using grafts of tumors spontaneously induced[4,13] or induced by viral,[14,15] or chemical[12] means, confirmed that prophylaxis with BCG could exert an inhibi-tory,[2-4,11,14,16] a neutral,[9,12,13] or, less often, a stimulatory[10,16,17] effect on tumor transplants. The advantage of a live viable organism such as BCG that multiplies in the body over non-viable products (c.parvum, MER, interferon, etc.) is that its action will remain operational over long periods of time to effect tumor surveillance.

BCG introduced into guinea pigs intravenously,[24] transcutaneously,[25] or by aerosol[26-28] produced not only specific response but also a nonspecific response which was related to the RES. The response to oral vaccination[29] was minimal. As little as one hour after intravenous introduction of BCG there was a specific response to the organism, as well as a nonspecific one, resulting in a swelling of the spetal cells of the lung, Kupffer cells of the liver, reticulum cells of the spleen, the resting histiocytes of the

Cancer: Etiology and Prevention, Ray G. Crispen, Editor

epicardium, and parivascular cells of the hilus of the kidney. The blood

responses mirrored the responses of the tissues.[24]

There is evidence that BCG vaccination at birth by the intradermal and intra-
cutaneous method reduces the mortality from cancer and leukemia. This evidence
stems from retrospective studies from Canada,[31] Europe[30] and the United
States.[32,33] Some reports, especially in older children, do not verify these
claims.[34-37] Dr. Robert N. Hoover, of the Epidemiological Branch of the
National Cancer Institute (NCI), reanalyzed the results of seven studies and
reported on the Chicago Study that ''allowing the calculation of an appropriate
denominator reduced the apparent protection (death rate) from the first
estimated 80-85 percent for leukemia and all cancers (actually 74 percent)[38]
to about 50 percent for both''.[39]

The object of this paper is to review the Chicago study to point out some
of the pitfalls of retrospective studies and the presentation of a hypothesis
that BCG vaccination at birth by stimulating the lymphoreticuloendothelial
system (RES) augments immune surveillance and may be one of the factors that
reduces the mortality to cancer and leukemia as children and adults.[23,33,38]

MATERIALS AND METHODS

Newborns in the maternity division of Cook County Hospital in Chicago were
vaccinated when two or three days of age. The vaccine used was made from
freeze-dried seed lots of a BCG substrain (Tice-Chicago) developed at the Tice
Laboratory of the University of Illinois and Research Foundation.[40,41] The
concentration of the vaccine was approximately 2 X 10^8 viable units per ml.
The multiple puncture disc (Rosenthal) was used for vaccinations. This began
as a service program for vaccination against tuberculosis. The number vaccinated depended largely on the personnel available. Thus about 40-50 percent of
the infants (97 percent black) born at the hospital were vaccinated. A certain
percentage of the infants returned to the clinic at regular intervals for
follow-up. There the reactions to the vaccine, the results of tuberculin

testing with typical and atypical tuberculins (OT, PPD-S, PPD-G, PPD-B*) and the general health of the children were determined. Revaccination was performed in the tuberculin-negative reactors, but this represents only a small fraction of the vaccinated population. Thus basically the results reported are for a single vaccination.

All cases of cancer deaths in the black population of Chicago under 20 years of age were obtained from death certificates, 1957-1969, at the Chicago Board of Health. The deaths were compared with the vaccination records of our clinic to determine the rate for the vaccinated as opposed to the non-vaccinated population. The total black population, 20 years of age and under, was determined by demographic means from the Chicago Board of Health birth records, adjusted for deaths during the period under study. The total black population in this study was 534,870, of which 85,356 were vaccinated at birth.[23]

RESULTS

Leukemia and Cancer Mortality

During the period 1957-1969, there were 306 deaths in the non-vaccinated, of which 106 were due to leukemia and 200 to other types of cancer. In the vaccinated, there were 13 deaths, of which six were due to leukemia and seven due to other forms of cancer (neuroblastoma, Wilms tumor, hypernephroma, lymphoma and sarcoma of bone). Leukemia (all forms) had the highest death rate in ages 1-9 years in both groups; in the vaccinated, five of the six cases were in the 1-4 year group. The death rates for all malignancies was 4.4/100,000/year for the non-vaccinated and 1.2/100,000/year for the vaccinated; the difference was statistically highly significant (p 0.001)(Table 1). There was a reduction of 74 percent in the mortality of the vaccinated as compared to the non-vaccinated as a group. As reported in an earlier study for

*OT=old tuberculin, PPD-S=purified protein derivative-standard, PPD-G=Gause or scotochrome, PPD-B=Battey.

leukemia the difference was approximately 85 percent.[32] Checking with the NCI revealed that there were no reported deaths due to cancer elsewhere in the country in our vaccinated population.

TABLE 1

CANCER DEATHS FOR ALL SITES - CHICAGO BLACK POPULATION (1957-1969)

		ALL SITES		
Age (Years)	No. of Deaths		Death Rate per 100,000		Reduction in vac.
	NV	V	NV	V	%
Under 1	7	0	2.3	0.0	100
1-4	77	8	6.6	3.2	50
5-9	81	4	5.7	3.0	48
10-14	67	0	6.2	0.0	100
15-20	74	1	9.7	5.3	45
Total	306	13	4.4	1.2	74

NV- Non-vaccinated = 534,870;   V- Vaccinated = 85,356

There was no death from leukemia or other malignancies under one year of age in the vaccinated group, whereas there were seven such deaths in the non-vaccinated (two from leukemia and five from other neoplasms). The rates were 0 versus 2.3/100,000/year, respectively. For the age group 1-4, the death rate for neoplasms was cut by 50 percent, and for the 5-9 group, by approximately 48 percent. At 10-14 years, there was no cancer death in the vaccinated, and 67 in the non-vaccinated (rates of 0 and 6.2/100,000/year, respectively). For the age group 15-20 years, there was approximately a 45 percent decrease in the death rate for malignancy in the vaccinated as compared to the non-vaccinated. The death rate from trauma was similar in the vaccinated and non-vaccinated populations.

Typical and Atypical Mycobacterial Infection

The population studies (vaccinated and non-vaccinated) were drawn from areas
of high incidence of tuberculosis in Chicago. For 1970, the new case rate
per 100,000 for Chicago was 72 for the non-white and 31.6 for the whites.
Reactors to PPD-G and PPD-B increased sharply with age. Thus, shortly after
birth (0-6 months) all non-vaccinated infants failed to react to 5TU of PPD-S
PPD-G and PPD-B. The first reactions to PPD-G and PPD-S were noted at seven
months to one year of age and to PPD-B at two to five years. The rise in
percentage of reactors were rapid so that at 13-16 years of age it was approximately 55 percent for PPD-G, 40 percent for PPD-B and 20 percent for PPD-S.[41]
(Figure 1) The tuberculin conversion in the vaccinated infants was manifest
as early as ten days after vaccination and by three months was 99.7% positive
using second strength tuberculin (controls 0.22% positive). The rates begin
to recede somewhat at one year and by 6 to 6½ years, 80% were still positive.

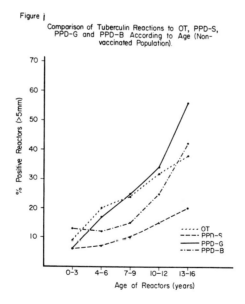

Figure 1

Comparison of Tuberculin Reactions to OT, PPD-S,
PPD-G and PPD-B According to Age (Non-
vaccinated Population).

Potency of Vaccine

The vaccine for the Chicago study was supplied by the Institution for Tuberculosis Research of the University of Illinois. The Tice-Chicago sub-strain has been proven to produce a highly effective vaccine against tuberculosis in guinea pigs, mice, monkeys, and human subjects (74% reduction in incidence of tuberculosis as compared to controls in a 23-year follow-up clinical trial).[23]

Source of Subjects for Study

The subjects were all black, living in similar community areas in the city of Chicago. The vaccinated and non-vaccinated groups were born in approximately the same years.

Diagnosis of Malignancy

The diagnosis of cancer death was determined from death certificates (1957-1969) at the Chicago Board of Health. Checking with the NCI revealed that there were no reported deaths due to cancer elsewhere in the country in our vaccinated population.[33,38]

DISCUSSION

The most promising results indicating a lowering of the mortality from cancer and leukemia come from populations BCG-vaccinated at birth.[30-32] Retrospective studies in such vaccinated populations should ideally be compared with non-vaccinated cohorts born in the same years and the immediate environment for both groups should be similar. The vaccine should be of proven potency, as determined for the time being in its efficacy in preventing tuberculosis and possible in the treatment of cancer and in immunoprophylaxis against cancer. The degree of infectivity to non-specific mycobacterial infection should be ascertained since the latter may mimic the response in the host to that of BCG.[23,33] The death rate from completely non-relative causes, for example, trauma, should be ascertained as a means of attesting to the similarity of the groups. All these requirements were met by the Chicago Study.

Neoplasia during childhood years is likely to be the result of a combination of factors, which up to now have been considered to be predominately genetic and enviornmental,[42] but recent evidence indicates that the immune system which is not at its full potential at infancy may play an important role.[43,44] Experimentally, it is known that carcinogenesis to chemicals is more effective in newborn animals than in the weanling or adults.[42,45] The incidence of malignancy in young persons with primary immunodeficiencies is many times greater than in the general age matched population.[44,46]

During fetal life the blood is produced primarily in the spleen and liver and to a lesser extent in other organs, but under ordinary conditions, after birth the bone marrow almost completely assumes this function.[47] However, extramedullary hematopoiesis in post-uterine life is not uncommon.[48] Hemato-poietic foci are most frequently seen in the spleen and liver, but falx cerebri, kidney, lymphnodes, thymus, broad legament are all also documented sites.[47] Certain pathological states associated with idiopathic anemia of children[47] or in myelofibrosis[49] are examples of extreme conditions of extra-medullary hematopoiesis. The possibility exists that poor immunologic sur-veillance in infancy may be related to the failure of the disappearance of embryonic hematopoiesis or other residual embryonic rests, and contributes to their proliferation and possible malignant transformation. The association of immunological deficiencies and malignancy is well documented.[46]

There has been a revival of the Cohnheim[50] concept that there may be an embryonic origin for malignancy. Abelev[51] of Russia isolated an alpha-feto protein, normally generated by a fetus' lung, from a cancerous liver of an adult; Gold and his group[52] of Canada described a protein in adult cancer of the colon-rectum that normally occurs in fetal intestines, now called carcinoembryonic antigen or CEA. Fishman[53] of the USA found placental phos-

phatase in the blood of patients with malignancy.

From the above data, a hypothesis is presented that states that:

a. Fetal rests are not uncommon in infancy;

b. Infants immune systems are not yet fully developed;

c. Immune deficient individuals have a rate of malignancy that is many
    times higher than the general population;

d. BCG stimulates the RES as demonstrated experimentally in animals and
    humans;

e. The stimulation of the RES enhances the immunological surveillance and
    fosters the sterilization and removal of embryonic rests as well as
    other abnormal cells that may be the source of malignancy early and
    late in life

Because the action of BCG on repressing cancer is through the RES (and the

NK cells) and is non-specific, a large antigen deposit is necessary at all

times; thus revaccination should be carried out at one or two year intervals

depending upon the response to tuberculin (if Mantoux reaction is over 15mm

to 5TU or 5 mm induration to the tine test defer revaccination).[23]

Two studies have indicated that BCG might enhance certain forms of cancer

after many years. In the New Zealand study, Skegg[54] reported that a higher

rate of deaths from non-Hodgkins lymphomas on North Island where BCG vaccin-

ation was continued than on South Island where BCG was stopped. Skegg noted

that "about 20 percent of the children of the North Island late cohorts were

not vaccinated, and migration between the two islands is not uncommon; both

these factors would tend to obscure any effect of BCG vaccination." Skegg

admits that his observations must be interpreted with caution because "it is

based on small numbers that could have been due to chance."

Kendrick and Comstock[55] report an excess among BCG vaccinees of the lymphoma-

Hodgkins disease-leukemia group, that did not become statistically significant

until the last few years of the 28-year follow-up (p = 0.05). Other reports

have not shown this result. In our study there were no deaths from lymphoma in the vaccinated groups and 50 in the non-vaccinated group[56].

CONCLUSIONS

There is compelling evidence that BCG vaccination at birth reduces the mortality from leukemia, as reported by two 5-year follow-up studies, and for all forms of cancer in a 20-year follow-up study.

A retrospective study is presented which involves some 85,356 BCG-vaccinated newborns who were followed over a 20-year period. There was an overall 74 percent reduction in all forms of cancer, including leukemia, as compared to 534,870 non-vaccinated cohorts--that is, infants born during the same period of time living in similar areas of Chicago, all black. The differences were highly significant statistically ($p < 0.001$). Traumatic deaths among the two groups were similar. Significantly, in the first year of life when immunity has not reached its full potential, there were no cases of cancer death in the vaccinated while the rate for the non-vaccinated was 2.31/100,000. After the first year there was more or less a 50% reduction in the mortality in the vaccinated as compared to the non-vaccinated. One possible explanation for the difference is that the protection by BCG in tuberculosis is specific, whereas the BCG effect in cancer is non-specific. For this reason, a large antigen deposit is necessary in cancer immunization so that the stimulating effect of BCG remains high at all times. Thus revaccination with BCG is recommended at one to two-year intervals. The advantage of a live viable organism such as BCG that multiplies in the body over non-viable products (c.parvum, MER, interferon, etc.) is that BCG has been proven to be clinically safe and its action will remain operational over long periods of time to effect tumor surveillance.

REFERENCES

1. Burnet, M. (1970) Immunological Surveillance, Pergamon Press, Oxford. Lon.
2. Old, L. and Clarke, D. (1959) Effect of Bacillus Calmette-Guerin Infection on Transplanted Tumors in the Mouse, Nature, 184:291.

3. Halpern, B., Biozzi, G., Stiffel, C. and Morton, D.L. (1959) Effet de la Stimulation du Systeme Reticuloendoethelial par Linoculation du Bacille de Calmette-Guerin sur le Development de Lepitheliome Atypique T-S de Guerin Ches le Rat, C R Soc. Biol. 153:919.

4. Inooka, S., Ebina, T., Tekase, Y., et al. (1962) Influence of BCG Vaccination on Erlich Ascites Tumor in Mice, Kekkaku 37:503-5.

5. Gillissen, G. and Nehring, G. (1969) Das Wachstum von Soliden Ehrlich-Ascites-Tumoren bei Mausen nach Immunisierung mit BCG, Beitr Klin Tuberk 139:206-10.

6. Wolf, M. and Wolf, C. (1971) Zur Frage Einer Wachstumsbeein flussung von UVT-Tumoren der Maus nach Vorheriger Immunisierung mit BCG, Arch Geschwulstforsch 37:210.

7. Viallier, J. and Pellet, M. (1959) Influence des Mycobacteries sur la Croissance de Tumeurs Experimentales Greffees, 1. Action des Injection de BCG, C R Soc. Biol. 153:1034.

8 Keller, R. and Hess, M. W. (1972) Tumour Growth and Nonspecific Immunity in Rats: The Mechanisms Involved in Inhibition of Tumour Growth, Br J Exp. Pathol 53:570.

9. Lemonde, P., Dubrenil, R., Guerdon, A., et al. (1971) Stimulating Influence of Bacillus Calmette-Guerin on Immunity to Polyoma Tumors and Spontaneous Leukemia, J Natl Cancer Inst. 47:1013.

10. Fortner, G.W., Hanna, M.G. and Coggin, J.R. (1974) Differential Effects of Two Strains on BCG in Transplantation Immunity to SV-40-Induced Tumors in Hamsters, Proc. Soc. Exp. Biol. Med. 147:62-67.

11. Schwartz, E. (1973) Effect of Mycobacterium Bovis BCG-Praha on the Growth of Transplanted Daels' Sarcoma in Guinea Pigs, Neoplasma 20:375.

12. Eilber, F.R., Holmes, E.C. and Morton, D.L. (1971) Immunotherapy Experiments With a Methyl-Cholanthrene-Induced Guinea Pig Liposarcoma, J. Natl. Cancer Inst. 46:803.

13. Hattori, S. and Matsuda, M. (1962) Relationship Between Cancer and Tuberculosis, 1. Effect of Tubercule Bacilli Infection on Transplanted Tumors in the Mouse, Kekkaku 37:41-46.

14. Amiel, J.L. (1969) Immunotherapie Active Nonspecifique par le BCG de la Leucemie Virale E Male G2 Ches des Receveurs Isogeniques, Rev. Eur Etud Clin. Biol. 14:685-88.

15. Lemonde, P. and Clode, M. (1962) Effect of BCG Infection on Leukemia and Polyoma in Mice and Hamsters, Proc. Soc. Exp.Biol. Med. 111:739-42.

16. Weiss, D.W. (1967) Immunology of Spontaneous Tumors, Proceedings of the Fifth Berkeley Symposium on Mathematical Statistics and Probability. Ed. by L. Lecam, J. Neyman. Berkeley: University of California Press, 657.

17. Sparks, F.C. and Breeding, J.H. (1974) Tumor Regression and Enhancement Results from Immunotherapy with Bacillus Calmette-Guerin and Neuraminidase, Cancer Research 34:3262-69.

18. Wolfe, S.A., Tracey, D.E. and Henney, C.S. (1977) BCG-Induced Murine Effector Cells 11. Characterization of Natural Killer Cells in Peritoneal Exudates, J. Immunol. 119:1152-1158

19. Tracy, D.E., Wolfe, S.A., et al. (1977) BCG-Induced Murine Effector Cells Cytolytic Activity in Peritoneal Exudates: An Early Response to BCG, J. Immunol. 119:1145-1151.

20. Djeu, J.Y., Heinbaugh, J.A., et al. (1979) Role of Macrophages in the Augmentation of Mouse Natural Killer Cell Activity by Poly I:C and Interferon, J. Immunol. 122:182-188.

21 Djeu, J.Y., Heinbaugh, J.A., et al. (1979) Augmentation of Mouse Natural Killer Cell Activity by Interferon and Interferon Inducers, J. Immunol. 122:175-181

22. Tagliabue, A., Mantovani, A., et al. (1979) Natural Cytotoxicity of Mouse Monocytes and Macrophages, J. Immunol. 122:2363-2370.
23. Rosenthal, S.R. (1980) BCG Vaccine, Tuberculosis-Cancer, Wright-PSG Publishing Co., Littleton, MA.
24. Rosenthal, S.R. (1936) Focal and General Tissue Responses to an Avirulent Tubercle Bacillus (BCG); Intracardiac Rout, Arch. Pathol. 22:348.
25. Rosenthal, S.R. (1937) Studies With BCG. IV. The Focal and the General Tissue Response and the Humoral Response; the Intradermal Route, Am. J. Dis. Child 54:296.
26. Rosenthal, S.R., McEnery, J.T. and Raisys, N. (1968) Aerogenic BCG Vaccination Against Tuberculosis in Animal and Human Subjects, J. Asthma Res. 5:309.
27. Rosenthal, S.R. (1974) BCG Vaccination and Leukemia Mortality, 1972 Paris Cancer Week, Paris, June, 1972, Recent Results in Cancer Res. 47:228-38.
28. Rosenthal, S.R. (1973) BCG and the Reticuloendothelial System, Conference on the Use of BCG in Therapy of Cancer, Washington, DC, Oct. 5-6, 1972, NCI Monograph No. 39, 91:106.
29. Rosenthal, S.R. (1937) Les Reactions Tissulaires et Humor Ales Consecutive a Labsorption du BCG par Voie Degestive, Ann. Inst. Pasteur 58:652.
30. Ambrosch, F., Krepler, P., and Weiderman, G. (1978) Zur Frage des Einflusses der BCG-Neugeborenen-Impfung auf die Leukamie-Hauflikeit, Munch. Med. Wschr, 120:243.
31. Davignon, L., Lemonde, P., St. Pierre, I.and Frappier, A. (1971) BCG Vaccination and Leukemia Mortality, Lancet 1:80.
32. Rosenthal, S.R., Crispen, R.G., Thorne, M.G., Piekarski, N., Raisys, N. and Rettig, P.G. (1972) BCG Vaccination and Leukemia Mortality, JAMA 222:1543.
33. Rosenthal, S.R. (1976) BCG Vaccination Against Cancer and Leukemia:Suggestions for Retrospective Studies, Symp.: Present Status of BCG in Cancer Immunotherapy, Montreal, Canada, April 22-23, 1976. In Lamoureux, G., et.al. (eds), BCG In Cancer Immunotherapy, New York: Grune and Stratton, 313-21.
34. Waaler, H.T. (1970) BCG and Leukemia Mortality, Lancet 2:686.
35. Hems, G. and Stewart, A. (1971) BCG and Leukemia, Lancet 1:183.
36. Kinlen, L.J. and Pike, M.C. (1971) BCG Vaccination and Leukemia, Lancet 2:398.
37. Comstock, G.W., Livesay, V.T. and Webster, R.G. (1971) Leukemia and BCG Lancet, 2:1062.
38. Crispen, R.G. and Rosenthal, S.R. (1976) BCG Vaccination and Cancer Mortality, Cancer Immunol. Immunother. 1:139-42.
39. Hoover, R.N. (1976) Bacillus Calmette-Guerin Vaccination and Cancer Prevention, A Critical Review of the Human Experience, Cancer Res. 36:652-654.
40. Rosenthal, S.R., Crispen, R.G., et al (1970) BCG Vaccination Against Tuberculosis Biennial Report 1967-68, Inst. TB Res., Dept. of Prev. Med., Univ. of IL, Chicago, Bd. of Health, Cook County Hosp. and Res Foundation, June 1, 1970.
41. Rosenthal, S.R., Crispen, R.G., et al (1972) BCG Vaccination Against Tuberculosis Biennial Report 1969-70, Inst. for TB Res., Dept. of Prev. Med., Univ. of IL, Chicago, Bd. of Health, Cook County Hosp. and Res. Foundation, Dec. 1, 1972.
42. Pitot, H.C. (1976) Carcinogenesis and Aging--Two Related Phenomena?, Am. Jr. Path. 87:444-472.
43. Rosenthal, S.R. (1976) The Present Status of the Role of the Immune System in Cancer and Leukemia, Cancer Cytology 16:8-16.
44. Gatti, R.A. and Good, R.A. (1971) Occurrence of Malignancy in Immunodeficiency Diseases, A Literature Review, Cancer, 28:89:98.

45. Schoental, R. (1974) Carcinogenicity as Related to Age, Ann. Rev. Pharmacol. 14:185-204.
46. Knudson, A.G., Strong, L.C. and Anderson, D.E. (1973) Heredity and Cancer in Man, Prog. Med. Genet. 9:113-158.
47. Brannon, D. (1927) Extramedullary Hematopoiesis in Anemia, Bull. John Hopkins Hosp. 41:104-136.
48. Wintrobe, M.M., et al (1974) Clinical Hematology, Philadelphia, Lea and Febiger, 57-79.
49. Wintrobe, M.M., et al (1974) Clinical Hematology, Philadelphia, Lea and Febiger, 1777-1788.
50. Cohnheim, J. (1889) Lecture on General Pathology: A Handbook for Practitioners and Students, Vol II, New Sydenham Soc., London, Trans. by A.McKee.
51. Abelev, G.L. (1968) Production of Embryonic Serum A-Globulin by Hepatomes, Review of Experimental Clinical Data, Cancer Research 28: 1344-1350.
52. Gold, P., Freedman, S.O. (1965) Demonstration of Tumor Specific Antigens in Human Colonic Carcinomata by Immunological Tolerance and Absorption Techniques, J. Exp. Med. 121: 439-462.
53. Fishman, W.H., Inglis, N.R. et al (1968) A Serum Alkaline Phosphatose Isoenzyme of Human Neoplastic Cell Origin, Cancer Res. 28:150-154.
54. Skegg, D.C. (1978) BCG Vaccination and the Incidence of Lymphoma and Leukemia, Int. J. Cancer 21:18-21.
55. Kendrick, M.A., Comstock, G.W. (1981) BCG Vaccination and the Subsequent Development of Cancer in Humans, JNCI 66:431-437.
56. Crispen, R.G.(1974) Immunoprophylaxis with BCG , Symp.: BCG Vaccination, Sept. 1973. In Crispen, R.(eds), Neoplasm Immunity: BCG Vaccination, Schori Press, Evanston, IL, 69-78.

BCG VACCINATION AND CHILD CANCER IN SWEDEN

ANDERS ERICSON, JAN GUNNARSKOG, DORAN GUSTAVSSON, BENGT KÄLLEN AND
BIRGITTA MALKER
National Board of Health and Welfare, Stockholm, Sweden

INTRODUCTION

Neonates used to be routinely BCG vaccinated in Sweden during their stay in
the delivery hospital - practically all births take place in hospitals. Due
to complications noticed this policy was changed on April 1, 1975, and since
then only risk infants were vaccinated. This situation gives us the possibility to compare child cancer rate in a population where the vast majority of
neonates were vaccinated, with that in a population where approximately 25%
were vaccinated, and with that in a population where only few were vaccinated.
Our analysis of this material does not support the notion that BCG vaccination
should affect the risk of developing a child cancer, at least not during the
first 4-5 years of life.

MATERIALS AND METHODS

Three birth cohorts were studied, born in 1974, 1975 and 1976, each cohort
representing the total number of deliveries in Sweden. The Medical Birth Register contains the computerized summary of the delivery records of all deliveries in Sweden and has a coverage of approximately 99.5%. This Register contains
information on diseases during pregnancy, diagnoses given during delivery and
possible operations performed, and diagnoses of infants and operations etc. performed. One item refers to if BCG vaccination was given or not. The death
date is given, if the infant dies in the neonatal period. The size of the cohorts at risk for developing child cancer was estimated as the number of infants without a death date in the Medical Birth Register.

Cases of child cancer were identified up to and including 1980 from three
sources: the Swedish Cancer Register, the Register of Death Certificates, and
a nation-wide Register of Child Leukemia. The function of and results from the

Cancer Register and the code system used have been published (1). The Death
Certificate Register is based on ICD codes given in death certificates. The
Register of Child Leukemia is run by a group of pediatric scientists working
on child leukemia and reports on these cases are obtained from the hospitals
(2). Each child is identified with its unique personal identification number
which makes it possible to individually check it against cases reported to the
other registers and to identify it in the Medical Birth Register.

Totally, 358 children with cancer and born in 1974-1976 were identified. In
six of them, however, death occurred within one month - five of them died in
the perinatal period - and these cases were excluded from the analysis.

For each child, the date of first diagnosis was taken from the Cancer Register and from the Register of Child Leukemia - if the two dates did not agree,
the earliest date was chosen. In cases only present in the Death Certificate
Register, no date of diagnosis was known. All but one of these had, however,
died before the age of one year - the single case which died later had a tumour
of the sympathetic nervous system and died at the age of 38 months - by comparing the time elapsed between diagnosis and death for other children dying
of that type of tumour, the time of diagnosis for that child was estimated as
25 months.

The rates of diagnosed cases of child cancer and the rates of dead cases of
child cancer were calculated cumulatively at the exact age of one year, two
years etc. The cumulative total death rate of children in Sweden after the
perinatal period and before the age of one is only 2 per 1.000 and before the
age of six 4 per 1.000. This change in the nominator was not compensated for.

RESULTS

Table 1 presents an over-view of the material. There were 139 children with
leukemia which should have appeared in both the Cancer Register and in the
Register of Child Leukemia - 13 were only in the former register, 14 only in

the latter, and one child was only in the Death Certificate Register under a leukemia diagnosis and in neither of the two other registers. 116 infants had died after one month's age - 109 had a diagnosis of malignancy in the Death Certificate register. Six had died before one month's age - 3 of them had no diagnosis of malignancy in the Death Certificate Register.

TABLE 1. OVERVIEW OF MATERIAL

DIAGNOSTIC GROUP	Year of Birth 1974	1975	1976	Total No.	Dead before 1 month
LEUKEMIAS, LYMPHOMAS	59	57	39	155	
among these:					
LYMPHOMAS	7	6	3	16	
ALL	40	38	32	110	
OTHER LEUKEMIAS	12	13	4	29	
NERVOUS SYSTEM TUMORS	38	31	24	93	4
EYE TUMORS	9	9	11	29	
KIDNEY TUMORS	16	6	5	27	
OTHER TUMORS	20	20	14	54	2
TOTAL	142	123	93	358	6

Table 2 presents the data on BCG vaccination among infants surviving the neonatal period and born 1974-1976, based on the information in the Medical Birth Register. It can be seen that in 1974 at least 96% of all infants were vaccinated, in 1975 at least 24%, but in 1976 only 0.6% were with certainty vaccinated. The relatively large proportions of infants where vaccination was not stated make these figures rather uncertain, but it is anyway a very marked difference between the three years.

Table 3 gives the cumulative numbers of infants with diagnosed cancer or cancer deaths according to year of birth. Thus, the column "-2" represents the number of infants in each group which had a diagnosed cancer before their second birthday (or died of cancer before that day, respectively). Figure 1 shows the cumulative rates. The graphs are based on the average values for the three birth cohorts. As can be seen, there is no significant difference between them.

TABLE 2. BCG VACCINATION OF INFANTS DISCHARGED FROM DELIVERY UNITS (SURVIVING NEONATAL PERIOD). DATA FROM MEDICAL BIRTH REGISTER.

BCG VACCINATION	No. of infants born			Percentage		
	1974	1975	1976	1974	1975	1976
YES	104,564	25,169	1,976	96.3	24.4	0.6
NO	980	66,509	85,329	0.9	64.6	87.5
NOT STATED	3,034	11,295	11,611	2.8	11.0	11.9

TABLE 3. CUMULATIVE NUMBER OF CANCER CASES ACCORDING TO AGE OF DIAGNOSIS OR DEATH IN THREE BIRTH COHORTS. TABULATION AFTER EACH INFANT'S ACTUAL AGE AT DIAGNOSIS OR DEATH.

CATEGORY	Year of birth	Number of cases at age of infant at diagnosis (death)					
		-1	-2	-3	-4	-5	-6
All cancers, age at	1974	26	54	71	92	122	133
	1975	25	46	68	86	111	
diagnosis	1976	18	38	60	83		
All cancers, age at	1974	10	21	23	31	42	47
	1975	6	13	21	31	40	
death	1976	5	9	15	20		
Leukemias or lym-	1974	5	17	27	36	48	52
phomas,	1975	6	18	28	38	53	
age at diagnosis	1976	4	10	21	43		

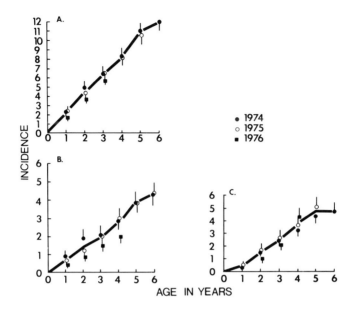

Figure 1. Diagram illustrating cumulative incidence of child cancer in cohorts born in 1974 (x), in 1975 (o), and in 1976 (.) at one to six years age. $\pm$ one standard deviation is given for each rate. Graphs connect mean values based on all three years. Rates are per 10,000 infants surviving the neonatal period - cases dead before one month's age are excluded.
A. all cancers according to age of diagnosis. B. all cancer deaths according to age at death. C. Leukemias and lymphomas according to age at diagnosis.

A total of 347 cancer cases were identified in the Medical Birth Register and searched for information on BCG vaccination. In 313, such information was present; 158 had been vaccinated as neonates, 155 had not. With knowledge of the year of birth and the proportion of infants each year with BCG vaccination according to the Medical Birth Register, the expected numbers of vaccinated and non-vaccinated cases can be calculated: they are 163.8 and 149.2 respectively, thus very close to the found figures.

DISCUSSION

This material does not support the notion that neonatal BCG vaccination influences the rate of childhood cancer in either direction. The three birth
cohorts studied show a very similar cumulative graph of diagnosed cancer up to
the age of 4 or 5 years (Figure 1 A). On the other hand, the rate of cancer
deaths is distinctly lower for the 1976 cohort than for the other two cohorts
(Figure 1 B). This could mirror a more intensive and successful therapeutic
approach to childhood cancer, especially for leukemia cases. When only cases
of diagnosed leukemia are studied (Figure 1 C), no statistically significant
difference is seen between the three cohorts, but the 1976 cohort (which had a
very low BCG vaccination rate) had a slightly higher rate at the age of 4 years
than the 1974 cohort had (which had a very high BCG vaccination rate). This
difference is probably random - and the 1976 2 and 3 years rates are lower than
the 1974 rates - but it is of course possible that a difference will emerge
when this cohort can be followed for a longer period. It can be noted that the
1975 cohort (which has about 25% vaccination rate) lies slightly above the 1974
cohort for all ages. The most likely explanation to these differences is random fluctuations. The distribution of vaccination and non-vaccination among
the cancer cases whose Medical Birth Register records contained information on
BCG vaccination was very close to the expected one, also indicating that the
present material gives no support for a protective effect of BCG vaccination
against cancer, at least during the first four years of life.

Only vaccination in the neonatal period was studied in this investigation.
It could be argued that in the majority of the 1976 cohort infants, a later
vaccination had been made which could give protection. The majority of child
vaccinations in Sweden occurs and are registered at Childrens Health Centers.
Romanus and Jonsell (unpublished report, 1981) made a study of all registered
child vaccinations using the records available at these centers. According

to this material 1.9% of all infants born in 1976 had had BCG vaccination -
thus some were vaccinated after the neonatal period but still the majority
were not vaccinated.

REFERENCES

1. Cancer Incidence in Sweden 1978. National Board of Health and Welfare.
    The Cancer Register, Socialstyrelsen, 1982.
2. Gustafsson, G. and Kreuger, H. Incidence of Childhood Leukemia in Sweden
    1975-1980, for the Swedish Child Leukemiagroup. Acta Peadr. Scand. 1982.

MASS BCG VACCINATION, TUBERCULOSIS INFECTION AND LEUKAEMIA RISK
REGISTER LINKAGE STUDY OF THE LONG-TERM EFFECTS

A. Sakari Haro
University of Helsinki, Finland

INTRODUCTION

The use of BCG vaccine as a therapy in malignancies with acute failure of the

immunity system is a much studied topic. Much less attention has been devoted

to the possible influences of BCG vaccination or long-term influences of natural

infection with mycobacteria on malignancies. At present when the incidence of

tuberculosis infection is rapidly decreasing in some countries, but remaining at

a high level in others, it is possible to measure such interrelationships - if

they exist. In some countries the BCG vaccination is still in full use having

full coverage and made repeatedly, while in other countries it has been abol-

ished as a routine procedure. Even a relatively weak correlation between myco-

bacterial infections and the incidence of malignancies is of marked theoretical

and even practical interest.

Tuberculosis is a disease in which the infectious microbe actively uses the

immunological mechanisms of the host organism to its own advantage. The primary

infection leads to a single or few isolated foci and the immunological mech-

anisms remain active during quite long periods. The reservoir of living bacilli

awaits a more favourable time to invade the tissues and spread the infection to

new hosts. The malignancies - at least in later stages - behave in the opposite

way. Accordingly it is natural to look for possible interactions.

The idea as such is not new. E.g. Magnus and Horwitz (1971) studied tuber-

culin allergy and cancer risk on the basis of material available at the Tuber-

culosis Register in Denmark, in which the age and size of tuberculin reaction

was recorded. About 425,000 persons, aged 20-44 years were studied during a

followup period of 12 years using cancer deaths as an indicator. Generally speaking, the results were negative, but the writers concluded that there is selection and trends which can not be controlled which might influence the results. "The negative results of this investigation do not necessarily preclude that a cellular immunity against cancer exists in the general population" is their final statement.

There are very different opinions on the influence of BCG vaccination preventing leukaemia. Some studies indicate positive effects, (Davignon et al., 1970, 1971; Rosenthal et al, 1972), but the human evidence is not persuasive (Hoover, 1976). In contrast, Comstock et al (1975) found that the vaccinated group in a large controlled trial of BCG vaccination against tuberculosis experienced an excess of Hodgkin's disease and other lymphomas. In their study, the extra risk of cancer was concentrated among people who were between 10 and 18 years old on entering the trial.

Skegg (1978) compared the Southern and Northern Islands of New Zealand. The similarity of disease rates in the early cohorts from the North and South Islands justifies the comparison of the two populations. After withdrawal of BCG vaccination in the South Island, mortality from leukaemia and Hodgkin's disease remained similar in the two islands, while the death rate from non-Hodgkin lymphomas became significantly higher in the North Island.

2. Hypotheses and materials. This study was limited to cases of leukaemia and the purpose was to have an answer to the following questions:

- do the BCG vaccinated persons have the same amount of leukaemia as the non-vaccinated ones?
- do the naturally infected (tuberculin positives) behave like the vaccinated?
- is this influence longstanding?

Two different registers covering in principle the whole of Finland (population approximately 5 million) were used as basis material. The cases of leukaemia are notified to the Cancer Register; the data about BCG vaccination and tuberculin positivity are available from a BCG roster, "Finnish Vaccination Index" (FVI), made during a national mass BCG vaccination campaign in 1946-49. The basic strategy is to have from the Cancer Register a list of cases of leukaemia in the birth year cohorts which participated in a mass BCG campaign during 1946-49. The followup period is about 30 years - up until the present years (1978). The birth year cohorts 1926-41 were selected for this study and the 422 cases of leukaemia found in the Cancer Register were located in the Finnish Vaccination Index (FVI). There are two subgroups in the FVI:

1.   Tuberculin positive, naturally infected and non-BCG vaccinated.

2.   Tuberculin negative and immediately BCG vaccinated.

There was no register of non-participants and any error in the matching naturally moves the case to the group of non-participants. A few words about the registers are justified for orientation purposes.

Finnish Cancer Registry. The Registry has been in full operation since 1953 and is based on compulsory notification of all malignant diseases in the country. In addition, the Registry collects information from hospital and laboratory records and from death certificates. As less than 2 percent of all cases become known from death certificates only, the notification rate is considered high and the data therefore quite representative. In 85 percent of cases the diagnosis has been confirmed by microscopy. The following information is available in the files of the Registry: patient's name, sex, date and place of birth and the type, site, distribution, main symptoms, duration and treatment of cancer.

The Finnish Vaccination Index (FVI). The construction of the Index started in 1949 when the Tuberculosis Research Office of WHO collected the field records of the mass BCG campaign in the whole of Finland. They were copied on to punch cards and then tabulated and arranged to form a Vaccination Index. The

index cards are combined registration and punch cards and have written and
punched information on: Identification data:name, sex, date of birth, place of
residence, Test data: type, date and result and Date of vaccination. The cards
are put in order according to sex, name (first two letters of the surname),
year, month and day of birth. The Index contains 849,694 cards. About 40 percent of the entire Finnish population born in 1923-49 is recorded in the Index,
very few born outside of this period. There are records for about 60 percent
of the children at school in 1945-49.

The critical issue in record linkage studies is the matching process. In
Finland, when women marry, they change their surname to that of their husband
which markedly complicates the linkage process mainly based on name. Due to
this, only males were studied on this occasion. The following table, Table I.
shows by cohort, the male population and the tuberculin vaccination/non-par-
ticipation status. The very few tuberculin negative non-vaccinated persons are
excluded from the FVI.

Table I. FVI Male Population by Birth Year Cohort 1926-41 by Tuberculin
Status (1949).

Birth year	Tuberculin positives	Tub. negatives BCG vaccinated	Non-participants Tub.status unknown	Together
1926	5120	987	26034	32171
1927	5381	1715	25046	32142
1928	3930	2019	27528	33477
1929	5994	4332	23057	33383
1930	6461	6014	21810	34285
1931	6283	7099	19535	32917
1932	6089	8793	16615	31497
1933	5853	9239	14762	29854
1934	4176	8193	18629	30998
1935	4733	10752	17164	32649
1936	4999	12429	14613	32049
1937	5187	13783	14206	33176
1938	5281	15838	14194	35323
1939	4758	17147	13751	35656
1940	3570	15247	11922	30739
1941	4157	21848	16536	42541
Together	82012	155435	295402	532849

Because there are numerous trends by calendar year, by age, time intervals from the vaccination or infection etc., the followup is a complicated process. In order to control at least some of these factors a cohort analysis was selected as the approach. The way of thinking is visualized in Figure 1 which shows how the persons belonging to selected birth year cohorts have passed some critical moments in their life and how this study is located in the framework of time. It also visualizes the idea of the "Lexis diagrammes" which give a three-dimensional picture of the situation for each birth year cohort by calendar year and by age. This is important because e.g. the age structure of the different groups in the FVI and the non-participants varies considerably and the number of leukaemia cases is too small to be studied using very narrow age-strata. In this case, 16 birth-year cohorts are followed. Figure 2 shows as an example such a table in reduced format. The numbers are actually cases of leukaemia recorded in the Cancer Register in 1949-78 and belonging to relevant male cohorts.

Using the population figures (Table I) and registered cases of leukaemia (Figure 1), one can calculate expected numbers of leukaemia separately for each group. These can be compared with actual findings. Due to long followup and numerous cohorts, the results are presented as summarized O/E ratios in the figures.

The critical issue in a material which is based on voluntary participation is the selection. As controls, general mortality, accidents, tuberculosis cases using the same type of analysis were used.

3. Matching errors. The first step in this kind of record linkage is to evaluate the exactness of the matching process. Very big registers and historical data can in addition have constructional abnormalities which have not been properly documented. This is especially relevant for the FVI, because it was established with quite different interests in mind - under postwar conditions - and

424

Figure 1. Age and calendar year data of the male birth-year cohorts born in 1926-41, in relation to mass vacination campaign, follow-up period.

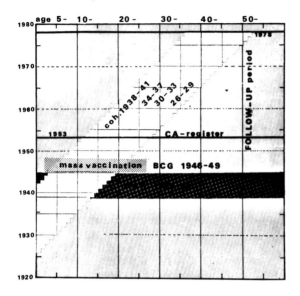

Figure 2. Cases of leukemia in Finland 1949-78 by calendar year and by birth-year cohorts (1926-41). Lexis diagram.

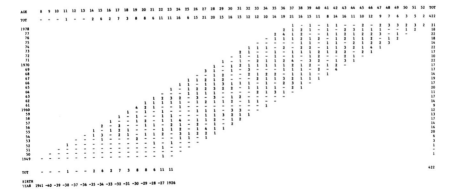

direct contact with the persons technically responsible is now no longer possible. Actually, the FVI was completely unused and abandoned during the period 1953-77.

The matching was done manually by an experienced person who has also previously made comparable analyses concerning tuberculosis (Haro, 1977).

In any case, matching errors are to be expected due to the fact that some persons who participated in mass campaigns are not found in the vaccination index for technical reasons such as a wrong birthday, a miswritten name, etc. Since no complete list of non-participants exists, any error in linkage raises the number of observations among non-participants. A matching error can be measured if the FVI population can be linked up with another register in which there is no selection. Closest to this ideal is the national population register, which in Finland exists as a computerized system. The whole population, listed on 461 microfilms (updated 1977) could be used for this project. A four percent sample, stratified by birth year cohorts, was taken from this register. The full name and birthday was available for each of the 2,131 male persons belonging to the sample. They were compared with the vaccination index manually, by the same persons and exactly in the same way as the cases have been done. The basic hypothesis was that if there were no matching errors, the relative distribution of individuals found and not found in the register should be the same as the population sizes: 621 BCG vaccinated and 329 naturally infected (tuberculin positive) participants should be found in the Index and 1,181 should not be found. Any disagreement with this distribution indicates that there are matching errors.

The results of the analysis are shown in Table 11. The matching error (ME) is generally speaking at an acceptable level of 11-16 percent, but the differences between cohorts are too great. Especially the cohorts 1926-29 are behaving abnormally - in the category of participants there are many more names than in the non-participant category. The same tendency was found when other material was linked to FVI. Obviously, the real number of participants in the cohorts 1926-29 is bigger than expected. There is reason to suspect that the opposite is true concerning cohorts 1938-41.

Table II. Matching a stratified representative sample of males from the national population register with the FVI. The sample size is 4 per cent of relevant population. The expected numbers are calculated on the basis of available data on participation, the observed numbers are persons actually found in the FVI

Year of birth	Tuberculin negative (BCG-vaccinated)			Tuberculin positive (naturally infected)			All participants			Non-participants			Whole pop.[2]
	obs.	exp.	o/e ratio[1]	obs.	exp.	o/e ratio[1]	obs.	exp.	o/e ratio[1]	obs.	exp.	o/e ratio[1]	
1941	72	87		7	17		79	104		91	66		170
1940	52	61	76.8	13	14	69.0	65	75	75.2	58	48	138.5	123
1939	45	69		13	19		58	88		85	55		143
1938	46	63		16	21		62	84		79	57		141
1937	41	55		17	21		58	76		75	57		133
1936	25	50	72.4	14	20	81.8	39	70	75.2	89	58	124.8	128
1935	38	43		26	19		64	62		67	69		131
1934	27	33		6	17		33	50		91	74		124
1933	28	37		19	23		47	60		72	59		119
1932	26	35	86.3	23	24	82.7	49	59	84.7	77	67	111.7	126
1931	25	28		23	25		48	53		83	78		131
1930	28	24		16	26		44	50		93	87		137
1929	22	17		27	24		49	41		84	92		133
1928	23	8	191.7	16	16	126.5	39	24	146.2	95	110	86.4	134
1927	10	7		21	22		31	29		98	100		129
1926	14	4		41	21		55	25		74	104		129
1926–1941	522	621	84.1	298	329	90.6	820	950	86.3	1 311	1 181	111.0	2 131
95 per cent conf. limits		(77–92)			(80–102)			(79–93)			(105–118)		

[1] Per cent [2] obs.=exp., o/e ratio=100

From Table II it is possible to calculate correction factors for matching error (ME). The following summary shows such factors as percentages. With these factors the numbers of participants observed should be multiplied in order to have a number of cases in each group which takes into account matching errors. The comparable amount in absolute numbers should be deducted from the figure of non-participants.

Year of birth	Tuberculin negatives (BCG vaccinated)	Tuberculin Positives (Naturally infected)
1941-1938	130	145
1937-1934	138	122
1933-1930	116	121
1929-1926	52	79
1926-1941	119	110

The correction factors are used in the presentation of results. Both the findings as such and the "Matching Error Corrected" (MEC) numbers are given. The method is relativley crude and can occasionally lead to biased results. Some of the errors are obviously due to inexact number of participants regis- tered. A "census" in the FVI must be made if the index is to be used in future for evaluative purposes. This was not possible at this stage due to time limitations.

4. Index cases of leukaemia

Another prerequisite for obtaining meaningful results is the representa- tiveness of notified cases of leukaemia. The Cancer Register covers the whole nation. Therefore the calculated rates by age of the list of cases and the national leukaemia death rates should be close to each other. Figure 3 shows the range of yearly death rates by age (male age groups 15-54) during 1954-77 in Finland. They vary quite markedly and the rates derived from the 422 leu- kaemia cases listed for this study are close to the medians. This is natural because the derived rates are average experiences of different years, e.g. the age-group 24-29 years is based on data collected during 1951-71. The comparable national rates in neighbouring countries such as Sweden, Norway and Denmark are also within the Finnish range of rates.

428

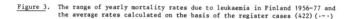

Figure 3. The range of yearly mortality rates due to leukaemia in Finland 1956-77 and the average rates calculated on the basis of the register cases (422) (·-·)

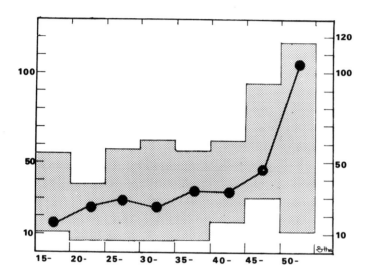

Figure 3.   The range of yearly mortality rates due to leukaemia in Finland 1956-77 and the average rates calculated on the basis of the register cases (422) (o-o).

The population figures in this study have not been adjusted for deaths, emigration etc. The size of the cohorts 1926-41 was checked in the census of 1960 and 1970. The size of cohorts diminished during 1950-70 by between 9.5 percent (cohort 1929) and 13.1 percent (cohort 1940); the average was 12.2 per cent. The trends during 1970-78 have not been estimated, but there is no

reason to expect that the relative size of age cohorts has changed very markedly during the Seventies. The crude population figures do not influence the
comparisons which are the main aim of this study, but the calculated rates e.g.
presented in Figure 3 are 10-15 percent too high in the older age groups.

5. Results

The results can be presented by age, by calendar year and by cohort. All
three are as such meaningful. In addition, a very critical issue in this con-
nexion is the fact that viewing the results from these different angles helps
to detect logical biases. The basic numbers are small and when summarized, the
different trends - both the known like age and the unknown or uncontrollable
like the environment - make the figures unreliable.

The observed (O) and expected (E) numbers of leukaemia in all tuberculin
negative (BCG vaccinated) and positive participants and in non-participants
were:

	O	E
Tuberculin negative, BCG vaccinated	36	66
Tuberculin positive	64	113
Non-participants	322	243
Together	422	422

The difference between the series is statistically significant
(N-2 x^2 = 60.567 p 0.001). On the other hand there are numerous sources of
logical errors and biases which require special attention.

The plan of presentation is as follows:

- In paragraph 5.1 the calendar year trends are presented.

- In paragraph 5.2 the experiences of different cohorts are examined.

- In paragraph 5.3 the problem is viewed by age.

In each paragraph the logical errors are especially underlined.

5.1 Yearly trends 1953-78

There are 480 "boxes" in the Lexis diagrammes used. The problem is how to generalize the findings. The available data make it possible to count expected values separately for each subgroup (tuberculin negative, BCG vaccinated; tuberculin positive; non-participants). The observed and expected numbers can be compared and the resulting O/E ratios presented as summarized indexes (the experience of the whole population = 100).

In Figure 4 the yearly trends between 1953-78 are presented separately for· each group. The 100 percent line is the experience by year of the whole male population born between 1926-41 and the differences between subgroups are relative ones. Each of the subgroups are represented by two lines, the thin one shows the recorded findings, the heavier line the calculated ones (MEC) using the matching error correction factors as presented previously. (Chapter 3).

The figure shows very clear   trends. If this study were to cover e.g. the time 1960-70, both the participating groups would have considerably fewer cases of leukaemia than the non-participants. In the years 1970-78 there are no obvious differences. If all the years are summarized the O/E ratios would be as follows:

	O/C ratio uncorrected	O/C ratio corrected (MEC)	Numbers of cases
Tuberculin negative, BCG vaccinated	55	61	36
Tuberculin positive	57	70	64
Non-participants	133	124	322
Together	100	100	422

The following conclusions can be drawn:

 -generally speaking the participants have much less leukaemia;

 -there is no marked difference between naturally infected and BCG vaccinated persons.

 -there is no clear indication of when this difference disappears;

 -there are abnormalities in the yearly experiences which are difficult to explain.

In the years when the curves behave in an unexpected way, the difference between uncorrected ratios and MEC ratios are relatively greater. This indicates

that the previously mentioned errors in denominators play a role and that the
MEC factors are too crude.

Figure 4. The yearly O/E ratios between 1953-78 for tuberculin positive (TUB+), BCG vaccinated and non-participants, (The whole population = 100). The thin lines are based on mathcing error corrected numbers (MEC).

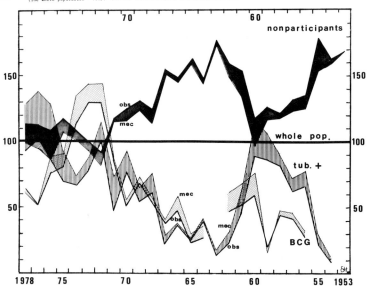

5.2 The experience by cohorts

The 16 participating cohorts followed, had vastly different histories at the
time of being tuberculin tested and vaccinated. The oldest ones had experienced wars and done military service, the youngest ones had lived their whole
life during a period of war and post-war economic shortage. It is possible
that these kinds of factors have a long-standing influence on health.

Accordingly all the cohorts should be studied separately.

Table III below is a summary of the findings of the four groups of cohorts:

1926-29, 1930-33, 1934-37, and 1938-41. The results are given as O/E and MEC/E

ratios. The years 1949-58, 1959-68 and 1969-78 are shown separately.

Table III O/E Ratios and MEC/O (corrected) Ratios of Leukaemia in Tuberculin
negative BCG-vaccinated (BCG), Tuberculin Positive (TUB+) and Non-participants
(NON) by Age-cohorts Separately for Ten Year Periods Starting 1949, 1959, 1969
and the Period 1949-78.

O/E RATIOS

Time	1949-1958			1959-1968			1969-1978			1949-1978		
Cohort	BCG	TUB+	NON	BCG	TUB+	NON	BCG	TUB+	NON	BCG	TUB+	NON
1926-29	19	81	118	17	180	112	104	191	91	56	157	105
1930-33	22	34	156	65	13	144	81	72	118	64	47	133
1934-37	45	19	174	18	22	185	78	25	158	46	23	172
1938-41	-	34	214	39	44	183	73	109	98	43	66	158
Together	21	36		35	41	150	86	82	112	54	57	133

MEC.O/E (CORRECTED)

Time	1949-1958			1959-1968			1969-1978			1949-1978		
1926-29	15	64	117	14	142	116	88	151	99	44	124	109
1930-33	26	41	151	79	16	134	98	87	106	77	57	124
1934-37	55	23	168	22	27	181	95	30	143	56	28	163
1938-41	-	50	194	56	64	153	106	158	27	63	95	115
Together	23	43	148	43	49	142	94	103	88	61	70	124

Table III shows that the two middle groups of cohorts behave systematically

as the overall results indicate. But the cohort 1926-29 is very irregular and

does not allow any exact conclusion to be made. The corrected ratios are some-

what closer to the whole experience, but the differences are still too great.

To some extent the same can be said about the youngest cohorts. In the cohorts

born 1930-37, the BCG vaccinated and tuberculin positive groups have much less

leukaemia than expected in all the 10 year periods. The two groups mentioned

had the greatest difference in the matching error control. One plausible ex-

planation for the "irregularities" can be that some denominators are unreliable.

5.3 The experience by age

The leukaemia rates by age derived from the available material as a whole are visualized in Figure 3. The calculated rates are, generally speaking, "normal". Accordingly, the calculated numbers of expected cases also reflect realistic incidences. In Figure 5, the comparison between different groups (BCG vaccinated, tuberculin positive, non-participants) is based on O/E and corrected MEC.E/O ratios. There is a very marked difference in age-groups from 15 to 34, but the relationships are not so clear in the ages 35 to 49. The influence of correction factors is relatively great in the older end of the age grouping. The oldest cohorts, born 1926-29, have a dominating role in these age-groups and this might introduce a considerable bias. In any case, the conclusions presented in paragraph 5.1 concerning the difference between participating/non-participating groups, the similarity of naturally and "artifically" infected groups and the longstanding effects can be repeated here as well.

Table IV presents the rates by age per 10^6, calculated both on the basis of observed and MEC numbers (corrected). The rates of BCG vaccinated participants are markedly lower than the comparable rates of tuberculin positives. Actually, the different sizes and varying yearly risks are reflected in this kind of presentation. The expected numbers are also low and the O/E ratios which are presented in Figure 5 show the differences in a more realistic way.

6. Tuberculosis infection during the followup period

There is no direct way of measuring the prevalence of tuberculosis in the group of non-participants, but it can be estimated. The "Tuberculosis Infection Incidence" (TII), commonly known as "risk of infection", has been calculated for Finland on the basis of a mathematical model by the Tuberculosis Surveillance Research Unit (TSRU), functioning under the International Union Against Tuberculosis. The yearly TII is given as a percentage rate, separately

434

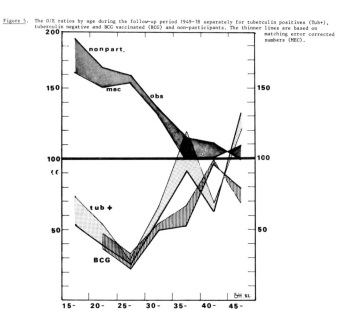

Figure 5. The O/E ratios by age during the follow-up period 1949-78 separately for tuberculin positives (Tub+), tuberculin negative and BCG vaccinated (BCG) and non-participants. The thinner lines are based on matching error corrected numbers (MEC).

for each calendar year. By using these numbers, one can calculate the accumulated prevalence of tuberculosis infectiion in this material as well. The
basic assumption is e.g. that in 1949 the non-participants had the same amount
of tuberculosis as the participants. The risk (TII) diminished very rapidly in Finland. In 1921, it was 10.15 percent yearly, in 1949 about 3.90,
in 1965 between 0.53 and 1.02 percent and in 1980 between 0.080 and 0.090 only.
In the sixties and seventies, the diminishing trend has been 16.7 percent

Table IV. Leukaemia Cases by Age per 10^6 Person Years During the Followup Period 1949-78 Separately for BCG Vaccinated, Tuberculin Positive Participants and Nonparticipants. Both observed (OBS) and corrected (MEC) Numbers are Presented. * based on 3 years, 50-52 only.

Age	BCG vaccinated		Tuberculin-positives		Non-participants		Together
	OBS	MEC	OBS	MEC	OBS	MEC	
15-19	-	-	24.5	35.5	22.7	19.7	14.6
20-24	3.9	5.0	18.4	25.5	31.8	29.1	24.7
25-29	3.9	5.0	12.2	16.0	46.1	44.4	28.9
30-34	6.4	7.1	24.4	27.8	34.5	33.2	24.4
35-39	9.8	12.3	55.3	71.6	39.1	33.3	33.5
40-44	27.4	27.1	23.6	25.8	38.4	37.9	33.7
45-49	51.2	32.1	42.4	38.6	22.6	48.3	44.7
(50-54)*	(-)	(-)	(33.9)	(26.8)	(51.4)	(40.6)	(103.0)

yearly, which is actually the most rapid national diminishing trend ever noticed (Haro 1982).

The TII rates were applied to the estimated negative groups of non-participants by birth year cohort. The "infected" persons were deducted from the groups and the same number of persons added to the comparable sub-groups of infected non-participants. The population by birth year cohort and calendar year could be defined both to tuberculin negatives and infected non-participants.

If the tuberculin positive non-participants behave like the tuberculin positive participants, the number of leukaemia among tuberculin negative participants which are not BCG vaccinated, can be estimated. Such calculations were made. In 1949-78 there would be about 4.9 million person years in the group of infected and about 3.9 million in the other groups. The number of cases among the infected group was calculated on the basis of the experiences of positive participants. There was only 36 cases scattered to different cohorts and calendar years. These numbers were applied to non-participating infected groups in four different ways:

1. assuming that the yearly rates are the same;

2. assuming that in each one year age group, the rates are comparable;

3. assuming that in each cohort the experiences are the same;

4. assuming that each "box" in the Lexis diagramme is behaving in the same way.

The calculated numbers of leukaemia of infected non-participants were 98.4 (using the first assumption), 98.0 (second), 119.0 (third) and 110.3 (fourth). The expected number of leukaemia among all non-participants is known to be 243. If the number of cases among infected non-participants (e.g. 110) is deducted from this, the non-infected non-participants should have about 133 cases of Leukaemia. The rates per 10^6 person years would be about 45 in the infected group and 30 among non-infected. Actually, the sizes of different cohorts in these two populations are like mirror images of each other. The cohorts 1926-29 dominate in the infected group and the cohorts 1938-41 in tne other. When applying the correction factors like in previous analyses, the differences in the cases of leukaemia become quite insignificant.

There is much evidence which indicates that the cohorts 1926-29 and to some extent 1938-41 are not giving correct results. The calculation is also based on assumptions which are difficult to verify. But on the other hand, these types of long-term studies have numerous fallacies and the 0-hypothesis is always a valid alternative. This exercise must be repeated when more exact data are available.

7. Some controls

The traditional recommendation in testing disease-registers is to use general mortality or accidents as the evaluation parameter. There is a consensus that BCG has at least limited preventive effect on tuberculosis and if the register is reliable this fact should be seen. All the three aspects mentioned have been checked.

General mortality

In 1977, the deaths - due to all causes - of birth-year cohorts 1926-41 were matched with the FVI, in principle in the same way as done in this study.

The years 1957-68 and 1973 were studied. The findings are presented below as yearly O/E ratios in Table V.

Table V. Deaths due to All Causes in 1957-68 and 1973 as Yearly Observed/ expected Ratios as Indexes (whole population in each year = 100) for Male Birth Cohorts 1926-41, separately for Tuberculin Negative (BCG-vaccinated) and Tuberculin Positive Participants, All Participants and Non-participants.

Year	Tuberculin negatives (BCG-vaccinated)	Tuberculin positives	All participants	Non-participants	Whole pop.
1973	81.1	88.8	84.3	109.5	100
—	.	.	.	.	.
1968	72.0	91.2	80.1	113.0	100
1967	73.7	82.0	77.0	114.7	100
1966	83.2	90.6	86.2	108.9	100
1965	82.1	89.6	78.6	109.8	100
1964	79.5	109.4	90.7	106.6	100
1963	66.1	92.3	76.3	115.8	100
1962	71.0	79.6	74.2	118.9	100
1961	66.9	74.1	69.6	122.3	100
1960	62.9	93.1	74.3	118.2	100
1959	69.3	83.7	74.7	118.3	100
1958	67.2	84.7	73.9	118.2	100
1957	71.5	82.8	75.8	117.4	100
TOTAL	70.8	88.2	77.6	114.0	100
M.E. corrected	84.2	97.0	89.8	106.1	100

There is a difference between participants and non-participants, but when applying ME corrections, it becomes relatively small. There is also a difference between tuberculin negatives (BCG vaccinated) and tuberculin positives. This is understandable because the tuberculosis infection, during early years of life, has been correlated with less favourable social conditions which obviously can have long-standing effects on health.

Traffic accidents

When FVI was initiated in 1946-49, it was recommended that the reliability of the register should be tested against accidents; the hypothesis was presented that "the accidents are a typical example of causes of death in which the mortality should be the same among registered groups and non-participants". Table VI shows the results based on traffic accidents in 1963, 1968 and 1973. The numbers indicate that there is a difference between tuberculin negatives and positives. When correction factors are applied, the difference becomes "reasonable". The non-infected children and adolescents have most likely come from socially better homes and one can postulate that this has a longstanding effect. In any case this control indicates that the vaccinated and non-vaccinated participants can behave differently and that the register reflects such circumstances.

Table VI. Mortality Due to Traffic Accidents as O/E Ratios in Tuberculin Negatives (BCG vaccinated), Tuberculin Positives and Non-participants (1963, 1968, and 1973).

Year	Tuberculin negatives			Tuberculin positives			Non-participants			Whole pop.[2]
	obs.	exp.	o/e[1]	obs.	exp.	o/e[1]	obs.	exp.	o/e[1]	
1973	25	39.7	63.0	24	22.9	104.8	99	85.3	116.1	148
1968	26	43.0	60.5	20	22.4	89.3	101	81.5	123.9	147
1963	22	45.6	48.2	19	25.6	74.2	123	92.8	132.5	164
TOTAL	73	128.3	56.9	63	70.9	88.9	323	259.6	124.4	459
95 per cent confidence limits			45–72			68–114			111–139	
M.E. corrected			67.7			97.7			116.6	100

[1] as per cent [2] obs.=exp., o/e=100

Tuberculosis

To be infected with virulent mycobacteria definitely introduces a considerable risk of becoming diseased. In a situation where the risk of infection is rapidly diminishing and later on becoming quite minimal, the real role of BCG

might be rather small in the age-groups covered by this study. <u>Table VII</u>
presents the O/E ratios for each birth year cohort in 1957-74.

<u>Table VII</u>. Observed/expected Ratios as Indexes (whole cohort = 100) of New
Cases of Pulmonary Tuberculosis in 1957-74 by Male Birth-year Cohorts 1926-41,
separately for Tuberculin Negative (BCG-vaccinated) and Tuberculin Positive
(naturally infected) participants and Non-participants. In addition Yearly
Case Rates per 100,000 for Whole Population.

Year of birth	Participants		Non-participants	Whole pop.	Case rate per 100 000
	Tub. negative	Tub. positive			
1941	58	152	143	100	99
1940	57	144	142	100	117
1939	55	138	143	100	126
1938	53	107	150	100	125
1937	59	108	138	100	130
1936	55	118	132	100	126
1935	64	112	120	100	126
1934	59	111	116	100	139
1933	49	92	135	100	134
1932	56	93	126	100	149
1931	54	100	117	100	133
1930	60	97	112	100	157
1929	64	100	107	100	156
1928	81	90	103	100	167
1927	79	74	107	100	188
1926	194	155	86	100	182
1926– 1941 M.E.	59	109	117	100	140
corrected	66	119	109	100	..

The findings correspond to the expectations and both the not-corrected as
well as the ME corrected ratios are much more favourable for the vaccinated
groups. As in all previous presentations, the cohort 1926 is behaving
"abnormally".

The presented controls give results which are understandable and indicate that the FVI in principle is functioning as expected and can be used for long-term evaluation. The oldest cohorts give unreliable results and introduce a varying amount of bias. This can be corrected by organizing a "census" which in this case - the register of about 900,000 persons is not in a computer - is a considerable, but not insolvable problem.

8. Conclusive remarks

The three basic questions presented in the beginning (chapter 2) can now be answered. There seems to be contructional weaknesses in some parts of the register which are difficult to correct. On the other hand, there is so much evidence of a positive effect of BCG that a hypothesis of preventive effect of vaccination is justified. To some extent it can be verified by repeating this study when the register is rearranged, and then also taking females into account. It would also allow for an analysis by type of Leukaemia. In this study the whole group of leukaemia (A59, ICD 8) was taken as an entity.

It is rather understandable that the naturally infected persons behave in the same way as the persons vaccinated with BCG. It can be postulated that as far as the unspecific immunological effects are concerned, the strains are close to each other. If the problem is human tuberculosis, the infection with virulent bacilli introduces a marked risk.

This material indicates that if there is some effect it is longstanding. Generally speaking, the natural tuberculosis infection introduces life-long changes in the specific immunological reactions. The opinions concerning BCG vary, but most likely it also has a rather longstanding specific effect against tuberculosis bacilli. There is no reason to deny the possibility that non-specific influences of mycobacterial infections are also effective for long periods of time.

These types of problems are difficult to study with reliable controls. The

natural history of disease is unclear, there is no information about the real
mechanism of intervention and there exists numerous - known as well as unknown-
trends and interactions, which are difficult to control. If this material had
been analysed only by age or calendar year using crude summarized rates as
basis of evaluation, evidence both in favour of or against could easily be
found. To evaluate the problem multidimensionally, at least by age, by calendar year and by using cohort structures as the foundation and also comparing
observed and expected numbers, the conclusions become more reliable, at least
one is obliged to formulate the statements more carefully.

There are many ways of checking these findings. There are ongoing "natural
experiments" which in the past were not feasible. The incidence of tuberculosis infection is negligible in some developed countries, whereas in others
BCG vaccination is still applied close to the 100 percent level. In rather
identical situations some countries do not vaccinate at all. Some give the
vaccine to healthy newborn in the third or fourth day of life, while other
countries vaccinate 6-7 year olds or even at a later stage and repeat the
process.

There is also reason to note that the tuberculin tests have an error rate of
about plus/minus 15 percent and that there are great numbers of strains of BCG
in general use. If the mycobacterial infections have some general influence
against immunological deficiencies there is much potentially useful information
accumulated in tuberculosis related research.

For the writer of this report, this was the first occasion to think that a
tuberculosis infection can have a longstanding positive unspecific effect on
immunological mechanism as a whole. At present, when an infectious agent intro-
ducing an acquired immunity deficiency (AID) can be postulated, it is quite
feasible to think that there exists microorganisms which rely on opposite
effect in their relationships to host organisms. Mycobacteria might belong to

442

this group, but there might be others which behave in a comparable way.

Summary

The information concerning Leukaemia in the Cancer Register in Finland was matched with a BCG vaccination index (FVI) constructed in 1946-49. Male birth-year cohorts 1926-41 were analyzed by comparing observed/expected ratios. There were 422 cases of Leukaemia (A59) in these cohorts during 1949-78 which was the follow-up period. The expected values were counted on the basis of the experience of the whole population of included cohorts. There were approximately 533,000 persons in the cohorts studied. About 295,000 participated in the mass BCG vaccination campaign. 82,000 were tuberculin positive, 155,000 were negative and BCG vaccinated.

The cohort analysis techniques were applied and the findings presented as Lexis diagrammes. A sample of population register was used in order to check the matching errors in FVI. The errors were generally at the level of 15 percent, but some cohorts were behaving abnormally. Obviously, the presented number of participants is not quite reliable. This is understandable because the register has not been in use from 1953-77 and contact with the organizers is no longer possible. With correction factors the errors can be adjusted. The register is functioning as expected in relation to general mortality and tuberculosis.

The results indicate that there is no marked difference between naturally T.B. infected and BCG vaccinated persons. The participants seem to have considerably less cases of leukaemia than the non-participants of which a great deal are not infected or vaccinated. Structural weaknesses in the FVI do not allow firm conclusions to be drawn. There is in any case so much evidence by age, by calendar year and by cohort that an hypothesis of the diminishing long-term effects on leukaemia is justified. The interrelationships are long-standing and noticeable during the whole followup period.

The structural weakness in the register can be corrected. The analysis can be broadened to cover females as well, which will also facilitate analysis by different types of leukaemia.

The possible longstanding effect of mycobacterial infections are discussed. Some strategies of further research are outlined.

Acknowledgements

This study was initiated due to a query from Professor R.G. Crispen. The Finish Cancer Register gave to the author the list of Leukaemia cases and the Finnish Association Against Tuberculosis took care of the expenses of linkage. This was made by Mrs. Elvi Ohman (National Board of Health, Finland). The typing of the text and diagrammes was done by Miss Vibeke Jahn (WHO EURO/ Copenhagen). Without the support and positive interest of these persons this study could not have been finalized.

References

1. Comstock, G.W., Martinez, J. and Livesay, V.T. Efficacy of BCG vaccination in prevention of cancer. J. Nat. Cancer J., 1975, 54, 835.

2. Davignon, L., et al. BCG vaccination and leukaemia mortality, Lancet 1970 (2), 638.

3. Hoover, R.N. BCG vaccination and cancer prevention: A critical review of the human experience. Cancer Res. 1976, 36, 652.

4. Haro, A.S. Long-term evaluation of mass BCG vaccination campaign: A study of thirty years of experience in Finland. Tub. and Resp. Diseases Yearbook (Finland), Vol 6, (9 Op) 1977 (Sept.).

5. Haro, A.S. Measuring and use of "risk of infection" indicators in BCG vaccinated populations. XXV World Conf. of IUAT, Buenos Aires, Proceedings (to be published). 1982.

6. Magnus, K. and Horwitz, O. Tuberculin allergy and cancer risk. J. Chron. Dis. 1971, 24, 635.

7. Rosenthal, S.R.; Crispen, R.G.; Thorne, M.G.; Piekarski, N.; Raisys, N. and Rettig, P.G. BCG vaccination and leukaemia mortality, AMA 1972, 222, 1543.

8. Skegg, D.C.G. BCG vaccination and the incidence of lymphomas and leukaemia. Int. J. Cancer. 1978, 21, 18.

PREVIOUS TUBERCULOSIS AND IMMUNOCOMPETENCE--FAVORABLE
PROGNOSTIC FACTORS IN LONG-TERM RESPONSE
TO CHEMOTHERAPY OF SOLID TUMORS

EZRA M. GREENSPAN, Mount Sinai School of Medicine
One Gustave L. Levy Place, York, New York, USA

We initially observed two Stage IIIB ovarian carcinoma patients, treated in the 1960's, apparently cured in 1975, 9 and 14
years, respectively, after receiving thio-TEPA and methotrexate
chemotherapy. Both patients previously had pulmonary and
systemic tuberculosis (TBC) as young adults. These index cases
led to a retrospective analysis [1] of the surviving residue of
some 600 heterogeneous Stage III-IV patients with breast and
ovarian cancer treated at our New York-based oncology group from
1954-74. An unusual 75% incidence of patients with extensive
previous TBC, Ghon foci, apical caps, pulmonary calcifications
and positive tuberculin tests was found among 42 patients
unexpectedly surviving 5 to 20 years, either disease-free or with
indolent breast cancer or occult ovarian cancer. Only 25% of
these 42 long-term survivors were PPD-negative with negative
chest x-rays. The precise denominator needed to precisely
interpret these findings is unattainable because of a large number of unavailable x-rays and records of deceased cases. Nevertheless, this "tip of the iceberg" observation showing
substantial incidence of previous TBC was highly provocative [2].
It was also noted that there were 4 patients with extensive
obviously old healed pulmonary TBC among 7 unexpected 5-year
survivors of gastrointestinal cancer with metastases.

Although the PPD is an important index of epidemiological exposure, clinical oncologists currently use the tuberculin test
merely as one of a battery of simple cutaneous procedures to measure immunocompetence. Strong individual local response to PPD
is often a significant clue to previous clinical TBC. The usual
PPD+ rate in primary operable Stage I-II carcinoma of the breast
was recently 44-45% at New York's Memorial Sloan-Kettering [3] and
41% in Quebec [4]. Normals without breast cancer show a 52% rate

in Quebec and a 45% rate in New York where it was found that large, bulky primary breast tumors are associated with a much higher PPD positivity (69%) than small primary tumors, with or without positive nodes [3,5,6]. As cancer progresses, as in visceral metastases, patients usually are expected to show declining rates of positivity to a 35% level. These diverse data indicate that some primary-tumor characteristics as well as metastatic patterns appear somehow related to PPD responses.

The favorable prognostic factor of good immunocompetence manifested by better survival in breast cancer [3,4,5,6,7,8] patients, and Mantoux Test positivity in lung cancer [9] has been established in the past few years. An "index of immunocompetence" as measured by the response to PPD and 3 or 4 cutaneous antigens as well as cellular humoral responses has been proposed by several investigators. In randomized trials the responsiveness of Stage III ovarian cancer patients [10] and Duke's C GI cancer patients after BCG plus chemotherapy [11] has been recently demonstrated. Even failed or untreated Duke's C+D patients live longer when they manifest good responses to BCG vaccination [12].

The high incidence of previous TBC in our cancer survivors suggests that previous TBC mediates either a better resistance to cancer characterized by an indolent clinical course, or a better chemotherapy response, or both. The indirect conclusion of immunocytologists could be that TBC acts to facilitate or trigger certain favorable lymphocytes and cellular humoral mechanisms after chemotherapy has induced a release of tumor antigens during a tumor-kill process. It is unlikely that a restoration of PPD responsiveness after chemotherapy in a self-selected population of TBC survivors could account for our findings, and it could not account for the data of Krown and others [3] which suggests that primary tumor characteristics, metastatic patterns and survival may be related to PPD response and other delayed antigens.

No epidemiological data [13] is available to suggest that exposure, per se, to TBC prevents cancer development. However, it could play a role in the gradual increase in slope of age incidence rates in European women and the flat rates in Japanese women. These contrast with the sharp rise and peak incidence rates of breast cancer at age 45 to 55 in the United States

(Clemmensen's Hook). The relative lack of TBC and other infections in the U.S. could be related to the epidemic of life-threatening breast cancer so common in the perimenopausal or premenopausal younger females. It is unfortunate that no data is yet available on the cancer age-incidence rate in any large group of TB patients treated after 1952 when modern chemotherapy replaced x-ray controlled chest-collapse procedures.

Our hypothesis is that prolonged survival from cancer may well be favorably influenced by previous TBC, especially in the presence of a good chemotherapy response in breast and ovary cancer and possibly in GI cancer. BCG immunization as an immuno-prevention agent has never been tested in any large number of high-risk women. A controlled randomized trial of repeated BCG vaccination over a 15- to 20-year period with approximately 20,000 patients would be required to define any such potential role.

REFERENCES

1. Greenspan, E.M. and Cohen, S.M. (1980) Proc. Am. Assoc. Cancer Res. & ASCO 21, 374.
2. Greenspan, E.M. (1982) Cancer Treatment Rep. 66, 206-208.
3. Krown, S.E., Pinsky, C.M., Wanebo, I.W. et al. (1980) Cancer 46, 1746-1752.
4. Mandeville, R. et al. (1982) Cancer 50, 1280-1288.
5. Adler, A., Stein, J.A. and Ben-Efraim, B. (1980) Cancer 45, 2074-2983.
6. Adler, A., Stein, J.A. and Ben-Efraim, B. (1980) Cancer 45, 2061-2073.
7. Bolton, P.M., Teasdale, G., Mauder, A.M. et al. (1976) Cancer Immunother. 1, 251-258.
8. Hortobagyi, G.N., Smith, T.L., Swenerton, K.D. et al. (1981) Cancer 47, 1369-1376.
9. Sewell, N.J.C.(1959) Thorax 34, 508-511.
10. Alberts, D.S., Moon, T.E., Stephens, R.A. et al. (1979) Cancer Treat. Rep. 63, 325-331.
11. Robinson, E., Bartal, A., Cohen, Y. et al. (1982) Cancer Chemother. Pharmacol. 8, 35-40.
12. O'Connell, M.J. et al. (1981) Cancer Clin. Trials 4, 439-449.
13. Potrakis, N.L. (1977) Cancer 39, 2709-2715.

Index

Virus leukemogenesis, 113

Vitamin E. See ∝-tocopherol

Von Recklinghausen's disease. See neurofibromatosis

Wilm's tumor, 71

Xeroderma pigmentosum, 73, 88